BREAST CANCER

Experimental and Clinical Aspects

EUROPEAN ORGANIZATION FOR
RESEARCH ON TREATMENT OF
CANCER (EORTC)

BREAST CANCER

Experimental and Clinical Aspects

Proceedings of the Second EORTC Breast Cancer Working Conference
held in Copenhagen, 30 May to 2 June 1979

Guest Editors

H. T. MOURIDSEN and T. PALSHOF

Finseninstitutet, Copenhagen

Published as a supplement to the
European Journal of Cancer. Supplement

PERGAMON PRESS

OXFORD · NEW YORK · TORONTO · SYDNEY · PARIS · FRANKFURT

U.K.	Pergamon Press Ltd., Headington Hill Hall, Oxford OX3 0BW, England
U.S.A.	Pergamon Press Inc., Maxwell House, Fairview Park, Elmsford, New York 10523, U.S.A.
CANADA	Pergamon of Canada, Suite 104, 150 Consumers Road, Willowdale, Ontario M2J 1P9, Canada
AUSTRALIA	Pergamon Press (Aust.) Pty. Ltd., P.O. Box 544, Potts Point, N.S.W. 2011, Australia
FRANCE	Pergamon Press SARL, 24 rue des Ecoles, 75240 Paris, Cedex 05, France
FEDERAL REPUBLIC OF GERMANY	Pergamon Press GmbH, 6242 Kronberg-Taunus, Hammerweg 6, Federal Republic of Germany

First edition 1980

British Library Cataloguing in Publication Data
EORTC Breast Cancer Working Conference, *2nd, Copenhagen, 1979*
Breast cancer
1. Breast - Cancer - Congresses
I. Title II. Mouridsen, H T
III. Palshof, T IV. European Organization for Research on Treatment of Cancer
616.9'94'49   RC280.B8   79-41496
ISBN 0-08-025886-7

Published as Supplement No. 1, 1980, to the *European Journal of Cancer*

In order to make this volume available as economically and as rapidly as possible the authors' typescripts have been reproduced in their original forms. This method has its typographical limitations but it is hoped that they in no way distract the reader.

Printed in Great Britain by A. Wheaton & Co. Ltd, Exeter

Contents

CELL KINETICS

PSYCHOLOGICAL ASPECTS OF BREAST CANCER

NEW ASPECTS OF PRIMARY TREATMENT

Introduction

The Second E.O.R.T.C. Breast Cancer Working Conference was held in Copenhagen, May 30 to June 2, 1979.

The conference assembled 375 participants and the subjects which were discussed included aspects concerning statistical planning of trials, diagnostic methods in early and advanced breast cancer, hormone receptors, local and systemic treatment of primary and advanced disease, cell kinetics and psychological and rehabilitation aspects.

This supplement to the *European Journal of Cancer* contains the invited lectures and the free communications presented at the conference.

As reported in these papers progress in the treatment of primary and of advanced disease continues. Among the subjects which in the near future require special efforts are screening methodology and methods of selecting patients for the specific treatment modalities.

The importance of cooperation on an international basis was reemphasized at this conference both in order to ensure rapid arrangement of new progress and to ensure the validity of the conclusions of large cooperative trials.

We are very greateful to the sponsors of the conference, ICI, Pharmaceuticals Division, Danish Cancer Society, Danish Medical Council, Ministry of Education, Handelsbanken and the Finsen Institute.

July 1979

H. T. Mouridsen and T. Palshof
Guest Editors

Clinical Trials

Exclusions from Clinical Trials

K. West Andersen

The National Health Service, Store Kongensgade 1, 1264 Copenhagen K, Denmark

Correspondence to K. West Andersen

Abstract—*It is well-known that in comparing the effect of two treatments it is necessary that the two groups of patients in the trial are "equal". Likewise the results of a clinical trial are not valid for all patients but only for patients "equal" to those included in the trial. To prevent misuse of the results of a trial patients not included should be characterized in relation to all patients and for the purpose one should record patients not fulfilling the entrance criteria and patients fulfilling the entrance criteria, but not included in the trial.*

In most clinical trials some patients fulfilling the entrance criteria must be excluded e.g. some doctors may consider one of the treatments in the trial less eligible to low-risk patients and since the randomization has to be respected, such patients cannot be included in the trial. One would get a biased comparison of the treatments in the trial, if e.g. low-risk patients were withdrawn from one of the treatment groups. This means that all such exclusions have to be done before randomization. It is sometimes said that all exclusions which take place before randomization are acceptable (1). This is in some sense correct: a patient who is not included in a clinical trial cannot cause any bias in the comparison of the treatments, but observe that a patient who is randomized to one treatment but does not get that treatment may cause bias in the comparison of the treatments.

Although exclusions from a clinical trial before randomization cannot bias the comparison of the treatments, exclusions before randomization may cause the trial to be of less value. The purpose of a clinical trial is to determine the better treatment and to use that treatment in the future. Even if the better treatment is determined by a proper clinical trial one cannot use that treatment for future patients without knowing something about the excluded patients. It is of very little value to determine the better treatment for a group of patients if one cannot describe these patients.

A hypothetical example may show the bias caused by exclusions before randomization. There are, say, 200 patients who fulfill the entrance criteria in a clinical trial. For some reason a number, say 100, of these patients are excluded before randomization. The reason may be that the patient will not participate in the trial or the patient is not considered eligible although the entrance criteria is fulfilled or some mistake has occurred. The trial is then carried out for the remaining 100 patients and treatment A and B are compared. The result of the trial may be as shown in Table 1.

Table 1. Hypothetical example of results to treatment A and B in selected patients.

Treatment	No. of patients	No. of cured patients
A	50	20 = 40%
B	50	10 = 20%

The result of the trial would probably imply that all patients fulfilling the entrance criteria will be treated by A, and one would forget that half of the patients fulfilling the entrance criteria were not included in the trial. And that would be very easy to forget as probably that fact will not be mentioned in the report of the trial. When applying treatment A to all patients fulfilling the entrance criteria for the original trial one could get the result shown in Table 2.

Table 2. Hypothetical example of results to treatment A in selected and unselected patients.

Patient group	Treatment	No. of patients	No. of cured patients
"Included"	A	100	40 = 40%
"Excluded"	A	100	10 = 10%
Total	A	200	50 = 25%

Patients in the "included" group are patients "equal" to those who were included in the original trial and "excluded" patients are patients "equal" to those excluded from the original trial although they fulfilled the entrance criteria, e.g. patients who would not participate in a clinical trial, if they were asked, or patients for whom treatment A (or B!) would be considered less eligible so that they could not be included in the original trial. For these patients who are "equal" to the excluded patients the effect of treatment A is not necessarily the same as for patients who were included in the original trial.

Another example where exclusions may cause serious bias is a multicenter trial where a standardized operation is followed by adjuvant chemotherapy. If in case of a slight deviation from the standardized operation the patient is neither included in the trial nor reported to a data collecting centre, one might, without knowing, perform a trial in which only highly selected patients are included (and the selection mechanism may be the same at all the participating hospitals). The report from the trial may recommend the standardized operation followed by the better adjuvant chemotherapy and that may cause damage if one is not aware of the fact that the patients for whom the operation were not completely successful are excluded from the trial.

When applying the result from a clinical trial one must have a patient group "equal" to those who were included in the trial. In order to make it possible to apply the results of a clinical trial in a proper way, the report from the trial should tell how many patients fulfilling the entrance criteria were not included in the trial and the reason why.

When performing a clinical trial it would therefore be of great importance to record all patients suffering from the disease and patients not included in the trial should be specially recorded, and the reason for not being included should be stated for every single patient (1,2).

The fact that the (good) results of many clinical trials are not achieved when applying the better treatment of the trial may be due to a difference between patients included in the clinical trial and patients for whom the result of the trial are applied. In order to make the results of clinical trials more useful one could propose that much effort should be done to characterize, quantitatively and qualitatively, the patients included in the trial in relation to all patients.

Another way to increase the usefulness of a clinical trial might be to include a treatment which is part of another clinical trial since that would make it possible to make a comparison of the results of the trials whatever the results of the two treatments are "equal" or not.

REFERENCES

1. R. Peto, M. C. Pike, P. Armitage, N. E. Breslow, D. R. Cox, S. V. Howard, N. Mantel, K. McPherson, J. Peto, and P. G. Smith, Design and Analysis of Randomized Clinical Trials Requiring Prolonged Observation of Each Patient. *Br. J. Cancer*, 34, 585 (1976).
2. Clinical trials of the treatment of breast cancer in Britain and Ireland, *Br. Med. J.* 1, 361 (1977).

On the Analysis of Response Rates in Studies of Advanced Disease*

R. Sylvester

E.O.R.T.C. Data Center, Institut Jules Bordet, 1 rue Héger-Bordet, 1000 Brussels, Belgium

Correspondence to R. Sylvester

Abstract—*Instead of simply comparing the percentage of responders in each treatment group in studies of advanced disease, this paper advocates the use of a well known statistic test which takes the ordering of all the response categories into account.*

INTRODUCTION

In analyzing the results of studies in advanced patients with measurable disease, it is common to group evaluable patients into different categories according to the degree of tumor response measured after the start of treatment. Hayward et al (1) have for example set forth criteria for the evaluation of treatment response in advanced breast cancer patients. For the purposes of this paper we shall assume that the response to treatment falls into one of the four following categories: complete remission (C.R.), partial remission (P.R.), no change (N.C.) or progression (Prog). Although results are often reported in this manner, it is customary to analyze the data from randomized trials by comparing only the percentage of responders (C.R. or P.R.) in each treatment group. In doing so all of the available information is not used since one ignores the distinction between complete and partial remission and between no change and progression. Important differences may be missed if the treatment differences depend on the inherent ordering of the response categories which reflect the degree of tumor change. In the next section a statistic test is presented which takes this ordering into account.

METHODS

Table 1 presents the results of a hypothetical study comparing the response rates of two treatments A and B in patients with advanced breast cancer. If one compares the percentage of responders (C.R. or P.R.) in each treatment group (45/75 = 60% on treatment A and 34/75 = 45% on treatment B) using the standard chi-square test with a continuity correction, it is found that the difference is not statistically significant (P = .10).

As stated previously the above analysis does not use all the available information. Using all four response categories, one can compute within each response category the percentage of patients who receive treatment A. These percentages are given in Table 1 for the example considered (63%, 55%, 48%, 38%). If there is no difference between the treatments, these proportions should differ from one another only due to random variation. The overall test for the equality of the four proportions is in fact not significant with P = .22. This last test does not however take into consideration the ordering of the response categories and lacks the power to detect specific deviations from the hypothesis of no treatment difference.

If the ordering of the categories is now taken into consideration, one would expect the percentage of patients receiving treatment A in each response category to increase as one goes from Prog to N.C. to P.R. to C.R. in that order if in fact treatment A is better than treatment B. One way to test this hypothesis is to assign a score (1, 2, 3, 4 for example) to each response category and then compute the linear regression of the percentage of patients receiving treatment A in each response category on the score in order to determine if there is a linear trend in the proportions as one goes across the table from C.R. to Prog. The overall chi-square statistic previously computed can now be broken down into two additive components, a chi-square which tests for linear trend and a chi-square which tests for departures from linear trend. In the example given, if one assigns the scores 4 for C.R., 3 for P.R., 2 for N.C., and 1 for Prog, the test for linear trend is significant (P = .04). This indicates that the percentage of patients receiving treatment A in each response category increases as one goes from Prog to N.C. to P.R. to C.R. It can be shown that the test for trend is equivalent to testing

*This work was supported by Grant Number 2R10 CA11488-10 awarded by the National Cancer Institute, DHEW.

5

Table 1. Response to treatment.

Treatment	C.R.		P.R.		N.C.		Prog		Total
A	12	63%	33	55%	15	48%	15	38%	75
B	7	37%	27	45%	16	52%	25	62%	75
Total	19	100%	60	100%	31	100%	40	100%	150

Comparison of treatments A and B	*P value*
Percent C.R. or P.R. (A: 60%, B: 45%)	.10
Overall (63%, 55%, 48%, 38%)	.22
Trend (63%, 55%, 48%, 38%)	.04

whether the average score on treatment A is equal to the average score on treatment B (2). Thus a significant test for trend can be interpreted as indicating that the average response on treatment A is higher than the average response on treatment B.

While the choice of a particular set of scores may be subjective and somewhat arbitrary, one has some leeway in choosing the set of scores to be used. If for example all response categories are considered a priori to be of equal importance then the scores should be chosen to be equally spaced and any set of equally spaced scores will give the same significance level for the test for trend. Examples of such scores might be 1, 2, 3, 4; -3, -1, 1, 3; or 7, 4, 1, -2 for example. Unless a priori one wishes to emphasize a particular response category or set of response categories, the scores should be chosen to be equally spaced.

The (uncorrected) chi-square test for the comparison of the percent responders (C.R. or P.R.) in each treatment group is just a special case of the test for linear trend where now the C.R. and P.R. categories are assigned one score and the N.C. and Prog categories are assigned another score. In practice, however, it is preferable to use the continuity corrected chi-square test when two proportions are being compared. The scores may be similarly modified if a priori one wishes to test other hypotheses.

DISCUSSION

In doing a test for trend one takes into consideration the ordering of the response categories. The test for trend is more powerful than the overall test for the detection of treatment differences if a linear trend is present, which may well be the case if the two treatments differ in efficacy. The decision however concerning choice of scores to be used should be made prior to the start of the study so that the choice of the hypothesis to be tested does not depend on the results of the study.

The formulas used in the above calculations can be found in the appendix which follows.

APPENDIX

The notation used in the appendix follows

that of Armitage (3). Suppose that you have k response categories for each of two treatments with a score X assigned to each category. Then a 2 × k contingency table of the treatment results can be constructed as shown in Table 2.

Where X_i = the score associated with response category i

r_i = the number of patients in response category i receiving treatment A

n_i-r_i = the number of patients in response category i receiving treatment B

n_i = the total number of patients in response category i

$P_i = r_i/n_i$ = the proportion of patients in response category i receiving treatment A

$R = \Sigma r_i$ = total number of patients receiving treatment A

$N-R = \Sigma n_i-r_i$ = total number of patients receiving treatment B

$N = \Sigma n_i$ = total number of patients

$P = R/N$ = overall proportion of patients receiving treatment A

where all summations are from i = 1 to k. Then for k > 2

$$X_{k-1}^2 = \frac{\Sigma(r_i^2/n_i)-R^2/N}{P(1-P)}$$

provides an overall test for the equality of the proportions P_i. Under the null hypothesis of no treatment difference, X_{k-1}^2 is approximately distributed as chi-square with k-1 degrees of freedom. If one wishes to ask whether there is a significant trend in the proportions P_i from response category 1 to response category k (a trend of P_i with x_i) then the statistic X_{k-1}^2 can be broken down into two additive components:

(1) a test for linear trend

$$X_1^2 = \frac{N(N\Sigma r_i X_i - R\Sigma n_i X_i)^2}{R(N-R)(N\Sigma n_i X_i^2 - (\Sigma n_i X_i)^2)}$$

which under the null hypothesis of no trend is distributed approximately as chi-square with 1 degree of freedom and

Table 2.

Group	1	2	...	i	...	k	
Score	X_1	X_2	...	X_i	...	X_k	Total
Treatment A	r_1	r_2	...	r_i	...	r_k	R
Treatment B	$n_1 - r_1$	$n_2 - r_2$	...	$n_i - r_i$	...	$n_k - r_k$	N–R
Total	n_1	n_2	...	n_i	...	n_k	N
Proportion Treatment A	P_1	P_2		P_i		P_k	$P = \dfrac{R}{N}$

(2) a test for departure from linear trend

$$X^2_{k-2} = X^2_{k-1} - X^2_1$$

which under the null hypothesis of no departure from linear trend is approximately distributed as chi-square with k-2 degrees of freedom.

For the case k = 2 the test for trend is equivalent to the uncorrected chi-square statistic for the comparison of two percentages. However, in this case it is preferable to use the following continuity corrected statistic:

$$X^2_1 = \frac{(|r_1(n_2-r_2)-r_2(n_1-r_1)| - N/2)^2 N}{R(N-R)n_1 n_2}$$

which under the null hypothesis of no treatment differences is asymptotically distributed as chi-square with 1 degree of freedom. For further details please consult Armitage (3,4), Cochran (2), Everitt (5), or Fleiss (6).

REFERENCES

1. J. L. Hayward, P. P. Carbone, J. C. Heuson, S. Kumaoka, A. Segaloff and R. D. Rubens, Assessment of response to therapy in advanced breast cancer. *Cancer* 39, 1289 (1977).
2. W. G. Cochran, Some methods for strengthening the common χ^2 tests. *Biometrics* 10, 417 (1954).
3. P. Armitage, *Statistical methods in medical research*, Blackwell Scientific Publications, Oxford (1971).
4. P. Armitage, Tests for linear trends in proportions and frequencies: *Biometrics* 11, 375 (1955).
5. B. S. Everitt, *The analyses of contingency tables*, Chapman and Hall Ltd., London (1977).
6. J. L. Fleiss, *Statistical methods for rates and proportions*, John Wiley and Sons, New York (1973).

Diagnostic Methods in Early and Late Breast Cancer

Scintigraphic Methods in Breast Cancer

C. S. B. Galasko

Department of Orthopaedic Surgery, University of Manchester, Hope Hospital,
Salford M6 8HD, U.K.

Correspondence to C. S. B. Galasko

Abstract—*Skeletal scintigraphy is the most accurate method, currently available, for the detection of skeletal metastases. It would also appear to be the most sensitive method of staging apparently early mammary carcinoma, skeletal metastases being found in approximately one-quarter of these patients. However, lower detection rates have been reported by some authors. Comparison of the different isotopes and detecting apparatus used does not fully explain this difference and it may be due to a difference in the size or the invasive properties of the tumour.*

The uptake of bone-seeking isotopes is not specific. It occurs in two phases; the earlier phase is a result of the increased bone blood flow, the later and more important phase is due to the selective concentration of the bone-seeking isotope in the reactive new bone. Any benign lesion associated with this type of osteoblastic response will be associated with an increased uptake of bone-seeking isotopes. Therefore high quality radiographs, tomographs or even C.T. scans of areas where there is a localised focus of increased uptake of bone-seeking isotope are required to exclude these benign lesions and minimise the risk of false positives.

What ideally is needed is a technique of detecting tumour at all sites, including the skeleton and the viscera but until such a technique becomes available, skeletal scintigraphy would appear to be a most useful method of staging mammary carcinoma.

INTRODUCTION

1. Skeletal Metastases in Advanced Breast Cancer

It is well accepted that scintigraphy is more accurate than other methods for the detection of skeletal metastases in patients with advanced mammary carcinoma. Galasko (1) reported an 84% detection rate with skeletal scintigraphy compared with a 50% detection rate with conventional radiography in the same patients. This incidence is similar to that reported by Jaffe (2) who found skeletal metastases at autopsy in 85% of patients who had died from mammary carcinoma. In contrast only 65% of patients with advanced mammary carcinoma and who had skeletal metastases evident on their X-rays complained of pain, and tenderness was elicited in only 16% (1). The alkaline phosphatase was raised in 66% of these patients. The urinary hydroxyproline (3,4,5) and the hydroxyproline/ creatinine ratio (5,6,7) are more accurate but are still associated with a high false negative rate. Radiographic examination is also inaccurate. Skeletal metastases develop in the medulla and only involve cortical bone at a late stage. Edelstyn and his colleagues (8) found that at least 50% of the medullary bone must be destroyed in the beam axis of the X-ray before the lesion will be seen radiographically, whereas lesions involving the cortex were detected when much smaller.

2. Skeletal Metastases in Early Breast Cancer

The use of scintigraphy for the detection of skeletal metastases in patients with apparently early mammary carcinoma is more controversial. If accurate, routine pre-operative skeletal scintigraphy would be extremely useful for staging the disease. In 1975 Galasko (9) reported the results of a 5 year follow-up of patients with apparently early mammary carcinoma and who had had a skeletal scintigram at the time of presentation, but whose treatment was not affected by the result of the scintigram. The results are shown in Table 1.

Twenty-four percent of the patients had skeletal metastases demonstrated on their scintigram. During the 5 year follow-up the scintigraphic findings were confirmed in all these patients either at autopsy or on subsequent X-rays, even though it took very many months and even years for these other manifestations of the skeletal metastases to appear in several of the patients (Table 2). Eighty-three per cent of patients with a

Table 1. Five year follow-up of patients with apparently "early"
mammary carcinoma.

	Scintigram		
	+ve	-ve	Total
No. patients	12 (24%)	38 (76%)	50 (100%)
No. developed advanced disease	12 (100%)	10 (26%)	22 (44%)
No. died from cancer	10 (83%)	8 (21%)	18 (36%)
No. died from other causes	0	3 (8%)	3 (6%)
No. alive at 5 years	2 (17%)	27 (71%)	29 (58%)
No. alive with metastatic disease	2 (17%)	2 (5%)	4 (8%)
No. alive with no evidence of recurrence	0	25 (66%)	25 (50%)

Table 2. Patients with apparently "early" mammary cancer:
the time taken for radiological or autopsy
confirmation of metastases demonstrated on the
pre-operative skeletal scintigram

Time taken	% of patients
3 months	33
6 months	42
12 months	50
18 months	50
2 years	83
3 years	83
4 years	92
5 years	100

positive scintigram died from mammary cancer during the five year follow-up whereas, of the patients with a normal scintigram, only 21% died from mammary cancer during this period, 8% died from an intercurrent illness with no recurrent or disseminated disease being found at autopsy and 5% had survived with advanced carcinoma which was being treated. At 5 years none of the patients with a positive scintigram was alive and apparently free from disease, compared with 66% of the patients with a negative scintigram.

This study has now been repeated in several centres. Many authors have described similar results reporting a 23-28% detection rate in patients with apparently early mammary carcinoma (Table IIIA).

Campbell and his colleagues (12) found that 86% of patients with positive scintigrams had developed signs of disseminated disease at 18 months follow-up compared with only 11% of those with negative scintigrams. However, some authors have reported a much lower detection rate (Table IIIB).

In 1978 the British Breast Group (14) reported the results of a survey of skeletal scintigraphy in women with apparently early disease. The results were obtained from eight centres in Britain. ^{99m}Tc diphosphonate

or phosphate compounds had been used in all the centres. Five centres had included T3 tumours, the others confining their study to patients with T1 and T2 tumours. Lymph node involvement was N0 or N1. The numbers of patients with positive scintigrams varied from 2 of 107 (1.9%) to 19 of 94 (20.2%). Four centres reported detection rates greater than 14%, one of 9% and three less than 5%. Technical variations may have accounted for some of their differences. One patient had a negative scintigram carried out in one centre but a repeat scintigram obtained in another centre within one week was positive. However, there were no apparent major differences in technique to account for the wide variation in results. There may be several possible explanations for the reported differences in detection rates.

1. The Isotope Factors in the Detection
   Rate

There are several bone-seeking isotopes currently available. ^{99m}Tc diphosphonate is associated with a higher detection rate than the ^{99m}Tc phosphate compounds, ^{85}Strontium or ^{87m}Strontium. ^{18}Fluorine is also associated with a high detection rate but its

Table 3. Detection of skeletal metastases, by skeletal
scintigraphy, in patients with apparently early
mammary carcinoma

A. Series associated with a *high* detection rate

Author	Year	Detection Rate
Galasko (1)	1972	24%
Blair (10)	1975	28%
Citrin et al (11)	1975	27%
Campbell et al (12)	1976	26%
Roberts et al (13)	1976	23%
British Breast Group (14)	1978	10.1% (1.9 - 20.2%)

B. Series associated with a *low* detection rate

Author	Year	Detection Rate
Green et al (15)	1973	10%
Charkes et al (16)	1975	9%
Davies et al (17)	1977	5%
Butzelaar et al (18)	1977	3.4%
British Breast Group (14)	1978	10.1% (1.9 - 20.2%)

availability is severely limited and it is
rarely used today. Although different isotopes have been used in different laboratories, the detection rates have varied even
when the same isotope was used.

2. Detecting Apparatus

The profile and rectilinear scanner are
not suitable for screening purposes. The
whole body scanner is more convenient than
a Gamma camera but is less sensitive, and
this may explain some of the differences. An
acceptable compromise may be to obtain
anterior and posterior scintigrams using the
whole body scanner and Gamma camera pictures
of any suspicious area.

3. The Tumour

Are patients presenting earlier as a result
of the publicity associated with the early
detection of mammary carcinoma? Burn (19)
observed an increasing incidence of patients
presenting with earlier tumours. In 1965/66
only 5% of patients with mammary carcinoma
presented with a T1 lesion, whereas in 1970/
71 T1 lesions accounted for 11%, in 1972/73
for 16% and in 1974 for 27%. During the same
period the incidence of T1 and T2 tumours
increased from 46% in 1965/66 to 64% in 1974.
It has been shown that the detection rate is
related to the stage of the disease (20,21).
Hoffman and Marty (22) found positive scintigrams in 20% of patients with Stage I mammary
cancer and 38% of Stage II cancers and
Campbell and his colleagues (12) reported an
18% incidence in Stage I and 41% in Stage II

mammary cancers. Gerber and his colleagues
(23) found that only 2 of the 110 patients
with early mammary cancer had abnormal scintigrams yet 27% developed scintigraphic evidence
of skeletal metastases at post-operative
follow-up examination. They stressed that
their patients tended to seek medical attention early as recipients of no-cost military
medical care. Schaffer and Kalisher (24)
examined 42 women whose cancers had been
detected by mammography but were not clinically suspected or demonstrable. Six patients
had presented with symptomatic metastases
from an unknown primary source. The scintigrams were normal in the other 36 patients.

CORRELATION TO PROSTAGLANDIN PRODUCTION

What may be more important than the size
of the tumour is its behaviour. Bennett and
his colleagues (25) have shown that the
greatest prostaglandin synthesis occurred in
those tumours associated with skeletal metastases. It has been suggested that prostaglandins and other humoral factors stimulate
osteoclast activity, osteoclast mediated bone
destruction follows and possibly as a result
of the latter, malignant cells are able to
seed and grow.

CONCLUSION

There may be a significant difference in
tumour population, either with respect to
size, invasiveness or other factors between
the different series and this may explain
the difference in results. Unfortunately,
these aspects of the primary tumour have not

been fully investigated; it is possible that if we were able to answer this question we would understand much more about the way in which mammary carcinoma metastasizes.

What cannot be denied is that in any group of patients with apparently early mammary carcinoma there are two populations: those who have a normal skeletal scintigram and a better prognosis and those with abnormal scintigram and hereby indicative of advanced disease. Because there are differences in the relative incidence between these two groups in different series, controlled trials evaluating adjuvant chemotherapy has to include skeletal scintigraphy as an essential part of their pre-operative assessment and grouping. Scintigram-negative patients should be matched with scintigram-negative patients and similarly for scintigram-positive patients.

Hammond and his colleagues (39) suggested that skeletal scintigrams should be performed prior to adjuvant treatment and that if the scintigram was abnormal more intensive and prolonged therapy appropriate for advanced mammary carcinoma should be instituted. They also suggested that the use of serial scintigrams may allow the selection of a sub-group of patients with a high risk of recurrence who might benefit from more intensive or more prolonged adjuvant therapy in an effort to reduce their risk of subsequent recurrence.

THE PATHOLOGICAL BASIS FOR SKELETAL SCINTIGRAPHY

It has been shown that the vast majority of skeletal metastases are associated with new bone formation as well as bone destruction (26). The exceptions tend to be many of the lymphomata, myelomata and rapidly growing highly destructive lesions which radiologically appear as large lytic deposits. This new bone has an increased avidity for bone-seeking isotopes, and autoradiographs using a variety of these isotopes have shown that the isotope is selectively concentrated in the reactive new bone (26).

The radiographic appearance of the metastasis is dependent on the net produce of the simultaneously occurring bone formation and bone destruction. Where the former predominates, for example in prostatic carcinoma the metastases are sclerotic, but where the destructive process predominates the lesion may appear to be purely lytic on X-ray, although on histological examination some new bone formation is present. Computer assisted tomographic scanning (C.T. scanning) of skeletal metastases frequently indicates areas of new bone formation in lesions which appear lytic on X-ray.

There is also an increased vascularity around the lesion (27) and this is probably due to the opening up of pre-existing capillary-arteriolar complexes. Bone-seeking isotopes pass freely across the bone capillary membrane (28) and an increase in vascularity will result in an increased concentration of the isotope in the bone extracellular compart-

ment. This phase occurs rapidly and probably explains why the skeleton is outlined on the scintigram within minutes of an intravenous injection of a bone-seeking isotope. During the ensuing hours the isotope is then selectively concentrated in the reactive new bone produced around the metastasis. During this period the isotope is cleared from the blood, and the background activity decreases. The isotope does not diffuse passively back into the circulation as it is now incorporated in the reactive new bone. This explains why it takes two to four hours (depending on the bone-seeking isotope being used) to see the differential uptake between normal and abnormal bone on the scintigram. This hypothesis of a two-phased uptake (27) has been supported by other studies (29,30).

FALSE NEGATIVES AND FALSE POSITIVES

1. False Negatives

There are at least three causes for false negatives. The first includes those tumours which do not evoke an osteoblastic response. The second group is associated with small deposits; although metastases of ½ cm. diameter can be detected scintigraphically lesions smaller than this are likely to be missed. In our study of patients with apparently early mammary carcinoma the majority of women with negative scintigrams and who developed disseminated disease, showed evidence of skeletal metastases. These lesions must have been present before mastectomy, but were not detected on the initial scintigram. Post-operative serial scintigrams show an increasing incidence of skeletal metastases (23,31).

Finally, lesions in the pubis and ischium may be very difficult to detect scintigraphically (32). Most bone-seeking isotopes are excreted in the urine and their concentration in the bladder tends to mask the pubis. With many techniques of scintigraphy the ischium is poorly visualised.

2. False Positives

The most important problem associated with skeletal scintigraphy is the question of false positives. The uptake of bone-seeking isotopes is non-specific and any abnormality associated with increased new bone formation and vascularity will appear as an area of increased uptake on the skeletal scintigram, for example, osteosarcoma, fractures, infections, the arthritides, Paget's disease of bone, many benign tumours and even the normal epiphyseal plate in a growing child (33). These lesions are usually obvious on X-ray. Therefore, skeletal scintigraphy should be the initial investigation and high quality X-rays and even tomograms obtained of any region where there is an area of increased uptake of bone-seeking isotope. If a benign lesion is present, corresponding to the area of increased uptake, the scintigram should be regarded as normal for that patient. The

C.T. scanner may have an important role to play in reducing this risk. C.T. scanning, in its current form, cannot be used for screening purposes, as it is impossible to examine the entire skeleton with this instrument. However, it is extremely useful in examining a localised area where a metastasis is suspected, either on scintigraphic or clinical grounds. It is difficult to demonstrate the apophyseal joint between the 5th lumbar and the first sacral vertebra on X-ray yet osteoarthritis occurs at this site. We have seen a patient with an apparently early mammary carcinoma and who had several areas of increased uptake of isotope on her scintigram. Radiographs were normal; C.T. scanning indicated that, although most of these foci were due to metastatic disease, an eccentric area of increased uptake in the lumbo-sacral region was due to osteoarthritis of an apophyseal joint.

DETECTION OF METASTASES AT OTHER SITES

Although skeletal scintigraphy is probably the most sensitive method of staging mammary carcinoma at this moment, it gives no indication of the extent of visceral involvement. Scintigraphic methods of examining the brain, lungs, and liver are available but the results obtained do not justify their use for screening purposes (34). However, they may be extremely useful in evaluating patients in whom there is a suspicion of metastatic involvement.

What is required is a technique of detecting tumour at all sites, including the skeleton and the viscera. Currently, much work is being carried out on the development of tumour localising isotopes and biochemical markers (35). The results have been disappointing with respect to staging of apparently early disease.

ASSESSMENT OF RESPONSE OF ADVANCED DISEASE TO THERAPY

The commonest site for distant metastases from mammary cancer is the skeleton and it may be the only site. The clinical and radiographic assessment of response of these lesions may be unreliable (36). Skeletal metastases from mammary carcinoma are commonly lytic although sometimes a combination of lysis and sclerosis is seen. With remission of disease, bones with lytic metastases may radiologically return to normal or the lytic areas may become sclerotic (37). The development of new lytic lesions or the enlargement of existing ones indicates progression of the disease. However, from radiographs it is impossible to differentiate sclerotic lesions due to progression of the disease from those due to healing. Galasko and Doyle (36) studied 30 patients with advanced mammary carcinoma, who had had a skeletal scintigram prior to commencement of treatment and again after an interval of a few months. They found that in 13 patients (43%) the serial scintigrams provided infor-

mation that was not available from serial clinical or radiological examinations and was of considerable value in the assessment of response to treatment. Lesions which have responded to treatment lose their increased avidity for bone-seeking isotopes, irrespective of their radiographic appearance whereas the increased uptake continues in those metastases which do not respond to treatment (27). Similar findings have been reported by other authors (38,39).

REFERENCES

1. C. S. B. Galasko, Skeletal metastases and mammary cancer. *Ann. Roy. Coll. Surg. Eng.* 50, 3, (1972).
2. H. L. Jaffe, *Tumours and Tumorous Conditions of Bones and Joints*. Lea and Febiger, Philadelphia (1958).
3. A. Cushieri, Urinary hydroxyproline excretion in early and advanced breast cancer – A sequential study. *Br. J. Surg.* 60, 800 (1973).
4. J. G. Roberts, M. Williams, J. M. Henk, A. S. Bligh and M. Baum, The hypronosticon test in breast cancer. *Clin. Oncol.* 1, 33 (1975).
5. T. J. Powles, Geraldine Rosset, C. L. Leese and P. K. Bondy, Early morning hydroxyproline excretion in patients with breast cancer. *Cancer* 38, 2564 (1976).
6. C. E. Guzzo, W. N. Pachas, R. S. Pinals and M. J. Krant, Urinary hydroxyproline excretion in patients with cancer. *Cancer* 24, 382 (1969).
7. F. Gielen, J. Dequeker, A. Drochmans, J. Wildiers and M. Merlevede, Relevance of hydroxyproline excretion to bone metastasis in breast cancer. *Br. J. Cancer* 34, 279 (1976).
8. G. A. Edelstyn, P. J. Gillespie and F. S. Grebbell, The radiological demonstration of osseous metastases. *Clin. Radiol.* 18, 158 (1967).
9. C. S. B. Galasko, The significance of occult skeletal metastases, detected by skeletal scintigraphy in patients with otherwise apparently "early" mammary carcinoma. *Br. J. Surg.* 62, 694 (1975).
10. J. S. G. Blair, Does early detection of bone metastases by scanning improve prognosis in breast cancer? *Clin. Oncol.* 1, 185 (1975).
11. D. L. Citrin, R. G. Bessent, W. R. Greig, N. J. McKellar, C. Furnival and L. H. Blumgart. The application of the $^{99}TC^m$ phosphate bone scan to the study of breast cancer. *Br. J. Surg.* 62, 201 (1975).
12. D. J. Campbell, A. J. Banks and G. D. Oates, The value of preliminary bone scanning in staging and assessing the prognosis of breast cancer. *Br. J. Surg.* 63, 811 (1976).
13. J. G. Roberts, A. S. Bligh, I. H. Gravelle, K. G. Leach, M. Baum and L. E. Hughes, Evaluation of radiography and isotope scintigraphy for detecting skeletal metastases in breast cancer. *The Lancet* 1, 237 (1976).

14. British Breast Group, Bone scanning in breast cancer. Preliminary statement by British Breast Group on bone scanning. *Brit. Med. J.* 2, 180 (1978).

15. D. Green, R. Jeremy, J. Towson and J. Morris, The role of fluorine 18 scanning in the detection of skeletal metastases in early breast cancer. *Aust. N.Z.J. Surg.* 43, 251 (1973).

16. N. D. Charkes, L. S. Malmud, T. Caswell, L. Goldman, J. Hall, V. Lauby, W. Lightfoot, W. Maier and G. Rosemond, Pre-operative bone scans. Use in women with early breast cancer. *J. Amer. Med. Assoc.* 233, 516 (1975).

17. C. J. Davies, P. A. Griffiths, B. J. Preston, A. H. Morris, C. W. Elston and R. W. Blamey, Staging breast cancer: role of bone scanning. *Br. Med. J.* 2, 603 (1977).

18. R. M. J. M. Butzelaar, J. A. van Dongen, J. B. van der Schoot and B. J. G. van Ulden. Evaluation of routine pre-operative bone scintigraphy in patients with breast cancer. *Europ. J. Cancer* 13, 19 (1977).

19. J. I. Burn - personal communication (1977).

20. A. A. El-Domeiri and S. Shroff, Role of pre-operative bone scan in carcinoma of the breast. *Surg. Gynec. Obstet.* 142, 722 (1976).

21. R. R. Baker, E. R. Holmes, P. O. Alderson, N. F. Khouri and H. N. Wagner, Jr., An evaluation of bone scans as screening procedures for occult metastases in primary breast cancer. *Ann. Surg.* 186, 363 (1977).

22. H. C. Hoffman and R. Marty, Bone scanning: its value in the pre-operative evaluation of patients with suspicious breast masses. *Am. J. Surg.* 124, 194 (1972).

23. F. H. Gerber, J. J. Goodreau, P. T. Kirchner and W. J. Fouty, Efficacy of pre-operative and post-operative bone scanning in the management of breast carcinoma. *New Eng. J. Med.* 297, 300 (1977).

24. D. L. Schaffer and L. Kalisher, Incidence of bone metastases in women with minimal and occult breast carcinoma. *Radiology* 124, 675 (1977).

25. A. Bennett, E. M. Charlier, A. M. McDonald, J. S. Simpson, I. F. Stamford, and T. Zebro, Prostaglandins and breast cancer. *The Lancet* 2, 624 (1977).

26. C. S. B. Galasko, The pathological basis for skeletal scintigraphy. *J. Bone Jt. Surg.* 57-B, 353 (1975).

27. C. S. B. Galasko, The mechanism of uptake of bone-seeking isotopes by skeletal metastases. In *Medical Radionucline Imaging Vol. 2* p. 125. International Atomic Energy Agency, Vienna (1977).

28. S. P. F. Hughes, D. R. Davies, J. B. Bassingthwaighte, F. G. Knox and P. J. Kelly, Bone extraction and blood clearance of diphosphonate in the dog. *Am. J. Physiol.* 232, H341 (1977).

29. S. Hughes, R. Khan, R. Davies and P. Lavender, The uptake by the canine tibia of the bone-seeking agent ^{99m}TC - MDP before and after an osteotomy. *J. Bone Jt. Surg.* 60-B, 579 (1978).

30. N. D. Charkes and C. M. Philips, A new model of ^{18}F - Fluoride kinetics in humans. In *Medical Radionuclide Imaging Vol. 2* p. 137. International Atomic Energy Agency, Vienna (1977).

31. D. L. Citrin, D. C. Tormey and P. P. Carbone, Implications of the ^{99m}TC diphosphonate bone scan on treatment of primary breast cancer. *Cancer Treat. Rep.* 61, 1249 (1977).

32. C. S. B. Galasko and F. H. Doyle, The detection of skeletal metastases from mammary cancer. A regional comparison between radiology and scintigraphy. *Clin. Radiol.* 23, 295 (1972).

33. C. S. B. Galasko, Skeletal scintigraphy in *The Scientific Basis of Medicine Annual Reviews 1973* p. 187 (Edited by I. Gilliland and M. Peden), Athlone, London (1973).

34. C. S. B. Galasko, Screening for the potentially curable patient in *Breast Cancer Management - Early and Late.* Edited by B. A. Stoll) p. 15. Heinemann, London (1977).

35. R. C. Coombes, T. J. Powles, J. C. Gazet, H. T. Ford, P. J. Sloane, D. J. R. Laurence and A. M. Neville, Biochemical markers in human breast cancer. *The Lancet* 1, 132 (1977).

36. C. S. B. Galasko and F. H. Doyle, The response to therapy of skeletal metastases from mammary cancer. Assessment by scintigraphy. *Brit. J. Surg.* 59, 85 (1972).

37. W. D. Graham, Metastatic cancer to bone. *S. Afr. Med. J.* 39, 936 (1965).

38. I. Gynning, P. Langeland, S. Lindberg and C. Waldeskog, Localisation with Sr 85 of spinal metastases in mammary cancer and changes in uptake after hormone and roentgen therapy. *Acta radiol.* 55, 119 (1961).

39. N. Hammond, S. E. Jones, S. E. Salmon, D. Patton and J. Woolfenden, Predictive value of bone scans in an adjuvant breast cancer program. *Cancer* 41, 138 (1978).

Tumor Associated Markers in Breast Cancer*

P. Franchimont*, P. F. Zangerle*, C. Colin, P. Osterrieth***, J. C. Hendrick*, J. R. van Cauwenberge** and J. Hustin****

*Radioimmunoassay Laboratory, Institute of Medicine, University of Liege, Belgium
**Obstetrics and Gynaecology Department, Institute of Medicine, University of Liege, Belgium
***Bacteriology and Virology Department, Institute of Medicine, University of Liege, Belgium

Correspondence to P. Franchimont, Radioimmunoassay Laboratory, Institute of Medicine, University of Liege, Belgium

Abstract—Amongst assayed tumor markers, human chorionic gonadotrophin (HCG) and its α and β subunits, alpha foeto protein, calcitonin, parathormone, prolactin were not of substantial clinical values. Two peptides extracted from MuMTV (GP47 and P28) were not detected either in serum of patients with breast cancer or in tumor extract. No antibody directed against them was detected in serum.

In contrast CEA, kappa casein and gross cystic disease fluid protein (G.C.D.F.P.) may be related to the local and systemic extension of the neoplasia and may be considered as a valid index of prognosis. G.C.D.F.P. might also constitute an index of breast cancer risk.

RESULTS OF INDIVIDUAL TUMOR MARKER

Oncofoetal Antigens

Two oncofoetal antigens were assayed: alpha foeto protein (αFP) (1) and carcino embryonic antigen (CEA) extracted from liver metastasis (2).

As described previously (3) αFP is never positive. Thus, αFP measurement has no clinical interest in breast cancer.

CEA determination is an useful criteria in the diagnosis, follow up and prognosis of breast cancer. In the serum of 935 blood donor, the detectable levels never exceed 10 ng/ml. The results obtained in a population of women with breast diseases (3) are illustrated in Table 1. CEA is discriminating between benign and malignant breast diseases and the incidence of positivity as the absolute concentration of CEA increases in advanced disease. Furthermore, abnormal postoperative CEA levels are associated with lymph node extension (Table 1).

Table 1. Incidence of abnormally high levels of CEA and casein in benign and malignant breast diseases.

Nature of the Disease	Total n	CEA > 10 ng/ml n	CEA > 10 ng/ml %	Casein > 25 ng/ml n	Casein > 25 ng/ml %
Benign breast diseases	55	0	0	1	1.7
Breast cancer:					
- Onset of the disease (T_1, T_2, T_3, N_0, N_1, M_0)	39	20	51	6	15
- With metastases (M+)	25	14	56	11	44
- After surgical removal:					
N-	30	0	0	1	1.7
M+	39	15	39	7	19

*Supported by Grant Number 20305 from National Foundation for Medical Research (F.R.S.M.) and by C.G.E.R. Foundation for Cancer Research.

Placental Antigens

HCG and its α and β subunits were assayed using specific radioimmunoassays (4). In the normal population native HCG, α and β subunit levels never exceeded 1 ng/ml, 3.5 ng/ml and 1.5 ng/ml respectively. The incidence of pathological values of α (> 3.5 ng/ml) and β (> 1.5 ng/ml) subunits is lower in breast cancer population than in non breast benign diseases. Native HCG levels were found elevated in 6 of 39 breast cancer patients (15%) at the onset of clinical symptoms (T_1, T_2, T_3, N_0, N_1) in absence of metastasis (HM_0) and before any treatment. Surprisingly, none of 25 patients with metastatic disease had elevation of HCG and its α and β subunits. Thus, there is a weak incidence of abnormal HCG levels in breast cancer and no discrimination between benign disorders and malignant breast diseases for α and β HCG subunits.

Milk Proteins

Amongst milk proteins, two were extensively investigated in our laboratory : casein (5, 6) and Gross Cystic Disease Fluid Protein (G.C.D.F.P.) (7, 8). Kappa casein may be considered as a good marker for the functional activity of the normal mammary gland (6). Thus, serum K casein levels increased during pregnancy and reached very high values when milk is produced during the first days of lactation.

In breast cancer, immunoreactive kappa casein is detected at higher concentration than in normal population (i.e. $\geqslant$ 25 ng/ml) as illustrated in Table 1. The metastatic extension increases both the incidence of positive casein values and the absolute levels (3).

Lung, digestive and urinary tract cancers can also release casein like substances in the blood which demonstrates the existence of an ectopic exocrine secretion (6).

As it will be demonstrated later on, casein level may provide a criteria of prognosis when assayed with CEA.

Haagensen et al. (7) recently described a glycoprotein isolated from breast gross cyst disease fluid (G.C.D.F.P.) with a molecular weight of 15.000. This G.C.D.F.P., believed to be an epithelial cell secretory product, is present in milk and saliva and is present in very high concentrations in the fluid of breast cysts.

With the radioimmunoassay carried out in our laboratory (8), G.C.D.F.P. levels were most often undetectable in the serum of 277 normal subjects. Only in three subjects of the normal population, G.C.D.F.P. levels were higher than 5 ng/ml (1%). In 1 of 30 (3%) lactating women, levels were higher than 5 ng/ml whereas no value as high as 5 ng/ml were detected in the serum of 17 pregnant women. In contrast with casein, G.C.D.F.P. does not appear as functional index of normal mammary gland.

G.C.D.F.P. levels were higher than 5 ng/ml only in 1.5% of patients with non breast benign diseases (251 cases).

In breast diseases, the incidence of G.C.D.F.P. levels higher than 5 ng/ml and the mean levels are elevated in benign cystic disease and in breast cancer independent of stage (Table 2) compared with the values observed in non-cystic breast benign diseases.

When metastasis exists, the incidence and the absolute levels of G.C.D.F.P. increase (8).

G.C.D.F.P. appears to be specific for breast diseases as it is very rarely detected in serum of patients with benign diseases or cancers of lung, digestive and other origins.

Hormones

Levels of calcitonin, parathormone, prolactin were always detected in the normal range when assayed with our radioimmunological methods in serum of patients with benign and malignant breast diseases (9).

Viral Peptides from MuMTV

Some publications have described that antigens extracted from human breast cancer cross reacted with peptides contained in MuMTV. Thus, Black et al. (10) described an antigen GP50 in breast cancer cross reacting with GP47 from MuMTV. Furthermore, a protein with a molecular weight of 27.000 was described in

Table 2. Incidence of Gross Cyst Disease Fluid Protein (G.C.D.F.P.) in Benign and Malignant Breast Diseases.

Breast Diseases	n	Incidence of G.C.D.F.P. Levels higher than 5 ng/ml		Mean Levels ng/ml ± SEM
		n	%	
Non cystic breast diseases	85	3	3.5	2 ± 1.04
Cystic breast diseases	53	30	58	12 ± 3.2
Breast carcinoma	98	64	66	44 ± 8.3

"virus core" prepared from human milk (11) and antibodies to antigens related to the core antigens of MuMTV were detected in the serum of breast cancer patients (12).

On that basis, we initiated a work on RIA of all the constituants of MuMTV and of antibodies against them.

Presently, two specific radioimmunoassays were carried out, one for GP47, the main envelope glycoprotein of MuMTV (13) and the other for P28 the main core protein of MuMTV (14).

Although GP47 and P28 were measured in several organs and serum of infected and tumor bearing mice, no substance immunologically related to GP47 and P28 were detected either in sera from 107 normal subjects, 65 women with benign mastopathy (9 fibroadenoma, 36 polycystic diseases, 20 considered to be a risk of developing breast cancer), 89 from women with breast cancer at different stages in 15 cystic fluids, in 12 milks and in 50 breast cancer extracts. Furthermore, no antibody against GP47 and P28 was detected in the same media.

More than ten different antisera for each antigen were used to exclude the possible selection of antibody only directed against antigenic groups specific for MuMTV.

Sporadic positive results could be interpreted by the fact that GP47 and P28 are damaged by proteases present either in the serum or in organ extracts. Thus, RIA may give false positive results.

Before concluding this work should be extended to the other components of MuMTV and to the whole virus. Some works seem to indicate that antibodies detected in serum of women with breast cancer are directed against the whole virus (15) and that antiserum against whole virus gives positive results by immunofluorescence when reacting with some breast cancer tissues (16).

II. CLINICAL INTEREST OF ASSAYING MARKERS

1. Factor of Risk

Till now, assays of tumor markers do not provide any indication on the risk for a woman to develop a breast cancer. But G.C.D.F.P. could be useful for that purpose as it is a specific breast marker and its incidence of positivity is high in Gross Cystic Disease. A long term evaluation of more than 2.000 patients with gross cyst disease has revealed that breast carcinoma developed at more than four times the frequency in normal women (7).

An epidemiological and histological study of women with breast cyst disease and positive G.C.D.F.P. in blood is needed to evaluate this epithelial protein as a biological index of risk.

2. Tumor Markers and Diagnosis

As previously stated (17), measurement of tumor markers is an useful diagnostic procedure which, however, is neither absolute nor specific.

Simultaneous assays of several tumor markers decrease the incidence of "false negative" cancer. In breast cancer, CEA is abnormally high in 51% of cases at the onset of clinical symptoms whereas abnormally high CEA or casein levels are detected in 65% of these cases.

Furthermore, the detection of abnormal levels of specific marker such as G.C.D.F.P. leads to the diagnosis of a breast disease.

3. Extension of the Tumor

As many authors and our group have already demonstrated (3), the incidence of positivity as the absolute levels of CEA, kappa casein and G.C.D.F.P. increase with extension of breast cancer (3).

4. Tumor Markers and Prognosis

Two retrospective studies have investigated the correlation between tumor markers and prognosis.

In 69 breast cancer patients the incidence of positivity of at least one of the two cancer antigens assayed (CEA and kappa casein) dropped from 65% to 33% after mastectomy. Thirty patients had no evidence of lymph node involvement or of distant metastases. Casein was found only in one case. The incidence of positivity of at least one antigen was therefore 1 out of 30.

In 39 N+ patients the frequency of appearance of casein and CEA was 7 and 15 on 39 cases respectively (Table 1). One case was positive for CEA and casein thus 21/39 were tumor marker positive (56%).

Two years later, local recurrence and/or metastases have appeared in 4 of 30 cases N–CEA–(one of the 4 patients was casein positive), in 10 of 24 cases N+CEA– (5 of them were casein positive) and in 10 of 15 patients N+CEA+. Local and distant recurrence was observed in 16/22 (72%) with abnormal high levels of casein or CEA and in only 8/47 (17%) in absence of these tumor markers.

Metastatic disease may be predicted when CEA or casein is detected in abnormally high levels in absence or in presence of lymph node invasion.

As casein and CEA, Gross Cyst Disease Protein Fluid is not detected in serum of women after removal of breast tumor when lymph nodes are not invaded (0/9) whereas 9/13 patients with lymph node metastasis are G.C.D.F.P. positive.

In a retrospective study, Colin (18) correlated the evolution of small breast cancer (T_1, T_2) after surgical removal with several parameters: number of invaded lymph nodes, invasion of mammary chain nodes, histological grade, thermographical and radiological stages and increased levels of CEA or casein.

No patient with a good prognosis i.e. alive without local or distant recurrence two years after mastectomy demonstrated high CEA or

kappa casein levels. No invasion of lymph
nodes and weakly evolutive aspects of histological, radiological and thermographical
investigations were observed in these cases.

In contrast, high CEA and/or casein levels
were measured in 11 of 16 patients with bad
prognosis, dying within two years following
the operation. Lymph nodes of these patients
were invaded and/or radiological, thermographical and histological investigations gave
highly evolutive results. Nine patients
with recurrence and/or metastasis but still
alive two years after breast cancer removal
were classified in the category of poor
prognosis. CEA or casein were detected in
the serum of three of them.

Thus, increased levels of CEA and casein
are always present in patients with poor
prognosis whereas absence of CEA and casein
are observed in patients of the three groups,
the incidence decreasing with aggravation of
the prognosis.

REFERENCES

1. P. Franchimont, P. F. Zangerle, M. L.
   Debruche, J. Proyard, M. Simon and
   U. Gaspard, Dosage radioimmunologique
   de l'alpha foeto protéine dans les
   différentes conditions normales et
   pathologiques. *Ann. Biol. Clin.*, 33, 139
   (1975).
2. P. Franchimont, M. L. Debruche, P. F.
   Zangerle and J. Proyard, Carcinoembryonic
   antigen (CEA). In: "Radioimmunoassay
   and Related Procedures in Medicine",
   Vol. II, *International Atomic Energy
   Agency*, Vienna, 267 (1974).
3. P. Franchimont, P. F. Zangerle, J. C.
   Hendrick, A. Reuter and C. Colin, Simultaneous assays of cancer associated
   antigens in benign and malignant breast
   diseases. *Cancer* 39, 2806 (1977).
4. P. Franchimont, A. Reuter and U. Gaspard,
   Ectopic production of human chorionic
   gonadotropin and its α and β subunits.
   In: "*Current Topics in Experimental
   Endocrinology*", L. Martini and V. H. T.
   James, Eds., Academic Press, New York,
   London, Vol. 3, 202 (1978).
5. J. C. Hendrick, A. Thirion and
   P. Franchimont, Radioimmunoassay of
   casein. In: "*Cancer Related Antigens*",
   P. Franchimont, Ed., North-Holland,
   Amsterdam, 51 (1976).
6. P. Franchimont, J. C. Hendrick, A. Thirion
   and P. F. Zangerle, Kappa casein: an
   index of normal mammary function and
   tumor associated antigen. In: "*Immuno-
   diagnosis of Cancer*", R. B. Herberman
   and K. R. McIntire, Eds., M. Dekker, Inc.,
   New York, Basel, Part I, 499 (1979).
7. D. E. Haagensen, Jr., G. Mazoujian,
   W. Holder, Jr., S. J. Kister and S. A.
   Wells, Jr., Evaluation of a breast cyst
   fluid protein detectable in the plasma
   of breast carcinoma patients. *Ann. Surg.*,
   3, 279 (1976).
8. P. F. Zangerle, J. Collette and
   P. Franchimont, Specific radioimmunoassay
   for gross cystic disease fluid protein
   (G.C.D.F.P.). Submitted for publication
   (1979).
9. G. Heynen, Discussion in "*Cancer Related
   Antigens*", P. Franchimont, Ed., North-
   Holland, Amsterdam, New York, 160 (1976).
10. M. M. Black, R. E. Zachrau, A. S. Dion,
    B. Shore, D. L. Fine, H. P. Leis, Jr.
    and C. J. Willams, Cellular hypersensi-
    tivity to GP55 of Rill-Murine Mammary
    Tumor Virus and GP55-like protein of
    human breast cancers. *Cancer Res.*, 36,
    4137 (1976).
11. P. Furmanski, C. P. Loeckner, C. Longley,
    L. J. Larson and M. A. Rich, Identifica-
    tion and isolation of the major core
    protein from the oncornavirus-like
    particle in human milk. *Cancer Res.*, 36,
    4001 (1976).
12. M. Muller, S. Zotter and C. Kemmer,
    Specificity of human antibodies to intra-
    cytoplasmic type A particles of the
    murine mammary tumor virus. *J. Natl.
    Cancer Inst.*, 56, 295 (1976).
13. P. F. Zangerle, C. M. Calberg-Bacq,
    C. Colin, P. Franchimont, C. Francois,
    L. Gosselin, S. Kozma and P. M. Osterrieth,
    Radioimmunoassay for glycoprotein GP47
    of murine mammary tumor virus in organs
    and serum of mice and search for related
    antigens in human sera. *Cancer Res.*, 37,
    4326 (1977).
14. J. C. Hendrick, C. Francois, C. M.
    Calberg-Bacq, C. Colin, P. Franchimont,
    L. Gosselin, S. Kozma and P. M. Osterrieth,
    Radioimmunoassay for protein p28 of
    murine mammary tumor virus in organs and
    serum of mice and search for related
    antigens in human sera and breast cancer
    extracts. *Cancer Res.*, 38, 1826 (1978).
15. N. K. Day, Communication at the XXVII
    Annual Colloquium on: "Protides of the
    biological fluids", Brussels (1979).
16. F. Loisillier, J. Saracino, D. Metivier
    and P. Burtin, Characterisation of an
    antigen associated to human mammary
    carcinoma. In: "*Protides of the biologi-
    cal fluids*", *XXVII Annual Colloquium*,
    Abstr. n⁰ 65 (1979).
17. P. Franchimont, P. J. Zangerle,
    J. Nogarede, J. Bury, F. Molter,
    A. Reuter, J. C. Hendrick and
    J. Collette, Simultaneous assays of
    cancer-associated antigens in various
    neoplastic disorders. *Cancer*, 38, 2287
    (1976).
18. C. Colin, submitted for publication
    (1979).

Biological Markers as Prognostic and Clinical Evaluation Tools

D. C. Tormey* and T. P. Waalkes**

*Departments of Human Oncology and Medicine, Wisconsin Clinical Cancer Center, Madison, USA
**The Johns Hopkins Hospital, Baltimore, USA

Correspondence to D. C. Tormey, Departments of Human Oncology and Medicine, Wisconsin Clinical Cancer Center, University of Wisconsin, 600 Highland Ave., Madison, WI. 53792, USA

Abstract—*The current status of the usefulness of biological markers in the clinical management of breast cancer patients is reviewed. It is suggested that there is no present role for such tests in screening settings. Their prognostic use preoperatively has not been evaluated and their postoperative prognostic use has only limited data available. Information with reference to the detection of recurrent disease with serial values or of prognosis at the onset of metastatic disease is fragmentary. Serial markers have been found useful for detecting changes in the tumor burden of advanced disease patients but the impact of this observation upon patient care remains undefined. Further advances with respect to the clinical use of markers will require an amalgamation of more incisive clinically relevant questions with appropriately designed clinical experiments.*

The identification of unique cancer-associated molecular species in body fluids has been a goal of biologists for decades. Thus far the discovery of such putative biological markers has been followed by the development of highly sensitive analytical methods that have shown the substance to also be present in "normal" individuals, albeit usually in lower concentrations, and frequently in some stage of embryogenesis. These observations have further supported the concept of a biological continuum existing between "normal" cells and their "malignant" counterparts. As a result the clinician has turned toward an analysis of how to utilize the quantitative differences that exist between normal and malignant states, and to the development of a matrix of tests. Utilizing these approaches the role of circulating cancer-associated biological markers can be assessed across at least seven defined clinical settings. Each of these settings will be described briefly with respect to the clinicians difficulties in utilizing biological marker assays. The discussion will focus upon breast cancer although examples will be drawn from other diseases.

Mass Screening of Normal Populations

The predictive value of a screening test is determined by the interaction of (1) the tests' sensitivity, (2) the tests' specificity, and (3) the disease prevalence in the population. Sensitivity is defined as the incidence of true positive results when patients with the disease are tested. Specificity is defined as the incidence of true negative results when persons free of the disease are tested. Sensitivity and specificity are inversely related. Focusing upon colorectal cancer as an example because of the greater data base and test sensitivity than for breast cancer, the use of >2.5 ng/ml as elevated for the plasma carcinoembryonic antigen (CEA) test of Hansen et al (1) provides an approximate 90% specificity and 67% sensitivity; defining >10 ng/ml as elevated increases the specificity to 99.9% but decreases the sensitivity to 6.4%.

The third term, the prevalence rate, defines the number of patients per 100,000 population who have the disease. For colorectal cancer, the prevalence rate for persons over age 35 is approximately 0.2% (2,3). Screening such a population of 100,000 persons with the CEA test would find 134 of the 200 colorectal cancer patients (i.e., 0.67 x 200); however, an additional 9,980 persons without the disease (i.e., 99,800 x 0.10) would also have an abnormal test result. Thus there would be 74 subjects with a false positive test for every one with a true positive test. A ratio of 69 to 1 was reported in a screening evaluation analyzed by Chu and Murphy (4).

Of interest is that raising the sensitivity to 100%, while detecting all the colorectal cancer patients, only decreases the ratio to 50 to 1. The specificity would need to be nearly 100% to yield a minimum number of false positives. From these considerations it appears that the prevalence rate may be the single most important factor with current assays and therefore only high risk populations are presently amenable to economical screening.

Screening of High Risk Populations

The development of high risk profiles for individual diseases is the most direct current method for isolating cohorts with an increased prevalence rate. Perhaps the most successful application of this principle is the use of calcitonin secretion under stimulation in family members of the autosomal dominant, variably expressed, familial medullary thyroid carcinoma (5-8). In this setting the sensitivity and specificity both are close to 100% and the prevalence rate approximates 50% making it economically feasible to test all suspect individuals. Such an approach for breast cancer detection might be considered using single tests and test matrices among high risk familial kindreds.

Disease Localization in Specific Sites

A relatively unexplored use for biological marker assays relates to their capability to aid in isolating the localization of metastatic disease. For example, in 106 patients with metastatic breast cancer we observed elevated hydroxyproline/creatinine ratios (OHP/Cr) above 2 standard deviations from normal in 20 (19%) and elevated CEA levels in 47 (44%) (9). A Venn diagram of these 106 patients demonstrated only OHP/Cr elevations in 6 (6%), only CEA in 33 (31%), and both in 14 (13%). When the data was further subsetted it was observed that 17 of the 20 OHP/Cr elevations (85%) were in the 58 patients with osseous involvement. In addition 6 of the 17 (35%) were associated with normal CEA levels. This contrasts with 30 of the 47 (64%) elevated CEA levels being associated with osseous involvement. Among the 54 patients with either or both tests elevated, OHP/Cr elevations were associated with osseous involvement in 17 (31%) and non-osseous disease in 3 (6%). Conversely, among the 47 patients with elevated CEA levels, concurrent elevated OHP/Cr ratios were present in 11 of 14 instances (78%) of associated osseous involvement. Thus, it would appear that the use of the OHP/Cr assay could aid in ascertaining the reason for a CEA elevation since 64% (30/47) of the patients' with a CEA elevation had osseous involvement whereas 78% (11/14) of the patients' with both elevated had osseous involvement. Similar evaluations with other cancer-associated biochemical tests could be similarly useful relative to other sites of involvement.

Prognostication in Patients with Either Localized or Metastatic Disease

There is a continuing need to identify preoperative and postoperative patients who are at high risk of having disseminated disease. Although high preoperative CEA levels have been associated with a poorer prognosis in colorectal carcinoma (10), there is only limited data available for breast carcinoma. The observation of an elevated postoperative CEA test in breast carcinoma has been associated with a higher short term relapse rate than is a normal test result (11,12). Similar observations have been reported for elevated urinary hydroxyproline/creatinine ratios (13) and for elevated serum ferritin levels (14). Clearly there is a need for improving the detection capability in this regard since less than 15% of axillary node negative and 20-25% of axillary node positive patients have elevated postoperative CEA values despite the fact that five year relapse rates approximate 20-26% with localized disease and 50% with regional disease (15). The addition of other tests such as human chorionic gonadotrophin (hCG), polyamines, and nucleosides has increased the axillary node positive postoperative detection rate to 67% (16). Unfortunately, the relationship of this observation and other matrix approaches to relapse rates is not yet clearly defined.

At the onset of overt metastatic breast cancer the major prognostic factors for therapeutic benefit include performance status, number of organ sites of disease involvement, dominant metastatic site, age, and estrogen receptor status. These factors appear to have become increasingly muted with the development of more effective therapeutic regimens. Recently, the chemotherapy response rate and time to treatment failure were both reported to be increased if the pretreatment CEA was ≤5 ng/ml (16). The response rate was 12/12 (100%) with CEA levels ≤5 ng/ml as compared to 14/23 (60.9%) with CEA levels >5 ng/ml. The time to treatment failure was 9.7 months as compared to 8 months. The effect was more pronounced if serum hCG measurements were also incorporated into the evaluation (16,17). The response rate with a CEA level >5 ng/ml and a hCG level >5 mIU/ml was 50%. The time to treatment failure was 10 months with either test below 5, and 6.3 months with both tests >5. The results appeared to be independent of other pretreatment variables. These data were subsequently supported by a report that patients with low CEA levels and metastatic disease survive longer than their counterparts with high CEA levels (18). Each of these observations is awaiting confirmation or refutation from other investigators. In addition, no information exists as to their value for selecting what type of systemic therapy to employ, a point that could be very relevant to the treatment of postoperative subclinical disease.

Recurrent or Residual Disease Detection Following Curative Therapy

The effectiveness of alpha-fetoprotein (AFP) and hCG assays in the followup and guidance of therapy in patients with hepatomas and female choriocarcinomas, respectively, has led to a search for similar markers in other diseases. The finding of rising postoperative CEA levels in colorectal disease and more recently in breast cancer has been shown to be associated with eminent relapse (19,20). The lead times vary up to 29 months in these studies (19). Unfortunately, not all patients breast tumors are associated with the production of CEA or any other single marker. Thus there is a need for additional markers to be studied in a serial manner to assess their role for recurrence detection in relation to CEA. Similarly, it is not yet known if the institution of therapy in the presence of a rising marker in these diseases will lead to an improvement in survival, although reports suggesting this effect in colorectal cancer have been published (21).

Assessment of Systemic Therapy Effectiveness

Data currently exists demonstrating good correlations between marker levels and clinical tumor burden. During the systemic therapy of metastatic breast cancer rising levels parallel disease progression and decreasing levels parallel disease regression. This is of particular use in hard to evaluate disease, such as osseous or intra-abdominal involvement. However, the survival impact of changing therapy based upon observing an increasing marker level is not known even though rising levels of CEA or polyamines can occur up to 3 months prior to overt clinical relapse (17, 22). There is at present no corresponding data published in the postoperative subclinical disease setting, although preliminary results suggest CEA levels can increase up to six months prior to recurrence (20). Markers shown to be useful in recurrent disease include CEA (16,23,24), the polyamines (17), and hydroxyproline/creatinine ratios (25). Recently, we have observed a similar effect with a serum fast-homoarginine-sensitive alkaline phosphatase (FHAP) isoenzyme. Details of the FHAP assay have been reported elsewhere (26). Utilizing an upper limit of normal with a 5% false positive rate, 67.9% of 103 metastatic breast cancer patients have elevations with a current range extending to 123 times the upper limit of normal.

The use of all current cancer-associated markers is clearly dependent upon the patients disease state being associated with their production. Since no marker has a 100% sensitivity for breast cancer, the development of a battery of tests continues to be under consideration with respect to measuring the impact of therapy and the status of the disease.

References

1. H.J. Hansen, J.J. Snyder, E. Miller, J.P. Vandevoorde, O.N. Miller, L.R. Hines, J.J. Burns. Carcinoembryonic antigen (CEA) assay: A Laboratory adjunct in the diagnosis and management of cancer. *Human Pathology* 5, 139 (1974).

2. S.J. Cutler, J.L. Young, Jr. *Third National Cancer Survey: Incidence Data*, Bethesda: DHEW Publication No. (NIH) p. 75-787 (1975).

3. P.C. Prorock. Cancers of the digestive system, in *Cancer Patients Survival: Report Number 5*, eds L.M. Axtell et al, Bethesda: DHEW Publication No. (NIH) p. 77-992 (1976).

4. T.M. Chu, G.P. Murphy. Carcinoembryonic antigen: Evaluation as screening assay in noncancer clinics. *NY State J. Med.* 78, 879 (1978).

5. A.H. Tashjian, Jr., H.J. Wolfe, E.F. Voelkel. Human calcitonin: Immunologic assay, cytologic localization and studies on medullary thyroid carcinoma. *AM. J. Med.* 56, 840 (1974).

6. G.W. Sizemore, V.L.W. Go. Stimulation tests for diagnosis of medullary thyroid carcinoma. *Mayo Clin. Proc.* 50, 53 (1975).

7. S.A. Wells, Jr., D.A. Ontjes, C.W. Cooper, J.F. Hennessy, G.J. Ellis, H.T. McPherson, D.C. Sabiston, Jr. The early diagnosis of medullary carcinoma of the thyroid gland in patients with multiple endocrine neoplasia type III. *Ann. Surg.* 182, 362 (1975).

8. K. Graze, I.J. Spiler, A.H. Tashjian, Jr., K.E.W. Melvin, S. Cervi-Skinner, R.F. Gagel, H.H. Miller, H.J. Wolfe, R.A. DeLillis, L. Leape, Z.T. Feldman, S. Reichlin. Natural history of familial medullary thyroid carcinoma: Effect of a program for early diagnosis. *N. Engl. J. Med.* 299, 980 (1978).

9. K.J. Pandya, D.C. Tormey, T.P. Waalkes, C. Gehrke, H. Hansen, J. Neifeld, J. Harberg. Hydroxyproline in breast cancer. *Proc. Am. Assn. Cancer Res.* 20, 223 (1979).

10. E.D. Holyoke, T.M. Chu, G.P. Murphy. CEA as a monitor of gastrointestinal malignancy. *Cancer* 35, 830 (1975).

11. D.Y. Wang, R.D. Bulbrook, J.L. Hayward, J.C. Hendrick, P. Franchimont. Relationship between plasma carcinoembryonic antigen and prognosis in women with breast cancer. *Europ. J. Cancer* 11, 615 (1975).

12. R.E. Myers, D.J. Sutherland, J.W. Meakin, J.A. Kellen, D.G. Malkin, A. Malkin. Carcinoembryonic antigen in breast cancer. *Cancer* 42, 1520 (1978).

13. A. Cuschieri. Urinary hydroxyproline in the management of breast cancer. *World J. Surg.* 1, 299 (1977).

14. A. Jacobs, B. Jones, C. Ricketts, R.D. Bulbrook, D.Y. Wang. Serum ferritin concentration in early breast cancer. *Br. J. Cancer* 34, 286 (1976).

15. L.M. Axtell, M.H. Myers. *End Results in Cancer, Report No. 4*, DHEW Publication No. (NIH) 767. U.S. Dept. Health, Education and Welfare, Washington, D.C., (1975).

16. D.C. Tormey, T.P. Waalkes. Clinical correlation between CEA and breast cancer. *Cancer* 42, 1507 (1978).

17. D.C. Tormey, T.P. Waalkes. Biochemical markers in cancer of the breast. *Recent Results in Cancer Research* 57, 78 (1976).

18. R.E. Myers, D.J.A. Sutherland, J.W. Meakin, D. Malkin, J. Kellen, A. Malkin. Clinical association of carcino-embryonic antigen in breast cancer. In: *Compendium of Assays for Immuno-Diagnosis of Human Cancer*. (Edited by R.B. Herberman) p. 381. Elsevier-North-Holland (1979).

19. J.J. Sorokin, P.H. Sugarbaker, N. Zam-
    check, M. Pisick, H.Z. Kupchik, F.D.
    Moore. Serial carcinoembryonic antigen
    assays. *JAMA* 228, 49 (1974).
20. H. Falkson, personal communication (1979).
21. J.P. Minton, E.W. Martin, Jr. The use
    of serial CEA determinations to predict
    recurrence of colon cancer and when to do
    a second-look operation. *Cancer* 42, 1422
    (1978).
22. D.C. Tormey, T.P. Waalkes, personal
    observations (1976).
23. A.M. Steward, D. Nixon, N. Zamcheck, A.
    Aisenberg. Carcinoembryonic antigen in
    breast cancer patients—serum levels and
    disease progress. *Cancer* 33, 1246 (1974).

24. N.M. Borthwick, D.W. Wilson, P.A. Bell.
    Carcinoembryonic antigen (CEA) in
    patients with breast cancer. *Eur. J.
    Cancer* 13, 171 (1977).
25. T.J. Powles, C.L. Leese, P.K. Bondy.
    Hydroxyproline excretion in patients with
    breast cancer and response to treatment.
    Brit. Med. J. 2, 164 (1975).
26. S.L. Ehrmeyer, B.L. Joiner, L. Kahan,
    F.C. Larson, R.L. Metzenberg. A cancer
    associated, fast, homoarginine sensitive
    electrophoretic form of serum alkaline
    phosphatase. *Cancer Res.* 38, 599 (1978).

The Value of Sequential Marker Estimations Following Mastectomy for Breast Cancer

R. C. Coombes[1], T. J. Powles[2], H. T. Ford[2], J.-C. Gazet[2],
C. W. Gehrke[3], J. W. Keyser[4], P. E. G. Mitchell[5], S. Patel[1],
W. H. Stimson[6], M. Abbott[1] M. Worwood[7] and A. M. Neville[1]

[1]Ludwig Institute for Cancer Research (London Branch), Royal Marsden Hospital,
Sutton, Surrey, SM2 5PX
[2]Royal Marsden Hospital, Sutton, Surrey
[3]Experiment Station Chemistry Laboratory, University of Missouri, Columbia,
Missouri 65201, USA
[4]The Royal Infirmary, Cardiff, CF2 1SZ
[5]Ninewells Hospital and Medical School, Dundee, DD1 9SY
[6]University of Strathclyde, 204 George Street, Glasgow, G1 1XW
[7]University Hospital of Wales, Heath Park, Cardiff, CF4 4XN

Correspondence to: R. C. Coombes Ludwig Institute for Cancer Research,
Royal Marsden Hospital, Sutton, Surrey, SM2 5PX

Abstract–*Ten markers have been measured at approximately 3-monthly intervals
in patients with breast cancer following mastectomy but before development
of overt metastatic disease. Only three markers (alkaline phosphatase,
carcinoembryonic antigen (CEA) and γ-glutamyl transpeptidase (γGT)) were
abnormal prior to the development of metastases in more than 1/23 patients.
These three markers were also found to be most frequently elevated at the
time of developing metastases.*

*In half the patients, a 'lead interval' of 3 months or more was obtained
using the markers examined, but identical lead intervals would have been
obtained had only alkaline phosphatase, CEA and γGT been used.*

INTRODUCTION

In the management of breast cancer there is
a major role for biochemical markers. At the
time of development of clinically obvious
metastases, often a large tumour bulk is
apparent and this may account for the relatively short remissions induced by chemotherapy and hormone treatment given at this
stage. Even when chemotherapy is given at
an early stage, before the development of
overt metastatic disease, results are
unfavourable in many patients (1) and this
may be due, at least in part, to the absence
of any clear method of quantitating disease
bulk to assess effectiveness and duration of
treatment.

For this reason, a study was undertaken two
years ago (2,3) to evaluate 19 biochemical
'markers' of disease activity of breast
cancer. The results showed, however, that
most elevations recurred only at the time of
metastasis and that, even at this late stage,
only 9/27 markers were abnormal in more than
50% of patients.

In the present study we have measured 10 of
the most commonly abnormal markers at regular
intervals before the development of overt
metastatic disease to determine the time or
'lead interval' that could be obtained before
the development of overt metastatic disease.

MATERIALS AND METHODS

1. Patients

Between 1975 and 1978, 152 sequential
patients were seen at the Medical Breast
Unit, Royal Marsden Hospital, Sutton, with
histologically confirmed, poor prognosis
(Grade 3 (4) and/or regional lymph node
involvement) primary breast carcinoma. They
were randomised to receive either benoral or
placebo following mastectomy to assess the
value of benoral as adjuvant therapy. By
August, 1978, there were 23 evaluable patients
who had developed metastases 8-42 months
(mean 21 months) after mastectomy.

To qualify for this study, full staging at
the time of mastectomy had to be carried out.
This involved full clinical examination,
full blood count, liver function tests,
serum urea, electrolytes, calcium phosphate
and urate, chest x-ray, bilateral mammography,
grey-scale liver ultrasound and/or liver
scan, technetium polyphosphate bone scan,
skeletal radiography and iliac crest marrow
aspirate. The presence of metastases as
disclosed by these tests excluded patients
from the study.

Blood and 'early morning' urine samples
for marker estimation were obtained between
4-6 months after mastectomy and at

approximately 3 monthly intervals thereafter.
The blood-sample was separated into plain
and E.D.T.A. tubes and spun at 2000 rpm for
10-15 minutes within 1 hour of removal. The
plasma or serum was then immediately placed
into 1ml containers and stored at -60°C until
required for assay.

On each occasion a patient was sampled and
at 6-monthly intervals, full clinical examination was carried out. Clinical examination,
chest x-ray, skeletal survey, bone scanning
and marrow aspirates were also performed in
most patients. In the first half of the
study period regular liver scans and liver
ultrasound examinations were carried out
(Table 1).

patients who remained disease-free for at
least 18 months; (c) 8 patients with benign
breast disease; (d) any transient elevations
that occurred in the study group followed by
a fall to within the normal range.

All samples were coded and sent in dry ice
to each laboratory. To assist in the determination of significant differences between
marker levels, the same sample was divided
into five aliquots and sent to each laboratory.

RESULTS

1. Abnormalities Found

Table 2 and Fig. 1a, b shows the incidence

Table 1. Physical tests carried out to monitor 23 patients.

Physical test	Number of tests carried out:				
	(a) before metastasis				(b) at metastasis
	> 8 mo.	5-8 mo.	1-4 mo.	Total	No % positive
Clinical examination (nodes, skin)	23	23	23	23	9 (39)
Liver scan	18	4	2	17	1 (6)
Liver ultrasound	20	4	2	16	4 (25)
Bone scan	24	18	8	21	8 (38)
Skeletal survey	23	19	7	22	9 (41)
Chest X-ray	23	20	7	23	9 (49)
Bone marrow aspirate	23	11	2	17	2 (12)

For the purpose of the present study, the
results of all markers and physical tests
have been examined at 3 periods before the
development of metastatic disease (Fig. 1a,b),
viz: >8 months, 5-8 months and 1-4 months
before metastases.

When symptoms or signs suggested the presence of metastasis, the patient was admitted
and full staging tests were carried out
together with marker estimation. With the
exception of those patients with solely bone
metastases, histological and cytological
evidence of metastasis was obtained from all
of the 23 patients.

As a control group, 6 patients who presented
with primary breast cancer but who have
failed to demonstrate any evidence of metastasis subsequently were also studied. These
were selected to compare with the original
staging, age and follow-up time of the
patients in the study group, and have been
subjected to identical staging tests and
blood and urine samples as the study group.

2. Markers

Ten putative markers were examined in
the present study and Table 2 lists the
markers with the methods used for their determination (5-10).

To derive the upper limit of normal for
each test, a level was found that was in
excess of (a) the normal range for the laboratory; (b) 23 pre-operative samples for

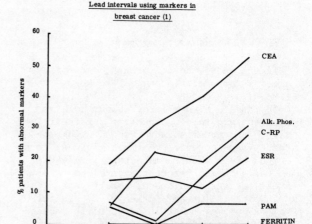

Fig. 1a. Abnormalities occurring before and
at the time of metastases in
breast cancer using CEA alkaline
phosphatase, C-reactive protein
(C-RP), erythrocyte-sedimentation-
rate (ESR), pregnancy associated-
macroglobulin (PAM) and Ferritin.

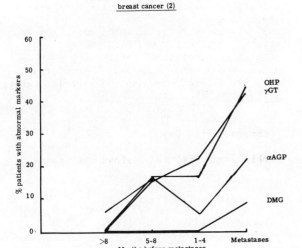

Fig. 1b. Abnormalities occurring before and
at the time of metastases in
breast cancer using γ-glutamyl
transpeptidase (γGT), hydroxyproline (OHP) α, - acid - glycoprotein
(α,-AGP) and dimethylguanosine
(DMG).

and degree of elevation of the ten markers
measured in 23 patients, and the overall percentage of abnormalities at each of the 4
periods studied (>8 months, 5-7 months, and
1-4 months before, and at the time of development of overt metastasis as disclosed in the
physical tests of metastasis outlined in
Table 1).

Persistent CEA elevations: antedated clinical evidence of recurrence in 8/23 patients;
alkaline phosphatase showed antecedent rises
in 4/23 patients and γGT in 2/16. 3 other
markers (C-reactive protein, $α_1$-AGP, and
hydroxyproline) each showed persistent rises
in a single patient. Overall 13/23 patients
developed antecedent marked rises whilst a
further 3 patients demonstrated a synchronous
rise at the time of detection of metastasis.
All 16 patients would have developed an
abnormal biochemical profile at the same
times had only alkaline phosphatase, CEA and
γGT been used.

Concerning the degree of elevations, it can
be seen from Table 2 that the markers showing
the greatest separation from normal were also
those having the highest incidence of abnormalities. Those displaying a rise in excess
of 100% before the development of metastasis
were CEA (5 patients), γGT (2 patients) and
C-reactive protein (1 patient). At the time
of metastasis those showing this degree of
elevation were CEA (7 patients), γGT (4
patients), alkaline phosphatase (4 patients),
and C-reactive protein (2 patients).

2. Lead Intervals

The lead intervals achieved by using all
ten markers are shown in Figs. 1 and 2.

Figure 2 shows that, by combining all
markers, persistently abnormal biochemical
profiles are found in half the patients
three months before the development of overt
metastatic disease. It can be seen from
Figs. 1 and 2 that only three markers, viz.
CEA, γGT and alkaline phosphatase appear to
be useful in predicting recurrence. The
remaining biochemical markers were not elevated in a significant percentage of patients.
Marker measurement compared favourably,
however, with physical methods for detecting
metastasis, since all of these, including
bone scanning, were normal within 8 months
of development of clinically obvious metastases.

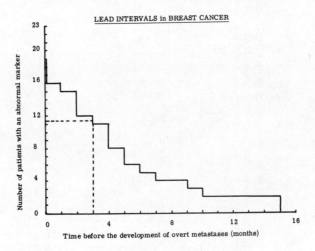

Fig. 2. Lead intervals found in breast
cancer by combining all the markers
studied. The interrupted line
indicates the time at which half
the patients show abnormalities,
i.e. at three months.

None of the six patients who were followed
sequentially and who failed to develop overt
metastases developed significant rises in
any marker.

3. Sites of Metastasis

Table 1 documents the sites of metastases
in the 23 patients as detected by physical
tests at time of presentation of metastases.
As previously documented (12) local, skeletal
and lung metastases are most commonly
detected. The inaccuracy of physical tests
(13) for liver metastases does not permit
accurate correlation but with this reserva-
tion, the 3/4 patients with liver metastases
at presentation had abnormal γGT or alkaline
phosphatase. The 3 patients with high urine
excretion of hydroxyproline all had skeletal
metastases. Otherwise, no correlation could
be found between site of metastases and
elevated markers.

Table 2. Markers evaluated showing degree of evaluation before metastases and at first metastasis.

Marker	Normal range	Units	Method of determination	Ref. no.	Elevated values before overt metastases†					Elevated values when first metastatic			Number paralleling outcome of treatment*
					No. of patients	Lead interval (mo.)		Abnormal values:		No.	Abnormal values:		
						Range	Mean	Range	Mean		Range	Mean	
1) ESR	0–40	mm/h	Westergren		0/18	–	–	–	–	3/18	50–76	61	0/6
2) Alkaline phosphatase	30–105	iu/l	Autoanalyser		4/23	4–10	5.7	110–175	139	7/22	110–500	260	5/11
3) PAM	0–164	g/l	Stimson and Sinclair 1974	5	0/23	–	–	–	–	1/16	220	–	0/6
4) C-reactive protein	0–1.6	g/l	Behringwerke kit		1/23	5	–	7.5	–	4/15	2.3–13.7	5.5	2/7
5) CEA	0–40	ug/l	Laurence et al. 1972	6	8/23	3–15	7.6	48.9–213	125	10/17	47.8–545	218	1/8
6) Ferritin	0–274	ug/l	Jones and Worwood 1973	7	0/23	–	–	–	–	0/18	–	–	0/7
7) α_1-acid glycoprotein	0–125	g/l	Roberts et al. 1975	8	1/23	3	–	1.68	–	3/17	1.3–2.0	1.62	1/7
8) Dimethyl-guanosine	0–2	nmoles/umoles creat.	Gehrke et al. 1979	9	0/11	–	–	–	–	1/11	2.88	–	0/4
10) Hydroxy-proline	1.0–3.0	mg/g creat.	Guzzo et al. 1976	11	0/11	–	–	–	–	2/13	3.1,4.7	3.9	1/5
11) γ-glutamyl transpeptidase	10–50	iu/l	Autoanalyser		2/16	1–5	3.0	85–380	232	7/17	52–270	150	4/8

ESR = Erythrocyte-sedimentation-rate
PAM = Pregnancy-associated-macroglobulin
CEA = Carcinoembryonic antigen

†ie. consistently elevated values, persisting with development of overt metastases

*ie. falling from elevated to normal after achieving response of metastases to treatment, or becoming elevated following response.

The seven patients who failed to demonstrate abnormal markers even at the time of metastasis did not differ from the other patients in respect of tumour-free-interval; further, only 2/4 patients who had only locally recurrent disease either in skin or lymph nodes, could therefore be considered as having a smaller tumour burden fell into the 'marker-negative' group.

4. Change following Treatment

Markers were quantitated in all 11 patients before and after 12 trials of therapy following the discovery of overt metastatic disease.
Five out of 12 treatments (3 of hormone therapy and 2 of chemotherapy) were succesful and the remainder resulted in no clinical or radiological evidence of response (5 hormone therapy and 2 of chemotherapy). In only 14 instances out of 75 did the marker values parallel the outcome of therapy and those more commonly found to do so were alkaline phosphatase and γGT (Table 2).

DISCUSSION

Most of the markers chosen for this study were those found to be most frequently abnormal in our previous studies (2,3). Using the present group of ten markers we have now shown that, at the time of first presentation with metastasis, 16/23 patients show abnormal levels of at least 1/11 markers but that only 13/23 patients showed any significant lead interval.

The most efficient combination of markers was that of alkaline phosphatase, CEA and γGT since by using these three markers one could obtain the same lead intervals as found by using all eleven markers.

The ESR has been previously shown to be non-specifically elevated in patients with metastatic cancer (13), although previous reports have supposed their measurement to be of more value than we have demonstrated. Total alkaline phosphatase is a well-known index of liver and/or skeletal metastasis and thus elevations (7/22) found in patients with overt metastasis is expected as is the relatively good correlation of level of alkaline phosphatase with outcome of treatment of metastases (Table 2). The reason for the lower percentage of elevated levels in this group than in our previous study (2) probably reflects an earlier stage of metastatic disease.

PAM estimations failed to distinguish those with metastases from those without and in no occasion did the level parallel outcome of therapy. C-reactive protein was only helpful in a single patient in predicting metastases, but was elevated in 4/15 patients at the time of development of metastases.

CEA is perhaps the most useful parameter studied and reflects the high percentage of abnormal values seen in metastatic breast cancer (2,6,14) and also confirms the lead interval that has been found before by our group (1) for this marker. The lead intervals were observed in a higher percentage of patients in this study (35% as compared with 11%) although the lead intervals so obtained were similar.

Of the remaining markers, both ferritin and hydroxyproline showed much lower detection rates than we have found previously (2). This may well be related to the different antiserum used, since the previous study was carried out using an antiserum raised against a tumour-derived isoferritin (16). The reason for the lower detection rate of hydroxyproline excretion is not clear but our results differ from those of Cuschieri (17) who found a 'lead interval' in 9 patients before the radiological demonstration of skeletal metastases. A possible reason for the reduced detection rate for α_1AGP as compared to previous studies (2,8) could be that we have elevated the upper limits of the normal range to include transient elevations that were found either in patients who subsequently developed metastases or in the six patients who did not.

The results of urinary dimethylguanosine are negative but may be due to the different method used to measure the nucleoside using high-performance liquid chromatography (9).

γGT appears to be elevated in a significant number of patients with metastatic disease in this study, although, as with most of the other markers, only 2/16 patients have high levels antedating overt metastasis.

Overall, therefore, regular alkaline phosphatase, CEA and γGT estimations appear to be capable of predicting overt metastases by 3 months or more in about half of the poor-risk patients with primary breast cancer in this study. The other markers may be useful in individual patients but do not appear to add to these three markers.

Some of the markers in blood and urine studied here may be of value in replacing the physical tests currently available to detect metastases. For example, a recent study from this Unit has demonstrated that alkaline phosphatase measurements should be used to select patients for physical imaging studies of the liver, since the latter are rarely, if ever, positive in the absence of a raised alkaline phosphase (12).

In this study, a screen of alkaline phosphatase, CEA and γGT together with clinical examination and chest x-ray would have alerted the physician to the possibility of metastatic disease in all the patients at the time metastases were detected.

Concerning the value of these markers in predicting the development of metastases, there are clearly some patients who have persistently high markers before physical tests are capable of detecting disease. It may be of interest to assess other staging techniques such as laparotomy in patients who develop such changes and thus obtain histological evidence of recurrence. Treatment at this earlier stage in the disease may prolong the palliative effect of chemotherapy or hormone treatment.

ACKNOWLEDGEMENTS

We thank the Biochemistry Department, Royal
Marsden Hospital for their assistance in
this study, Miss M. Jones for statistical
help and advice and Mrs. L. Bush for typing
the manuscript.

REFERENCES

1. G. Bonadonna, P. Valagussa, A. Rossi,
   R. Zucali, G. Tancini, E. Bajetta,
   C. Brambilla, M. De Lena, G. Di Fronzo,
   A. Banfi, F. Rilke and U. Veronesi,
   Are Surgical Adjuvant Trials Altering
   the Course of Breast Cancer. *Seminars in
   Oncology* 5, 450 (1978).
2. R. C. Coombes, T. J. Powles, J. C. Gazet,
   H. T. Ford, A. G. Nash, J. P. Sloane,
   C. J. Hillyard, P. Thomas, J. W. Keyser,
   D. Marcus, N. Zinberg, W. H. Stimson
   and A. Munro Neville, A Biochemical
   Approach to the Staging of Human Breast
   Cancer. *Cancer* 40, 937 (1977).
3. R. C. Coombes, Biochemical Markers in
   Human Breast Carcinoma, *Invest. Cell
   Pathol.* I, 347 (1978).
4. H. J. G. Bloom, W. W. Richardson and
   E. J. Harries, Natural History of
   Untreated Breast Cancer (1805-1933):
   Comparison of Untreated and Treated
   Cases According to Histological Grade of
   Malignancy. *Br. Med. Journal* 2, 213
   (1962).
5. W. H. Stimson and J. M. Sinclair, An
   Immunoassay for a Pregnancy-Associated
   α-Macroglobulin Using Antibody Enzyme
   Conjugates. *FEBS Letters* 47, 190 (1974).
6. D. J. R. Laurence, U. Stevens,
   R. Bettleheim, D. Darcy, C. Leese,
   C. Turbeville, P. Alexander, E. W. Johns
   and A. M. Neville, Role of Plasma CEA
   in Diagnosis of Gastrointestinal, Mammary
   and Bronchial Carcinoma. *Br. Med. Journal*
   III, 605 (1972).
7. B. M. Jones and M. Worwood, An Automated
   Immunoradiometric Assay for Ferritin.
   Journal Clin. Path. 28, 540 (1975).

8. J. G. Roberts, J. W. Keyser and M. Baum,
   Serum α-I-Acid Glycoprotein as an Index
   of Dissemination in Breast Cancer.
   Br. Journal Surg. 62, 816 (1975).
9. C. W. Gehrke, K. C. Kuo, T. P. Waalkes
   and E. Borek, Patterns of Urinary
   Excretion of Modified Nucleosides.
   Cancer Research 39, 1150 (1979).
10. C. E. Guzzo, W. N. Pachas, R. S. Pinels
    and M. J. Krant, Urinary Hydroxyproline
    Excretion in Patients with Cancer.
    Cancer 24, 382 (1966).
11. J. M. Thomas, W. H. Redding, R. C.
    Coombes, J. P. Sloane, H. T. Ford,
    J-C. Gazet and T. J. Powles, Failure to
    Detect Intra-Abdominal Metastases from
    Breast Cancer: A Case for Staging
    Laparotomy. *Br. Med. Journal* 2, 212
    (1975).
12. L. De Rivas, T. J. Powles, H. T. Ford,
    J-C. Gazet, A. M. Neville and R. C.
    Coombes, Test for Liver Metastases in
    Breast Cancer: Evaluation of Liver Scan
    and Liver Ultrasound. Clinical Onlology:
    submitted.
13. A. M. Neville and E. H. Cooper, Biochemi-
    cal Monitoring of Cancer. A Review. *Ann.
    Clin. Biochem.* 13, 283 (1976).
14. D. C. Tomey, T. P. Waalkes, D. Ahmann,
    C. W. Gehrke, R. W. Zumwatt, J. Snyder
    and H. Hansen, Biological Markers in
    Breast Cancer. Incidence of Abnormality
    of CEA HCG, three Polyamines and three
    Nucleosides. *Cancer* 35, 1095 (1975).
15. A. M. Neville, E. H. Cooper, R.Bettelheim,
    R. C. Coombes, D. J. R. Laurence,
    C. Turberville and J. H. Westwood, The
    Role of Plasma CEA Assays in the Manage-
    ment of Colorectal and Mammary Carcinomas.
    Protides in Biological Fluids, p. 671
    (1977).
16. D. M. Marcus and N. Zinberg, Measurement
    of Serum Ferritin by Radioimmunoassay:
    Results in Normal Individuals and Patients
    with Breast Cancer. *Journal Nat. Cancer
    Inst.* 55, 791 (1975).
17. A. Cuschieri, Urinary Hydroxyproline
    Excretion in Early and Advanced Breast
    Cancer - A Sequential Study. *Br. Journal
    Surg.* 60, 800 (1973).

Needle Biopsy and Aspiration Cytology in the Diagnosis of Malignancy in Clinically Suspicious Breast Masses: A Rational Approach

M. M. Shabot*, I. M. Goldberg*, P. M. Schick*, R. Nieberg**, M. R. Coates*, J. R. Benfield* and Y. H. Pilch***

*Department of Surgery, Harbor/UCLA Medical Center, Torrance, California, UCLA School of Medicine, Los Angeles, California
**Department of Pathology, Harbor/UCLA Medical Center, Torrance, California, UCLA School of Medicine, Los Angeles, California
***Surgical Oncology Service, Department of Surgery, University of California at San Diego, San Diego, California

Correspondence to M. M. Shabot, M.D., Assistant Professor of Surgery, Los Angeles County Harbor/UCLA Medical Center, 1000 West Carson Street, Torrance, California 90509, U.S.A.

Abstract—*Two sequential series of patients were evaluated to determine the accuracy of physical examination, mammography, needle biopsy and aspiration cytology in establishing the diagnosis of breast masses. All but three of the 378 biopsies were performed under local anesthesia. In the first series of 297 consecutive cases, physical examination was correct in 92% of cases, mammography in 89%, and needle biopsy in 88%. The second series of 81 consecutive patients with highly suspicious breast masses yielded correct diagnoses by physical examination in 85%, mammography in 52.8%, needle biopsy in 78.9% and thin needle aspiration cytology in 96.2%. Combining the results of aspiration cytology and needle biopsy provided a diagnosis of frank malignancy in 45 of 50 patients with breast cancer. Based on the efficacy of aspiration cytology and needle biopsy, we propose an algorithm for the management of breast lesions which eliminates general anesthesia for biopsy and facilitates rapid outpatient confirmation of the diagnosis of malignancy.*

INTRODUCTION

Over the past several years, interest in establishing the diagnosis of malignant breast masses prior to definitive surgery has markedly increased (1). Diagnostic modalities evaluated include physical examination, mammography, xeroradiography, thermography, needle biopsy, thin needle aspiration cytology and excisional biopsy under local anesthesia (2-10). The following reasons have been advanced to explain this interest:

1. An increasing number of women no longer wish to consent for "frozen section - possible mastectomy", i.e., they want to participate in the decision for mastectomy prior to receiving a general anesthetic (11).
2. Surgeons now wish to avoid the risks of general anesthesia for the 80% of patients who come to excisional biopsy for benign disease (10).
3. There is increased appreciation among clinicians for the need to survey the patient for evidence of metastatic disease prior to definitive surgical therapy for cancer (10).

4. Newer, alternative methods of dealing with the primary tumor, such as segmental mastectomy, are best performed with the mass in situ as a landmark.

While mammography, xeroradiography and thermography serve to confirm suspicion for palpable breast lesions and initiate suspicion for certain nonpalpable ones, these modalities, by themselves, cannot definitely establish the diagnosis of malignancy. For this purpose surgeons have relied upon excisional biopsy, now frequently performed under local rather than general anesthesia. In an attempt to construct an algorithm to establish the diagnosis of cancer in an even less invasive manner, we have evaluated needle biopsy and aspiration cytology in two sequential series of patients.

MATERIAL AND METHODS

All patients were evaluated in the Harbor-UCLA Medical Center Breast Clinic, a referral clinic for patients with breast masses or symptoms. Most patients receive mammography prior to their first attendence in the clinic.

Details pertaining to the patient populations and diagnostic criteria have been published separately (10,12).

In case Series I, 297 consecutive biopsies
were performed, all but three under local
anesthesia. The diagnostic accuracy of
physical examination, mammography and needle
biopsy were compared. Thin needle aspiration
cytology was added to the aforementioned
diagnostic modalities for Series II, in
which 81 patients were studied prospectively.
These patients differed from those in the
first series in that they were selected for
inclusion only if the clinical impression
indicated greater than 50% chance of malignancy. Concurrent patients with less suspicious lesions simply received breast
biopsy under local anesthesia, a technique
well proven by our first study. For all
patients receiving breast biopsy under local
anesthesia, a one gram portion of the biopsy
specimen was rapidly frozen in liquid nitrogen for estrogen and progesterone assay if
malignancy was proven on tissue section.
In all patients in both series, negative or
inconclusive needle biopsy and aspiration
cytology was rapidly followed with excisional
biopsy.

	Needle Biopsy			
	Malignant	Atypical	Benign	Not Done
Malignant	27		10	1
Suspicious	5		3	
Atypical	2	1		
Benign				
Unsatisfactory			1	

45/50 cases = 90% combined diagnosis rate

Fig. 1. Combined diagnosis of malignancy
in 50 cases.

cancer, concurrent needle biopsy identified
an additional 7 patients who had either
suspicious or atypical cytology. Thus frank
malignancy was proven in 45 of 50 patients
(90%) by needle alone. No mortality and no
significant morbidity resulted from biopsy
techniques in the entire group of 378
patients.

RESULTS

Comparative diagnostic accuracy of the
various methods is given in Table 1.

Table 1. Accuracy of diagnostic methods.

Diagnostic method	% Correct		% False positive		False negative		Total no. cases	
Series	I	II	I	II	I	II	I	II
Physical examination	92	85	1	12.5	7	2.5	297	80
Mammography	89	52.8	5	15.7	6	31.5	246	57
Needle biopsy	88	78.9	0	0	12	21.1	44	72
Aspiration cytology	-	96.2	-	0	-	3.8	-	78

Case selection for only highly suspicious
lesions in Series II probably accounts for
most of the observed differences. Physical
examination was quite accurate (85-92%) in
both groups. Mammography proved to be less
accurate in the second subset of patients
with highly suspicious lesions. Needle
biopsy was highly reliable (79-88%) in both
series. However, the most accurate diagnostic modality proved to be thin needle
aspiration cytology, which yielded correct
diagnoses in 75 of 78 patients (96.2%) with
satisfactory specimens, with 3.8% false
negatives and no false positives. The value
of combined aspiration cytology and needle
biopsy in patients with suspicious masses is
demonstrated in Fig. 1.

While cytology yielded diagnoses of frank
malignancy in 38 of the 50 patients with

DISCUSSION

Based on the results of our two breast
biopsy studies over the past 5½ years, we
propose that an algorithmic or flow chart
approach may be formulated for orderly, rapid,
efficient and cost-effective management of
breast masses (Fig. 2).

The results of mammography, xeroradiography
and thermography, as indicated, are taken
together with the physical examination and
history to form a clinical impression. If
the impression is not suspicious for cancer,
the patient may be scheduled for followup
as appropriate. Aspiration cytology alone
should be considered for screening these
clinically benign lesions for occult malignancy.

If the impression is suspicious but there

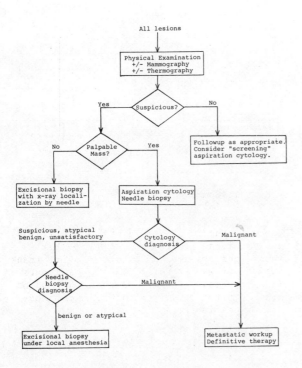

Fig. 2. Algorithm for management of breast
masses.

is no palpable mass (i.e., the suspicion is
based on mammo-, xero- or thermography),
excisional biopsy under local anesthesia
should be performed with x-ray needle localization or confirmation of the suspicious
tissue.

Most patients with clinically suspicious
lesions have a palpable mass and are therefore
candidates for needle biopsy and thin needle
aspiration cytology. These tests are performed in the outpatient clinic at the conclusion of the initial visit, assuming that
mammography has already been obtained. Within
24 to 48 hours of the clinic visit, pathology
results should be available. Cytology is
considered first due to its accuracy. If
frank malignancy is proven, the patient is
scheduled for evaluation for evidence of
metastatic disease (currently chest x-ray,
liver function profile and bone scan) and
scheduled for definitive therapy. If the
cytologic diagnosis is suspicious, atypical,
benign or unsatisfactory, needle biopsy
results may show malignancy and the patient
is directed towards the metastatic workup.
If both needle biopsy and aspiration cytology
are negative or inconclusive, excisional
biopsy under local anesthesia is scheduled.

In conclusion, we have presented an algorithmic approach to the evaluation of breast
masses which eliminates general anesthesia,
frozen section tissue examination, and
consent for "possible mastectomy". This
method represents a rapid, accurate and cost-
effective means of establishing the diagnosis
of malignancy in clinically suspicious breast
masses.

REFERENCES

1. C. Davies, C. Elston, R. E. Cotton and
   R. W. Blamey, Preoperative diagnosis in
   carcinoma of the breast. *Brit. J. Surg.*
   64, 326 (1977).
2. S. A. Feig, G. S. Shaber, G. F. Schwartz,
   A. Patchelfsky, H. I. Libshitz,
   J. Edeiken, R. Nerlinger, R. F. Curley,
   and J. D. Wallace, Thermography, mammography, and clinical examination in
   breast cancer screening. *Diagnostic
   Radiol.* 122, 123 (1977).
3. R. L. Egan, G. T. Goldstein and M. M.
   McSweeney, Conventional mammography,
   physical examination, thermography and
   xeroradiography in the detection of
   breast cancer. *Cancer* 39, 1984 (1977).
4. C. J. Davies, C. W. Elston, R. E. Cotton,
   R. W. Blamey and R. G. Wilson, "Tru-cut"
   needle biopsy versus fine needle aspiration cytology in the diagnosis of primary
   breast cancer. *Clin. Oncol.* 3, 123
   (1977).
5. T. S. Kline and H. S. Neal, Role of
   needle aspiration biopsy in diagnosis of
   carcinoma of the breast. *Obstet. and
   Gynecol.* 46, 89 (1975).
6. W. J. Frable, Thin-needle aspiration
   biopsy, A personal experience with 469
   cases. *A.J.C.P.* 65, 168 (1976).
7. T. S. Kline and H. S. Neal, Needle
   aspiration of the breast - Why bother?
   Acta Cytol. 20, 324 (1976).
8. J. Zajicek, T. Caspersson, P. Jakobsson,
   J. Kudynowski, J. Linsk and M. Us-Krasovec,
   Cytologic diagnosis of mammary tumors
   from aspiration biopsy smears, Comparison
   of cytologic and histologic findings in
   2,111 lesions and diagnostic use of
   cytophotometry. *Acta Cytol.* 14, 370
   (1970).
9. G. Kreuzer and E. Boquoi, Aspiration
   biopsy cytology, mammography and clinical
   exploration: A modern set up in diagnosis
   of tumors of the breast. *Acta Cytol.* 20,
   319 (1977).
10. M. R. Coates, Y. H. Pilch and J. R.
    Benfield, Changing concepts in establish-
    ing the diagnosis of breast masses.
    Amer. J. Surg. 134, 77 (1977).
11. R. R. Baker, Out-patient breast biopsies,
    Ann. Surg. 185, 543 (1977).
12. M. M. Shabot, I. M. Goldberg, P. Schick,
    R. Nieberg, Y. H. Pilch, Aspiration
    cytology is superior to Tru-cut needle
    biopsy in establishing the diagnosis
    of clinically suspicious breast masses.
    Cancer (submitted for publication).

The Possibility of Accurate Prediction of Recurrence Rates after Mastectomy

R. D. Bulbrook*, D. Y. Wang*, R. R. Millis** and
J. L. Hayward***

*Department of Clinical Endocrinology, Imperial Cancer Research Fund, London,
U.K.
**Hedley Atkins Unit, New Cross Hospital, London, U.K.
***Breast Unit, Guy's Hospital, London, U.K.

Correspondence to R. D. Bulbrook, Department of Clinical Endocrinology, Imperial
Cancer Research Fund, Lincoln's Inn Fields, London WC2A 3PX, U.K.

Abstract—*A clinical trial has been established to assess the possibility of
accurate prediction of recurrence rates after mastectomy. Recurrence rates
have been calculated for various categories of the 390 patients who entered
the trial in the first three years.*
*These rates are such that unless highly selected patients are studied
(which can lead to bias) it may be necessary to accumulate large numbers of
serial patients (≈1000) followed for long periods of time, if definitive
statements about new predictors are to be made.*

INTRODUCTION

It is only in the last decade that so many
alternative treatments have become available
for the treatment of patients with early
breast cancer. When radical mastectomy (or
a minor variant of this treatment) was the
only option, prediction of response to
treatment was relatively unimportant. Now
that the choice of primary treatment ranges
from X-ray alone to super-mastectomy, and
chemotherapy, immunotherapy or endocrine
therapy may be used for adjuvant therapy an
accurate estimation of the probability of
recurrence for a particular patient is much
to be desired. Intensive combination
chemotherapy after primary radical surgery
might very well be considered for a patient
with a 90% chance of recurrence within, say,
2 years, but might be considered wholly
inappropriate for patients with small, highly
differentiated tumours with no nodal involvement, since the majority of these patients
will be alive and well ten years after
mastectomy.

In spite of a considerable literature on
tests for the prediction of recurrence, it
is noticable that the methods used to treat
early breast cancer are rarely determined
by the results of such tests. Prediction
of response and hence, treatment, is still
largely decided by the pathological stage
of the tumour, particularly the number of
nodes involved. Surprisingly, tumour size
and grade are rarely used as determinants of
treatment in spite of the fact that both are
well-established as predictive indices.

MATERIAL AND METHODS

In February, 1975, a collaborative experiment was set up between the Breast Unit at
Guy's Hospital and the Department of Clinical
Endocrinology in the Imperial Cancer Research
Fund. The former undertook to supply blood
and urine specimens from serial patients, in
each of whom a detailed pathological investigation was carried out. The latter undertook
to check the value of a variety of predictive
tests which had been either devised within
the Department or taken from the literature.
The criteria for selecting these was that
they should have at least some semblance of
credibility.

The design of the experiment was simple.
A 24h. urine specimen was obtained from
each patient before mastectomy and 10 days
after operation. The pH of the urine was
adjusted to pH 6.5 before storage at -20°.
Serum was prepared from the blood specimens,
aliquoted to 2ml portions and stored at -20°.

An extensive history was obtained from each
patient in which details of reproductive
history, family history of breast disease,
previous breast and other diseases, menstrual
status and use of steroidal contraceptives
were obtained.

Clinical and pathological stage were determined; the latter involved examining an
average of 23 nodes in each patient, with a
count of the number involved.

As a preliminary screen, the "markers"
under test at the moment are; various aspects
of endocrine function, hydroxyproline, CEA,
ferritin, tryptophan metabolism, sialyltrans-
ferase activity and SHBG.

During the first three years of the experiment, 390 patients with operable breast
cancer accrued to the trial. Of these, 19
did not fit the protocol (lost to follow-up;
insufficient blood and urine specimens; no
data on menopausal status; nodal status
unavailable, etc.) and these were rejected.

RESULTS

For the purpose of this paper the follow-up
on the remaining patients was taken to April
1979.

There were 93 pre-menopausal patients with
Stage 1 disease entered into the trial during
this 3 year period. Of these 12 had a recurrence of their disease. The comparable
figures for menopausal and post-menopausal
Stage 1 patients are 116 entered:13 recurred.

For patients with Stage II disease there
were 60 pre-menopausal patients entered, with
14 recurrences and 102 menopausal and postmenopausal patients with 32 recurrences.

The rates of recurrence are shown in
Figure 1.

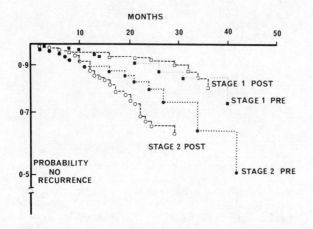

Fig. 1. Recurrence rates after mastectomy
        by pathological stage and meno-
        pausal status. The term post refers
        to both menopausal and post-meno-
        pausal women: pre refers to pre-
        menopausal women.

DISCUSSION

Even the most cursory examination of these
data indicates the first problem in establishing new predictive tests: very large
numbers of patients are required if a substantial number of recurrent cases are to be
obtained, especially if patients have no
nodal involvement. But there is no way of
establishing the reliability of a test without
obtaining relatively large numbers of recurrent cases within each major stratification
(stage certainly, possibly also grade, tumour
size, menopausal status, age).

The slopes of the curves shown in Figure 1
make it possible to calculate the approximate
number of recurrences that will occur with a
given rate of accrual to the trial, over a
given time (assuming log-linearity of
recurrence). For patients with Stage 1
tumours, an entry of 1,000 patients and a
follow-up of 10 years might be necessary.

These considerations lead to another
problem. The almost universal custom is to
take all the patients with recurrence and to
compare the levels of a particular tumour
marker in these cases with the levels in a
small sample of the non-recurrent cases.
This may lead to an over-estimate of the
usefulness of the predictive test.

The only way to obtain an unbiased estimate
of the potential usefulness of a test is to
carry out the test on serial patients or at
least not to bias the results by over-
selecting recurrent patients. The problem
becomes more complicated when multiple marker
assays are used.

Finally, there is the problem of validating
the test or tests. The simple solution
would be to carry out a prospective trial
on serial patients, and under routine clinical
conditions, so that an estimate might than
be made on how the test works in practice.
Another possibility would be to use the
results of a predictive test as an additional
stratification parameter, as is almost
invariably done with stage and is often
done with estrogen receptor. Whatever
strategy is adopted, the establishment and
validation of new tests of prediction of
recurrence is a formidable undertaking.

Hormone Receptors

The Usefulness of Steroid Hormone Receptors in the Management of Primary and Advanced Breast Cancer

W. L. McGuire

*Department of Medicine/Oncology, University of Texas Health Science Center,
7703 Floyd Curl Drive, San Antonio, Texas 78284, U.S.A.*

Correspondence to W. L. McGuire

Abstract—*Estrogen receptor status is a valuable prognostic guide for recurrence and survival in early breast cancer. Its role in endocrine therapy of advanced breast cancer is well established. Conflicting data exists regarding receptor and response to chemotherapy; a prospective trial is indicated. The presence of progesterone receptor signals a very likely response to endocrine therapy.*

INTRODUCTION

In this invited manuscript, I will provide a brief overview of the role of steroid receptor assays in the management of breast cancer patients. For a more historical account with detailed bibliographies, I refer the reader to several more complete reviews (1-3).

1. Estrogen Receptor as a Prognostic Factor in Early Breast Cancer

The theoretical correlation between estrogen receptor (ER) and the state of tumour differentiation has led investigators to examine the relationship between ER and prognosis of patients with primary breast cancer. Since ER negative tumors tend to be more undifferentiated histologically and have a higher growth fraction as determined by thymidine labeling index, one might hypothesize that these tumors have a more rapid rate of proliferation resulting in a worse prognosis and several studies have confirmed this (4-9). More important, however, the relationship between ER and prognosis is independent of other variables such as axillary nodal status, age or menopausal status, size or location of the tumor, and the degree of histological differentiation (grade) of the tumor. From a study in San Antonio, we found that the number of axillary node negative patients with recurrent disease 20 months after mastectomy was 3 times higher if the tumor was ER negative (22%) compared to ER positive (7%) (6). Similarly, 50% of ER negative, node positive patients had recurred at 20 months compared to 25% of the ER positive group. These observations have obvious implications for clinical trials. It is clear that both axillary nodal status and ER status must be included in the stratification of all patients undergoing surgical and/or adjuvant chemotherapy trials since they are independent prognostic variables of

similar power. Furthermore, the ER status is important in planning new adjuvant treatment protocols both for selecting patients for hormonal adjuvant therapy and for selecting poor prognosis patients with a high risk of recurrence (ER negative) who may benefit from more aggressive management.

2. Estrogen Receptor as a Guide in the Management of Advanced Breast Cancer

The value of the ER assay in predicting tumor response to endocrine therapy has been established. Numerous independent studies have now confirmed the results presented at the international workshop on estrogen receptors in breast cancer held in 1974 (10). These cumulative data from 14 institutions world-wide using different assay methods and with independent review of all clinical correlations provided the most convincing evidence for the usefulness of the ER assay (Table 1).

Table 1. Tumor ER and response to endocrine therapy.

ER Status	Response to Endocrine Therapy (%)	
	Additive	Ablative
Positive	55	60
Negative	8	9

Adapted from reference 10.

About 55 to 60% of patients with ER positive tumors respond to endocrine therapy. Although 40% of ER positive tumors fail to regress with endocrine therapy, the response rate is double that seen when clinical criteria alone are used to select patients (30%). Recent efforts have been aimed at improving the predictive index in the ER positive group (see below).

A more striking relationship exists for ER negative tumors. A response rate of less than 10% is consistently observed in this group. Thus physicians will be correct more than 90% of the time in their decision to avoid hormone therapy in ER negative patients.

One attempt to improve the selection in ER positive patients has been to quantitate the ER content in the tumor sample, reasoning that tumors with a high ER level might contain a high proportion of ER positive cells resulting in a larger reduction in tumor burden with endocrine therapy. Recent data from several laboratories supports this hypothesis (Table 2).

Table 2. Percent response to endocrine
therapy as a function of ER
concentration.

| | ER concentration | | |
Study	High	Medium	Low
McGuire (2)	81	46	6
Allegra (11)	78	45	9
DeSombre (5)	70	50	5

For the purposes of comparison we have adapted the data from each of these studies into table form by arbitrarily dividing the tumors into high, medium, or low to undetectable ER content. As noted previously, tumors with low or absent ER respond infrequently (5-9%). About 45 to 50% of tumors with an intermediate ER content respond to endocrine therapy, whereas tumors with high ER levels have high response rates (70-81%). Thus, quantitating ER in the breast tumor sample further improves our ability to select patients for endocrine therapy.

It is important to point out that ER simply serves as a marker for the endocrine dependence of the tumor, and is not helpful in choosing a specific type of endocrine therapy for a given patient. The presence of ER predicts response to all forms of hormonal manipulation including the administration of high dose estrogens, androgens, progestins glucocorticoids, antiestrogens, or ablative procedures such as ovariectomy, adrenalectomy and hypophysectomy. The choice of a particular therapy for an individual patient is based on established clinical guidelines and physician preference.

3. Progesterone Receptor in the Management
   of Advanced Breast Cancer

In normal target tissues such as uterus, progesterone action requires estrogen priming. This observation is explained by the fact that synthesis of progesterone receptor (PgR), which is required for progesterone activity, is induced by estrogen. Thus, the presence of PgR, an end product of estrogen action, may indicate that the estrogen response mechanism is functionally intact. Horwitz

et al. hypothesized that measurement of PgR in human breast cancer specimens might therefore be a better marker for hormone dependence than the presence of ER (12). First, the hypothesis that PgR synthesis may be regulated by estrogen in human breast cancer is strengthened by the observation that specimens rarely contain PgR in the absence of ER. Second, about one-third of tumors have neither receptor and would be expected to be hormone independent. Another third contain both receptors and would be expected to be hormone dependent by the above hypothesis. Finally, about one-third contain ER but no PgR, suggesting that despite the presence of ER, these tumors might have a defect in the estrogen response mechanism resulting in a hormone independent cell population.

The data in Table 3 correlating the objective response to endocrine therapy with the presence of ER and PgR in several studies further supports the hypothesis. Tumors containing both receptors have a high response rate (77%), as predicted, whereas tumors with neither receptor respond infrequently (8%). There are insufficient ER negative, PgR positive tumors to draw firm conclusions, but the response rate (35%) suggests that many of these are hormone dependent. The most perplexing group is the ER positive, PgR negative tumors. This group has a low response rate (32%). If the above hypothesis is correct one might ask why any of these PgR negative tumors respond to treatment, since the absence of PgR should indicate hormone independence. An obvious explanation is that the hypothesis is not fully correct, i.e., that the mechanisms for estrogen induced growth of some tumors are at least partially those for PgR regulation. A second possibility is a false negative PgR assay. One could speculate that certain patients (particularly postmenopausal) have a negative PgR assay because of insufficient endogenous estrogen to stimulate PgR synthesis and not because of a defect in the estrogen response mechanism. This has been demonstrated in a few patients by G. A. Degenshein et al. (personal communication). Alternatively, high circulating progesterone levels in premenopausal patients during the luteal phase of the menstrual cycle might occupy and translocate receptor sites, also resulting in a negative PgR assay. In fact, Saez et al. reported an inverse relationship between plasma progesterone and PgR in human breast cancer specimens, and no measurable PgR was observed when plasma progesterone exceeded 100ng/100ml (13). These data indicate the need for additional studies to determine if plasma steroid hormone levels or nuclear exchange assays should be part of the interpretation of PgR assays.

Thus, either quantitating ER or measuring PgR improves the clinician's ability to select patients for endocrine therapy. It is not clear whether the added time and expense of performing both assays is beneficial; since tumors with high levels of ER are more likely to contain PgR, these assays may be selecting the same group of patients.

Table 3. Objective remission of metastatic breast cancer
as a function of ER and PgR (316 patients)

Series	ER-, PgR-	ER-, PgR+	ER+, PgR-	ER+, PgR+
A	0/11	-	7/17	13/16
B	0/7	1/1	1/9	13/16
C	1/5	1/2	1/7	8/9
D	-	0/1	1/3	1/3
E	4/34	1/4	12/37	20/30
F	-	-	0/3	4/5
G	1/7	-	1/3	3/4
H	3/30	2/3	2/6	9/12
I	1/8	1/2	1/7	12/14
J	0/4	-	1/4	5/5
K	0/12	0/4	8/14	11/14
Totals	10/118 (8.4%)	6/17 (35%)	35/110 (32%)	99/128 (77%)

Series (A) McGuire and Osborne. Other series represent personal communica-
tions: (B) Degenshein and Bloom; (C) King, Redgrave, Rubens, Millis, and
Hayward; (D) Leclercq and Heuson; (E) Nomura, Takotani, Sugano, and Matsumoto;
(F) Singhakowinta; (G) DeSombre and Jensen; (H) Skinner, Barnes, and Ribeiro;
(I) Young, Einhorn, Ehrlich, and Cleary; (J) Jonat and Maass; (K) Allegra,
Lippman, and Thompson.

It is interesting that the response rates of
tumors with high ER are strikingly similar to
those of tumors with ER and PgR (about 80%).
Further study will be necessary to define the
exact role of each of these assays in the
management of patients with breast cancer.

4. Estrogen Receptor and the Response to
   Chemotherapy

There is now a considerable body of data
showing a relationship between the ER status
of a human breast cancer and certain other
biochemical, histological, and clinical
parameters. Recently, several studies have
asked whether these differences between ER
positive and negative tumors might be
reflected in their sensitivity to cytotoxic
chemotherapy (Table 4).

The available data cannot define a correlation between ER and response to chemotherapy
since an entire spectrum of results is
observed. Several studies suggest that ER
negative tumors respond better to chemotherapy; in support of their results, these
investigators emphasize that ER negative
tumors proliferate more rapidly based on
cell kinetic and clinical observations, and
that chemotherapy generally is more effective
in rapidly dividing cells. On the other hand,
several other studies report the opposite
result: ER positive tumors are more sensitive
to chemotherapy. Still other studies find
no association between these two parameters.
The explanation of these contradictory
results is not readily apparent. However,
all of these studies were retrospective

analyses; chemotherapy was not uniform even
within individual studies; and the chrono-
logical sequence of the ER assay and the
chemotherapy trial was variable. In fact,
some investigators studied only those
patients with an ER assay performed on metastatic tissue immediately prior to the
initiation of chemotheraphy; others used the
ER assay obtained earlier from the primary
tumor; and others accepted patients for
study who had the ER status determined after
completion of the drug trial. Perhaps these
or other as yet undefined methodologic or
prognostic variables account for these
disparate results. A prospective clinical
trial is needed to answer this question,
which has important ramifications in the
planning of the new approaches to treatment.

ACKNOWLEDGEMENTS

The work from the authors laboratory was
partially supported by the National
Institutes of Health CA11378, CB23682, and
the American Cancer Society. I thank the
investigators who provided data to me prior
to publication.

Table 4. Estrogen receptor and objective response rate to
chemotherapy

Series	ER–		ER+	
Lippman (14)	34/45	(76%)	3/25	(12%)
Jonat (15)	20/28	(71%)	6/14	(43%)
King (a)	8/12	(67%)	11/19	(58%)
Bonadonna (16)	7/16	(44%)	14/28	(50%)
Sama (a)	35/69	(51%)	24/37	(65%)
Webster (17)	17/45	(38%)	12/20	(60%)
Nomura (a)	3/22	(13%)	6/14	(42%)
Kiang (18)	14/40	(35%)	16/20	(80%)
Block (19)	0/11	(0%)	3/4	(75%)
Total	138/288	(48%)	95/181	(52%)

(a) Personal communication.

REFERENCES

1. W. L. McGuire, Physiological principles underlying endocrine therapy of breast cancer. In *Breast Cancer: Advances in Research and Treatment*. (Edited by W. L. McGuire) Vol. I, p. 217. Plenum Press, New York (1977).

2. W. L. McGuire, K. B. Horwitz, D. T. Zava, R. E. Garola, and G. C. Chamness, Hormones in breast cancer. *Metabolism* 27, 487 (1978).

3. W. L. McGuire, Hormone receptors: Their role in predicting prognosis and response to endocrine therapy. *Seminars in Oncology* 5, 428 (1978).

4. A. Singhakowinta, H. G. Potter, T. R. Buroker, B. Samal, S. C. Brooks, and V. K. Vaitkevicius, Estrogen receptor and natural course of breast cancer. *Ann. Surg.* 183, 84 (1976).

5. E. R. DeSombre, G. L. Green, and E. V. Jensen, Estrophilin and endocrine responsiveness of breast cancer. In *Hormones, Receptors, and Breast Cancer*. (Edited by W. L. McGuire) p. 1. Raven Press, New York (1978).

6. W. A. Knight III, R. B. Livingston, E. J. Gregory, and W. L. McGuire, Estrogen receptor is an independent prognostic factor for early recurrence in breast cancer. *Cancer Res.* 37, 4669 (1977).

7. M. A. Rich, P. Furmanski, and S. C. Brooks, Prognostic value of estrogen receptor determinations in patients with breast cancer. *Cancer Res.* 38, 4296 (1978).

8. P. V. Maynard, R. W. Blomey, C. W. Elston, J. L. Haybittle, and K. Griffiths, Estrogen receptor assay in primary breast cancer and early recurrence of the disease. *Cancer Res.* 38, 4292 (1978).

9. J. C. Allegra, M. E. Lippman, R. Simon, E. B. Thompson, A. Barlock, L. Green, K. K. Huff, H. M. T. Do, S. C. Aitken, and R. Warren, The association between steroid hormone receptor status and disease free interval in breast cancer. *Cancer Treat. Rep.*, in press (1979).

10. W. L. McGuire, P. P. Carbone, M. E. Sears, and G. C. Escher, Estrogen receptors in human breast cancer: an overview. In *Estrogen Receptors in Human Breast Cancer*. (Edited by W. L. McGuire, P. P. Carbone, and E. P. Vollmer) p. 1. Raven Press, New York (1975).

11. J. C. Allegra, M. E. Lippman, E. B. Thompson, R. Simon, A. Barlock, L. Green, K. K. Huff, H. M. T. Do, S. C. Aitken, and R. Warren, Estrogen receptor status is the most important prognostic variable in predicting response to endocrine therapy in metastatic breast cancer. *Europ. J. Cancer.*, in press (1979).

12. K. B. Horwitz, W. L. McGuire, O. H. Pearson, and A. Segaloff, Predicting response to endocrine therapy in human breast cancer: A hypothesis. *Science* 189, 726 (1975).

13. S. Saez, P. M. Martin, and C. D. Chauvet, Estradiol and progesterone receptor levels in human breast adenocarcinoma in relation to plasma estrogen and progesterone levels. *Cancer Res.* 38, 3468 (1978).

14. M. E. Lippman, J. C. Allegra, E. B. Thompson, R. Simon, A. Barlock, L. Green, K. K. Huff, H. M. T. Do, S. C. Aitken, and R. Warren, Lack of estrogen receptor predicts response to chemotherapy in breast cancer. *N. Eng. J. Med.* 298, 1223 (1978).

15. W. Jonat and H. Maass, Some comments on the necessity of receptor determination in human breast cancer. *Cancer Res.* 38, 4305 (1978).

16. G. Bonadonna, G. DiFronzo, and G. Tancini, Estrogen receptors (ER) and response to chemotherapy in advanced and early breast cancer. *Proc. Am. Soc. Clin. Oncol.*, in press (1979).

17. D. J. T. Webster, D. G. Bronn, and J. P. Minton, Estrogen receptors and response of breast cancer to chemotherapy. *N. Engl. J. Med.* 299, 604 (1978).

18. D. T. Kiang, D. H. Frenning, A. I. Goldman, V. F. Ascensav, and B. J. Kennedy, Estrogen receptors and responses to chemotherapy and hormonal therapy in advanced breast cancer. *N. Engl. J. Med.* 299, 1330 (1978).

19. G. E. Block, R. S. Ellis, E. DeSombre, and E. Jensen, Correlation of estrophilin content of primary mammary cancer to eventual endocrine treatment. *Ann. Surg.* 188, 372 (1978).

Specific Binding of Prolactin in Human Mammary Tumors

S. M. Thorpe and J. L. Daehnfeldt
with the technical assistance of L. Huusom, U. Haerslev,
B. Reiter, T. Rignes and U. Thomsen

The Fibiger Laboratory, 2100 Copenhagen 0, Denmark

Correspondence to S. M. Thorpe, The Fibiger Laboratory, Ndr. Frihavnsgade 70,
2100 Copenhagen 0, Denmark

Abstract—*Specific binding of 125-I-ovine prolactin has been investigated in 58 human mammary tumor biopsies. The majority of tumors were found to specifically bind very small amounts of prolactin. Specific binding of greater than or equal to 10% of the total prolactin cpm incubated/mg membrane protein was observed in 7 biopsies. No correlation was observed between amounts of estrogen and prolactin specifically bound, nor was there a correlation between the patients' age and amount of prolactin specifically bound.*

INTRODUCTION

It is well established that prolactin plays a major role in carcinogenesis in rodents (see reviews in 1-3). A multitude of experiments have been conducted in different strains of both mice and rats demonstrating that increased prolactin levels can both induce tumors and promote tumor growth (4-14). Conversely, tumor induction in rodents can be inhibited (9,15-16) and tumors can be made to regress (17-19) when prolactin levels are lowered by administration of ergot alkaloids.

Experiments investigating re-growth of experimental tumors that were regressing due to endocrine ablation suggest that both prolactin and estrogen are necessary to stimulate tumor growth (12-14).

One of the important interactions between estrogen and prolactin in mammary cancer has been shown to occur at the tissue level. Prolactin has been demonstrated to induce or activate the estrogen receptor in DMBA induced mammary tumors both *in vivo* (20) and *in vitro* (21), and in a human mammary tumor cell line (22).

Prolactin receptors have been demonstrated in many hormone-responsive mammary tumors of rodents, while prolactin receptor levels usually are lower or not measurable in hormone independent tumors (23-27). However, Holdaway and Friesen (28) found that consideration of the prolactin receptor level in DMBA tumors could not reliably predict which tumors responded to treatment with CB-154.

While it is well known that estrogen is important in some human mammary cancers, it is still controversial whether prolactin plays a definite role in human mammary cancer (see also reviews 29-33). Serum prolactin levels in breast cancer patients have been subject to several investigations (34-38). Generally, levels in breast cancer patients have been found to correspond to those found in controls. In a few studies, serum prolactin has been found to be higher in daughters of breast cancer patients (36-38). In all studies of serum prolactin levels, the difficulties inherent in obtaining what could be considered to be valid serum prolactin profiles must be borne in mind. Secretion of prolactin from the pituitary has both a sleep-dependent circadian pattern (39) and a cyclic pattern in menstruating females (40-41). Furthermore, the half-life of prolactin in the blood is very short; the initial decay constant has been reported to be of the order of 3-16 minutes (42-45).

While hypophysectomy is known to bring about remissions in some breast cancer patients, remissions have also been shown to occur in patients with pituitary stalk section where serum prolactin levels are increased (46). Furthermore, CB-154, an ergot alkaloid known to decrease prolactin levels (47), has shown to be ineffective in causing remissions (48-49).

Thus it appears that if serum prolactin levels are important in human mammary cancer, the role that the hormone level plays is not easily definable.

Recently, prolactin receptors have been detected in human breast cancer biopsies (50-55). The data from our own study of prolactin binding in human mammary tumors are presented here.

x Sponsored by the Danish Cancer Society.

MATERIALS AND METHODS

1. Chemicals

Ovine prolactin was the generous gift of Ferring AB, Malmö, Sweden. Carrier-free Na^{125}I was purchased from Radiochemical Centre, Amersham, Bucks, England. Lactoperoxidase was obtained from Calbiochem-Behring Corp. All other reagents were purchased from Merck, and were of analytical grade.

2. Tissue Storage

Biopsies from primary tumors and metastases from pre- and postmenopausal women were stored at -80°C until homogenization, which usually occurred within two weeks of the operation.

Mammary gland tissue from 1-2 day lactating rabbits was stored at -20°C for up to four months until homogenization. The prolactin receptor is stable under these conditions (S. Thorpe, unpublished data).

3. Tissue Preparation

Tumors were homogenized and the cytosol was prepared as previously described (56). The pellets obtained were kept at -80°C for a maximum of 3 months until isolation of the crude membrane fraction. The crude membrane fraction was isolated using the method of Shiu et al. (57). Following ultracentrifugation, the pellet with the membrane fraction was resuspended in 500 µl assay buffer (25 mM Tris-HCl, pH 7.6, 25 mM CaCl$_2$, 0.1% (w/v) bovine serum albumin (Sigman, Fraction V), and was stored at -80°C for up to 7 months before the prolactin binding assay was performed.

Crude membrane fractions from the lactating mammary gland of the rabbit have been stored at -80°C for up to 6 months before use with no demonstrable change in the prolactin binding (S. Thorpe, unpublished data).

Protein was determined according to the method of Lowry et al. (58).

4. Iodination of Prolactin

Ovine prolactin was iodinated with lactoperoxidase using a slightly modified method of Thorell and Johansen (59). 1 mCi 125-I$^-$, 5 µg prolactin, and 10 µg lactoperoxidase were mixed for 75 seconds at room temperature. The reaction mixture was diluted with 1 ml 50 mM sodium phosphate buffer, pH 7.2, and layered on a 1.5 × 50 cm Sephadex G-100 column precoated with 1 ml 1% bovine serum albumin in elution buffer (Tris-HCl, pH 7.6). Elution was performed at 7°C into tubes containing 250 µl elution buffer with 0.1% BSA. Prolactin eluted in three peaks. The descending shoulder of the third peak was used for binding experiments. The specific activity of the iodinated prolactin was approximately 70 µCi/µg.

5. Prolactin Binding Experiments

Final volumes of 500 µl assay buffer containing ca. 0.3 ng 125-I-prolactin and tumor membrane preparations with or without 100 ng radioinert ovine prolactin were incubated in duplicate at 25°C with shaking for approximately 18 hours.

Incubations were carried out at a median protein concentration of 250 µg (range 168-392 µg) crude membrane protein. After incubation, 1 ml ice-cold assay buffer was added, and samples were centrifuged for 2 minutes at 10.000 × g in a Beckman microfuge. Supernatant was aspirated, the tip of the tubes containing the membrane pellet was cut off, and pellets were counted in a Nuclear Chicago γ-counter with a counting efficiency of 50%. The difference between the 125-I-prolactin bound in the presence and absence of the unlabelled prolactin was taken to be the amount of prolactin specifically bound. When this value was less than twice the background of the γ-counter (30 cpm), the sample was arbitrarily considered to be unmeasurable and is designated as being prolactin receptor negative (Prl R -). In the prolactin receptor positive (Prl R +) samples, the median number of cpm 125-I-prolactin specifically bound was 246 cpm (range 81-1661). For comparative purposes, binding in the Prl R + samples was expressed as procent of total prolactin cpm specifically bound per mg membrane protein.

For analysis of binding of 125-I-prolactin to the lactating rabbit mammary gland, approximately 0.3 ng 125-I-prolactin was incubated with 130 µg membrane protein and with increasing amounts of unlabelled ovine prolactin (0.05 ng to 25 ng). Samples were incubated in triplicate for each hormone concentration, and the results were analyzed according to the method of Scatchard (60) and corrected for unspecific binding according to Chamness and McGuire (61).

Due to the small amount of tumor membranes available and the low specific binding, it has not been possible to perform satisfactory Scatchard analysis of the binding of prolactin to the human mammary tumors.

6. Steroid Hormone Receptor Determinations

The cytoplasmic estrogen receptor concentration in the specimens was evaluated using the DCC technique as previously described (56). The cut-off limit between receptor positive and receptor negative samples was arbitrarily set at 20 fmol/mg cytosol protein.

7. Statistical Analysis

The Wilcoxon Rank Sum Test for unpaired data was used to analyze the data.

RESULTS

A Scatchard plot analysis of the binding of 125-I-prolactin to the crude membrane fraction of the lactating rabbit mammary gland is shown in Fig. 1.

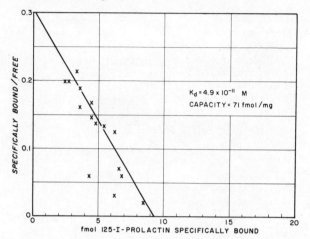

Fig. 1. Scatchard analysis of binding of 125-I-prolactin to the crude membrane fraction (130 µg membrane protein) isolated from the lactating rabbit.

The same batch of 125-I-prolactin has been used for the binding experiments in the human mammary tumors. A total of 58 biopsies has been investigated, and 76% of these have been found to specifically bind prolactin. The distribution of the specific binding of prolactin/mg membrane protein in all biopsies is shown in Fig. 2.

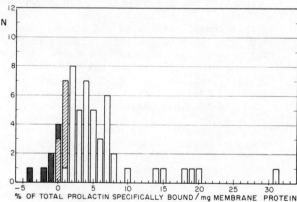

Fig. 2. Distribution of specific binding of prolactin per mg membrane protein (per cent of total prolactin cpm specifically bound/mg membrane protein) in 58 human mammary tumor biopsies. Open bars indicate tumors designated as prolactin receptor positive (Prl R +). Single cross-hatched bars indicate tumors classified as prolactin receptor negative (Prl R -) due to the cut-off limit between positive and negative samples. Double cross-hatched bars denote tumors classified as Prl R - where the difference between samples incubated with and without an excess of unlabelled prolactin (H - (H+C)) resulted in a negative number.

The amount of prolactin specifically bound to the human tumor membranes is extremely low. A median of 1.2% of the total prolactin cpm incubated has been found to bind specifically (range 0.4-6.9%). In comparison, the lactating rabbit mammary gland shown here specifically bound 15% of the total cpm prolactin incubated. Occasionally the difference between the cpm bound with and without unlabelled prolactin (Hot - (Hot + Cold)) in the human mammary tumors was a negative number. These samples are denoted in Fig. 2, and are considered to be representative of the experimental variation in the binding assay.

Estrogen receptor assays have been performed on all except one biopsy. The amount of prolactin bound (per cent of total prolactin cpm bound specifically/mg membrane protein) in ER + and ER - tissues did not differ significantly (P > 0.1). A scatter diagram of prolactin specifically bound vs. estrogen receptor level is shown in Fig. 3.

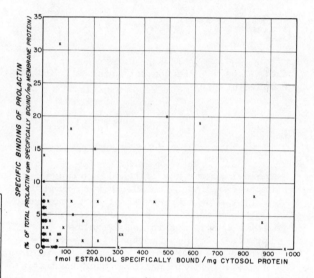

Fig. 3. Scatter diagram of binding of prolactin versus binding of estradiol in individual tumor biopsies.

There is no correlation between amounts of prolactin and estrogen bound in each biopsy.

The amount of specific binding of prolactin to biopsies was also considered in relation to the patient's age. No correlation was present (data not shown).

DISCUSSION

Although the amount of specifically bound prolactin is extremely low in human mammary tumor biopsies compared to nonprimate target tissues such as the lactating rabbit mammary gland, it is apparent from Fig. 2 that a major proportion of the biopsies investigated specifically bind prolactin. Because the cut-off level for positive and negative prolactin binding has been arbitrarily set, a number of biopsies could be falsely classified as negative or positive.

S. M. Thorpe and J. L. Daehnfeldt

Table 1. Prolactin binding in human mammary cancer.

Author (ref.)	Method iodination	Specific activity of 125-I-prolactin	Preparation assayed	PrlR+	%PrlR+	K_d
Holdaway and Friesen (53)	lactoperoxidase	∿130μCi/μg	differentially centrifuged 100.000 × g particulate membrane fraction or tissue slices	20/63	32%	4×10^{-10}M
Morgan et al. (52)	lactoperoxidase	–	100.000 × g particulate fraction	15/55	27%	$\sim 10^{-8}$M
Partridge and Hähnel (55)	chloramine-T	10-40μCi/μg	15.000 × g subcellular fraction	3/9	33%	6.8×10^{-12}M
Pearson et al. (54)	lactoperoxidase	130-170μCi/μg	5.000 × g particulate fraction	57/11!	51%	5.4×10^{-10}M
Stagner et al. (51)	–		100.000 × g particulate fraction	14/20	70%	–
Thorpe and Daehnfeldt	lactoperoxidase	70μCi/μg	differentially centrifuged 100.000 × g particulate membrane fraction	44/58	76%	

Table 1 summarizes this and other prolactin binding experiments conducted with human mammary tissue. Great variation is apparent in both percentage of prolactin receptor positive tumors and in the K_d values. A great deal of this discrepancy in percent prolactin receptor positive tumors is inherent in the selection of criteria used to distinguish between prolactin receptor positive and negative tumors. The most relevant cut-off limit for prolactin receptor positive and negative tumors would be based on presence or absence of a biological or clinical response – a parameter that has not been assessed at the present time. Pearson et al. (54) note that had they not considered the Scatchard analysis of binding, approximately 25% more tumors would have been classified as being prolactin receptor positive. Aside from difference in cut-off limit between receptor positive and negative samples, there is also variation in the quality (iodination method, specific activity) of the iodinated prolactin used for the binding assays, the cell fraction investigated for binding of prolactin, and the incubation time during the binding experiment. Thus it appears that although the absolute percentage of prolactin receptor positive tumors varies in these investigations, the important fact is that specific binding, albeit in very low levels, is found in each investigation.

In all of the three investigations with the greatest number of biopsies investigated for prolactin and estrogen binding (53,54, and present investigation), there is no correlation between amounts of prolactin and estrogen bound in the individual biopsies. In this investigation, of the seven biopsies with high specific prolactin binding (≥ 10% of the total cpm incubated specially bound/mg membrane protein), two are estrogen receptor negative, one has a low estrogen receptor value (40 fmol/mg cytosol protein), and the remaining four have high estrogen receptor levels (120-625 fmol/mg cytosol protein). Likewise, some biopsies have high estrogen receptor levels and do not demonstrate specific binding of prolactin.

Fifty to sixty percent of the patients with advanced breast cancer and an estrogen receptor positive biopsy respond to endocrine manipulations. It has been reported that when progesterone receptor content is also taken into consideration, an even higher rate of response to endocrine therapy is observed in the group of patients with an estrogen receptor positive and a progesterone receptor positive tumor (62). Whether inclusion of investigation of prolactin binding will improve the prediction of the rate of response remains to be determined.

ACKNOWLEDGEMENTS

Tumor specimens were received from the following hospitals: Surgical Dept. R, Københavns Amts Sygehus, Gentofte, (K.A.S. Gentofte), Dept. of Thoracic Surgery,

Københavns Amts Sygehus, Glostrup (K.A.S. Glostrup), Surgical Dept. D, Københavns Amts Sygehus, Herlev (K.A.S. Herlev), Surgical Dept. L, Bispebjerg Hospital, Copenhagen (B.B.H.), Dept. of Surgery, Finseninstitutet, Copenhagen, and the Departments of Surgery in Frederiksborg Amts Sygehuse in Hillerød (F.A.S. Hillerød), Helsingør (F.A.S. Helsingør), and Frederikssund (F.A.S. Frederikssund). Dr. T. Palshof's help in collecting the tumor specimens is gratefully acknowledged. We would also like to thank the personell in these departments for their participation and co-operation.

The fruitful discussions with Drs. P. Briand and C. Rose during preparation of the manuscript are gratefully acknowledged. We are indebted to Ms. A. Methling for excellent secretarial assistance in preparation of the manuscript.

REFERENCES

1. C. W. Welsch and J. Meites, Prolactin and Mammary Carcinogenesis, in *Endocrine Control in Neoplasia*. (Edited by R. K. Sharma and W. E. Criss) p. 71. Raven Press, N.Y. (1978).
2. M. E. Costlow and W. L. McGuire, Prolactin Receptors and Hormone Dependence in Mammary Carcinoma, in *Endocrine Control in Neoplasia*. (Edited by R. K. Sharma and W. E. Criss) p. 121. Raven Press, N.Y. (1978).
3. A. R. Boyns and K. Griffith, eds., *Prolactin and Carcinogenesis*, Alfa Omega Alfa Publishing, Cardiff (1972).
4. O. Mühlbock and L. M. Boot, The mode of action of ovarian hormones in the induction of mammary cancer in mice. *Biochem. Pharmacol.* 16, 627 (1967).
5. O. H. Pearson, O. Llerena, L. Llerena, A. Molina, and T. Butler, Prolactin-dependent rat mammary cancer: a model for man? *Trans. Assoc. Am. Physicians* 82, 225 (1969).
6. C. W. Welsch, J. A. Clemens, and J. Meites, Effects of hypothalamic and amygdaloid lesions on development and growth of carcinogen-induced mammary tumors in the female rat. *Cancer Res.* 29, 1541 (1969).
7. L. M. Boot, Prolactin and mammary gland carcinogenesis: the problem of human prolactin. *Int. J. Cancer* 5, 167 (1970).
8. C. W. Welsch and J. Meites, Effects of reserpine on development of 7,12-dimethyl-benz(a)anthracene induced mammary tumors in female rats. *Experentia* 26, 1133 (1970).
9. R. Yanai and H. Nagasawa, Inhibition of mammary tumorigenesis by ergot alkaloids and promotion of mammary tumorigenesis by pituitary isografts in adreno-ovariectomized mice. *J. Nat. Cancer Inst.* 48, 715 (1972).
10. P. A. Kelly, C. Bradley, R. P. C. Shiu, J. Meites, and H. G. Friesen, Prolactin binding to rat mammary tumor tissue. *Proc. Soc. Exp. Biol. Med.* 146, 816 (1974).
11. B. S. Leung and G. H. Sasaki, On the mechanisms of prolactin and estrogen action in 7,12-dimethyl-benz(a)anthracene-induced mammary carcinoma in the rat. II. In vivo tumor responses and estrogen receptor. *Endocrinology* 97, 564 (1975).
12. P. Briand, S. M. Thorpe and J. L. Dæhnfeldt, Effect of prolactin and bromocriptine on growth of transplanted hormone-dependent mouse mammary tumors. *Br. J. Cancer* 35, 816 (1977).
13. C. W. Welsch, L. Lambrecht, and C. Hassett, Suppression of mammary tumorigenesis in C3H/He mice by ovariectomy or treatment with 2-bromo-α-ergocryptine: a comparison. *J. Natl. Cancer Inst.* 58, 1135 (1977).
14. A. Manni, J. E. Trujillo, and O. H. Pearson, Predominant role of prolactin in stimulating the growth of 7,12-dimethyl-benz(a)anthracene-induced rat mammary tumor. *Cancer Res.* 37, 1216 (1977).
15. H. Stähelin, B. Burckhardt-Vischer, and E. Fluckinger, Rat mammary cancer inhibition by a prolactin suppressor 2-Bromo-α-Ergokryptine (CB-154). *Experientia* 27, 915 (1971).
16. C. W. Welsch and C. Gribler, Prophylaxis of spontaneously developing mammary carcinoma in C3h/HeJ female mice by suppression of prolactin. *Cancer Res.* 33, 2939 (1973).
17. J. C. Heuson, C. Waelbroeck-van Gaver, and N. Legros, Growth inhibition of rat mammary carcinoma and endocrine changes produced by 2-Br-α-Ergocryptine, a suppressor of lactation and nidation. *Eur. J. Cancer* 6, 353 (1970).
18. J. E. Clemens, and C. J. Shaar, Inhibition by ergocornine of initiation of growth of 7,12-dimethylbenz(a)anthracene-induced mammary tumors in rats: effect of tumor size. *Proc. Soc. Exp. Biol. Med.* 139, 659 (1972).
19. H. Nasr and O. H. Pearson, Inhibition of prolactin secretion by ergot alkaloids. *Acta Endocrinol.* 80, 429 (1975).
20. F. Vignon and H. Rochefort, Regulation of estrogen receptors in ovarian-dependent rat mammary tumors I. Effects of castration and prolactin. *Endocrinology* 98, 722 (1976).
21. G. H. Sasaki and B. S. Leung, Prolactin stimulation of estrogen receptor *in vitro* in 7,12-dimethyl-benz(a)anthracene-induced mammary tumors. *Res. Commun. Chem. Pathol. Pharmacol.* 8, 409 (1974).
22. S. Shafie and S. C. Brooks, Effect of prolactin on growth and the estrogen receptor level of human breast cancer cells (MCF-7). *Cancer Res.* 37, 792 (1977).
23. R. W. Turkington, Prolactin receptors in mammary carcinoma cells. *Cancer Res.* 34, 758 (1974).
24. M. E. Costlow, R. A. Buschow, N. J. Richert, and W. L. McGuire, Prolactin and estrogen binding in transplantable hormone-dependent and autonomous rat mammary carcinoma. *Cancer Res.* 35, 970 (1975).
25. M. E. Costlow, M. Sluyser, and P. E.

Gallagher, Prolactin receptors in mammary tumors in GR mice. *Endocr. Res. Commun.* 4, 285 (1977).

26. E. R. DeSombre, G. Kledzik, S. Marshall, and J. Meites, Estrogen and prolactin receptor concentrations in rat mammary tumors and response to endocrine ablation. *Cancer Res.* 36, 354 (1976).

27. R. Smith, R. Hilf, and A. E. Senior, Prolactin binding to R3230 AC mammary carcinoma and liver in hormone-treated and diabetic rats. *Cancer Res.* 37, 595 (1977).

28. I. M. Holdaway and H. G. Friesen, Correlation between hormone binding and growth response of rat mammary tumor. *Cancer Res.* 36, 1562 (1976).

29. H. G. Friesen, The role of prolactin in breast cancer, in *Recent Results in Cancer Res.* 57, 143 (1976).

30. W. L. McGuire, G. C. Chamness, K. B. Horwitz, and D. T. Zava, Prolactin and estrogen receptors in breast cancer. *Pathobiol. Annu.* 7, 191 (1977).

31. A. C. W. Montague, Prolactin in breast cancer. *Prog. Clin. Biol. Res.* 12, 155 (1977).

32. H. Nagasawa, Prolactin and human breast cancer: a review. *Eur. J. Cancer* 15, 267 (1979).

33. F. Smithline, L. Sherman, and H. D. Kolodny, Prolactin and breast carcinoma. *N. Eng. J. Med.*, 292, 784 (1975).

34. A. R. Boyns, E. N. Cole, K. Griffiths, M. M. Roberts, R. Buchan, R. G. Wilson, and A. P. M. Forrest, Plasma prolactin in breast cancer. *Eur. J. Cancer* 9, 99 (1973).

35. R. G. Wilson, R. Buchan, M. Roberts, A. P. Forrest, A. R. Boyns, E. N. Cole, and K. Griffiths, Plasma prolactin and breast cancer. *Cancer* 33, 1325 (1974).

36. H. G. Kwa, M. DeJong-Bakker, E. Engelsman, and F. J. Cleton, Plasma prolactin in human breast cancer. *Lancet* 1, 433 (1974).

37. H. G. Kwa, F. Cleton, M. de Jong-Bakker, R. D. Bulbrook, J. L. Hayward, and D. Y. Wang, Plasma prolactin and its relationship to risk factors in human breast cancer. *Int. J. Cancer* 17, 441 (1976).

38. B. E. Henderson, V. Gerkins, I. Rosario, J. Casagrande, and M. C. Pike, Elevated serum levels of estrogen and prolactin in daughters of patients with breast cancer. *N. Eng. J. Med.* 293, 790 (1975).

39. J. F. Sassin, A. G. Frantz, E. D. Weitzman, and S. Kapen, Human prolactin: 24-hour pattern with increased release during sleep. *Science* 177, 1205 (1972).

40. E. N. Cole, R. A. Sellwood, P. C. England, and K. Griffiths, Serum prolactin concentrations in benign breast disease throughout the menstrual cycle. *Eur. J. Cancer* 13, 597 (1977).

41. J. Meites, Relation of estrogen to prolactin secretion in animals and man. *Adv. Biosci.* 15, 195 (1975).

42. C. E. Grosvenor, Disappearance rate of exogenous prolactin from serum of female rats. *Endocrinology* 80, 195 (1967).

43. H. G. Kwa, C. A. Feltkamp, A. A. van der Gugten, and F. Verhofstad, The rate of

elimination of prolactin as a determinant factor for plasma levels assayed in rats. *J. Endocrinol.* 48, 299 (1970).

44. Y. Koch, Y. F. Chow, and J. Meites, Metabolic clearance and secretion rates of prolactin in the rat. *Endocrinology* 89, 1303 (1971).

45. M. Birkenshaw and I. R. Falconer, The localization of prolactin labelled with radioactive iodine in rabbit mammary tissue. *J. Endocrinol.* 55, 323 (1972).

46. R. W. Turkington, L. E. Underwood, J. J. Van Wyk, Elevated serum prolactin levels after pituitary stalk section in man. *N. Eng. J. Med.* 285, 707 (1971).

47. E. del Pozp, R. Brun del Re, L. Varga, and H. Friesen, The inhibition of prolactin secretion in man by CB-154. *J. Clin. Endocrinol. Metab.* 35, 768 (1972).

48. J. C. Heuson, A. Coune, and M. Staquet, Clinical trial of CB-154 in advanced breast cancer. *Eur. J. Cancer* 8, 155 (1972).

49. A. Barrett, L. Morgan, R. P. Raggatt, and J. R. Hobbs, Bromocriptine in the treatment of advanced breast cancer. *Clin. Oncol.* 2, 373 (1976).

50. L. de Souza, J. R. Hobbs, L. Morgan, and H. Salih, Localization of prolactin in human breast tumors. *J. Endocrinol.* 73, 17P (1977).

51. J. I. Stagner, P. R. Hochimsen, and B. M. Sherman, Lactogenic hormone binding to human breast cancer: correlation with estrogen receptor. *Clin. Res.* 25, 302A (1977).

52. L. Morgan, P. R. Raggatt, I. de Souza, H. Salih, and J. R. Hobbs, Prolactin receptors in human breast tumors. *J. Endocrinol.* 73- 17P (1977).

53. I. M. Holdaway and H. G. Friesen, Hormone binding by human mammary carcinoma. *Cancer Res.* 37, 1946 (1977).

54. O. H. Pearson, A. Manni, M. Chambers, J. Brodkey, and J. S. Marshall, Role of pituitary hormones in the growth of humanbreast cancer. *Cancer Res.* 38, 4323 (1978).

55. R. K. Partridge and R. Hähnel, Prolactin receptors in human breast carcinoma. *Cancer* 43, 643 (1979).

56. J. L. Daehnfeldt and P. Briand, Determinations of high-affinity gestagen receptors in hormone-responsive and hormone-independent GR mouse mammary tumors by an exchange assay, in *Progesterone Receptors in Normal and Neoplastic Tissues*. (Edited by W. L. McGuire, J. Raynaud, and E. Baulieu) p. 59. Raven Press, N.Y. (1977).

58. O. H. Lowry, N. J. Rosebrough, A. L. Farr, and R. J. Randall, Protein measurement with the folin phenol reagent. *J. Biol. Chem.* 193, 265 (1951).

59. J. I. Thorell and B. G. Johansson, Enzymatic iodination of polypeptides with 125-I to high specific activity. *Biochim. Biophys. Acta* 251, 363 (1971).

60. G. Scatchard, The attractions of proteins for small molecules and ions. *Ann. N.Y. Acad. Sci.* 51, 660 (1949).

61. G. C. Chamness and W. L. McGuire, Scatchard plots: common errors in correction and interpretation. *Steroids* 26, 538 (1975).

62. K. B. Horwitz and W. L. McGuire, Estrogen and progesterone: their relationship in hormone-dependent breast cancer, in *Progesterone Receptors in Normal and Neoplastic Tissues* (Edited by W. L. McGuire, J. Raynaud, and E. Baulieu) Raven Press, N.Y. (1977).

Estrogen Receptors in Early Breast Cancer

T. Cooke*, D. George*, R. Schields*, P. V. Maynard** and K. Griffiths**

*Department of Surgery, Royal Liverpool Hospital, U.K.
**Tenovus Institute for Cancer Research, University Hospital of Wales, Cardiff, U.K.

Correspondence to T. Cooke, Department of Surgery, Royal Liverpool Hospital, U.K.

Abstract—In a prospective study the oestrogen receptor content of early breast cancers from 421 patients was related to the development of disease recurrence. The patients were followed for a mean of 21.6 months. Fifty two per cent of the tumours contained oestrogen receptors, but tumours in premenopausal women were less likely to contain receptors than those in post-menopausal women. The presence or absence of oestrogen receptors was independent of tumour size and axillary lymph node histology. Tumours with oestrogen receptors were associated with significantly longer disease-free periods, irrespective of menopausal status. Patients without lymph node metastases whose tumours did not contain oestrogen receptors were found to have the same poor prognosis as those with lymph node involvement. Levels of oestrogen receptor in tumours that had re-occurred were similar to those of tumours that remained disease-free.

INTRODUCTION

Estimation of the oestrogen receptor content of advanced carcinomas of the breast is now widely used in the prediction of response to endocrine therapy (1). Much less is known of the role of oestrogen receptor analysis in early breast cancer. Recent reports have suggested that the presence or absence of receptors for oestrogen is a guide to prognosis in early cancer of the breast (2,3,4). These studies indicate that the presence of oestrogen receptor was associated with a more favourable prognosis, and that this effect was independent of other prognostic factors (2).

The aim of the present study was to investigate the role of oestrogen receptor analysis in primary cancer of the breast, with particular reference to prognosis following local treatment.

MATERIALS AND METHODS

This investigation is part of a larger study of several aspects of cancer of the breast which is being carried out in the Liverpool area and receives patients from 15 contributing surgeons.

A total of 421 patients with primary cancer of the breast were studied. All tumours were staged clinically by the international TNM system. Distant metastases were screened for by skeletal survey or bone scan, chest X-ray and liver function tests. Only patients with clinically localised cancer of the breast ($T_{1-3}N_{0-1}M_0$) were included in this study.

Clinical data was obtained pre-operatively and listed on a standard pro-forma. All the patients were treated by mastectomy with either axillary biopsy or dissection. The diagnosis of breast cancer was confirmed by histology, as was the presence or absence of axillary metastases and the clinical staging was reviewed in the light of this information.

Regular postoperative review of all patients was carried out at the hospital in which they received their original treatment, and follow-up data was recorded on pro-formas. The women have been followed up for periods between 3 and 42 months with an average of 21.6 months. The emergence of local or nodal recurrence was confirmed by biopsy and the presence of distant metastases only accepted on unequivocal radiological evidence.

1. Oestrogen Receptor Assay

Tumour biopsies were placed on ice at the time of mastectomy and were subsequently stored in liquid nitrogen prior to assay for oestrogen receptors. All the procedures of the assay were carried out at a temperature not exceeding 4°C.

Frozen tumour tissue was powdered in a Thermovac tissue pulveriser and homogenised 10-20% (w/v) in 10 mM-tris HCl buffer (pH 7.4) containing 1 mM EDTA and 3 mM sodium azide. A cytosol was obtained by centrifugation at 100,000 g for 60 min and its protein content was determined (5).

Eight 200 µl aliquots of the cytosol were incubated with an equal volume of tris HCl buffer containing tritiated oestradiol (specific activity 96 Ci/m mol) in amounts ranging from 10 to 500 p g for 18 hours. Four hundred microlitres of a suspension of charcoal (0.5% w/v) in tris HC1 buffer containing gelatin (0.1 w/v) and dextran T70 (0.05 w/v) was then added and the tubes agitated for 90 mins. The charcoal was precipitated by centrifugation and the radioactivity in 50 µl of the supernatant determined.

An estimate of the binding site concentration was made by the Newton-Raphson iterative curve fitting technique (6). Non-specific binding was accounted for by the inclusion of a saturating concentration of 3 {H} oestradiol in one tube and this was used as a correction to the other points. Tumours were considered positive for oestrogen receptors only when the association constant was higher than 10^9/mol and the binding site concentration was greater than 5 fmol/mg cytosol protein.

2. Statistical Methods

The follow-up data was analysed by life table methods and is presented in the form of graphs. The curves on each graph were compared by the log rank test, which evaluates differences between entire curves rather than individual points on the curves (7). The presence or absence of receptors for oestrogen in the primary tumour was related to the rate of recurrence, first for all patients studied, secondly for patients sub-divided by menopausal status, and lastly for patients with or without axillary lymph node metastases.

RESULTS

A total of 421 patients with primary cancer of the breast were studied. Of the 421 tumours, 219 (52%) contained receptors for oestrogen, and 202 (48%) did not. The patients were followed up for periods between 3 and 42 months with a mean follow-up of 21.6 months. To date 84 (20%) of the 421 patients have developed proven recurrence of their disease. Of the 84 patients with recurrence 58 (69%) had tumours which did not contain receptors for oestrogen.

1. Tumour Stage and the Presence of Oestrogen Receptors

No correlation was found between the presence or absence of receptors for oestrogen and either the clinical stage of the disease, or the histology of the axillary lymph nodes. The proportion of cancers with or without receptors for oestrogen was similar in all groups when patients were separated by clinical staging ($T_{1-3}N_{0-1}$). In the same way, of 171 patients with histological evidence of lymph node metastasis 86 had receptors for oestrogen in the primary tumour and 85 did not.

2. Menopausal Status and the Presence of Oestrogen Receptors

The presence or absence of receptors for oestrogen in the primary tumour was affected by the menopausal status of the patient. Tumours in pre-menopausal women were less likely to contain receptors for oestrogen than those in patients who were past the menopause. Of 114 tumours in pre-menopausal women, 47 (42%) contained receptors compared with 171 (56%) of 307 tumours in post-menopausal women.

3. Rates of Recurrence and the Presence of Oestrogen Receptor

The rate of recurrence was affected by the presence or absence of receptors for oestrogen. In 219 patients whose tumours contained receptors, the rate of recurrence was significantly lower ($P < 0.001$) than that in 202 patients whose tumours did not contain receptors (Fig. 1). This relationship remained true when patients were sub-divided by menopausal status or by the presence or absence of axillary lymph node metastases.

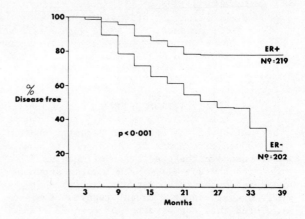

Fig. 1. Rates of recurrence in tumours with and without oestrogen receptors.

4. Menopausal Status

Although the number of tumours which contained receptors for oestrogen was lower in pre-menopausal patients than post-menopausal ones, the rate of recurrence for tumours with or without receptors was not influenced by menopausal status. In both pre- and post-menopausal patients the rate of recurrence for tumours which contained receptors for oestrogen was significantly lower ($P < 0.001$) than that for those which did not contain receptors (Figs. 2 and 3).

5. Axillary Lymph Node Histology

Of the 171 patients with axillary lymph node metastases at the time of mastectomy, 85 had tumours which did not contain receptors for oestrogen. Although the rate of recurrence for these patients did not differ significantly from that for the 86 patients with receptors for oestrogen (Fig. 4) they had the highest rate of recurrence of any of the groups studied.

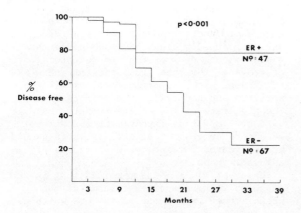

Fig. 2. Rates of recurrence for premeno-
        pausal patients with and without
        oestrogen receptors in their
        tumours.

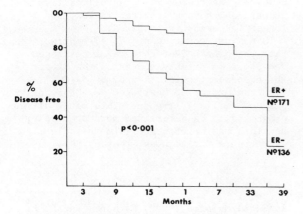

Fig. 3. Rate of recurrence for post-
        menopausal patients with and
        without oestrogen receptors in
        their tumours.

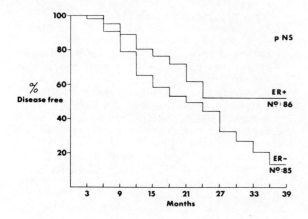

Fig. 4. Rates of recurrence for patients
        with axillary lymph node
        metastases.

Of the 250 patients without axillary lymph
node involvement, the rate of recurrence in
the 134 patients whose tumours contained
receptors for oestrogen was significantly
lower (P < 0.001) than that in the 116

patients whose tumours did not contain
receptors for oestrogen (Fig. 5). Despite
the more favourable prognosis usually
attributed to patients without axillary lymph
node metastases, the absence of oestrogen
receptors in such patients was associated
with an unexpected high rate of recurrence.
The rate of recurrence for the 116 patients
without axillary node metastases and without
receptors for oestrogen was equal to that of
the total group of 171 patients with axillary
node metastases (Fig. 6).

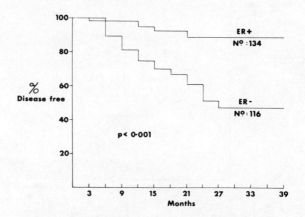

Fig. 5. Rates of recurrence for patients
        without axillary lymph node
        metastases.

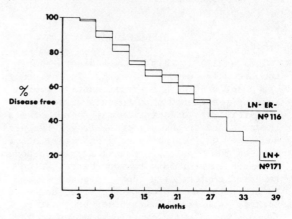

Fig. 6. Rates of recurrence in patients
        without axillary node metastases
        and without oestrogen receptors
        in their tumours (LN-, ER-) and
        in all patients with axillary node
        metastases (LN+).

6. Recurrence and Levels of Oestrogen
   Receptor

Of the 84 patients who developed recurrent
disease, 26 (31%) had tumours which contained
receptors for oestrogen. The levels of
receptor protein in these tumours did not
differ from the levels of receptor protein
found in tumours which to date have not
recurred (Fig. 7).

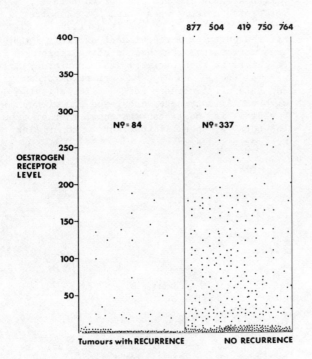

877 504   419 750 764

400 —

350 —

300 —

OESTROGEN
RECEPTOR
LEVEL

N⁹ = 84   N⁹ = 337

250 —

200 —

150 —

100 —

50 —

Tumours with RECURRENCE   **NO RECURRENCE**

Fig. 7. Levels of oestrogen receptor in
tumours that have developed recurrence and those that remained
disease-free.

DISCUSSION

The results of this study indicate that
tumours which contain receptors for oestrogen
are associated with a significantly lower
rate of recurrence than tumours without such
receptors. No association was found between
the presence or absence of oestrogen receptors
and other well-established prognostic factors
such as tumour size, and axillary lymph node
metastases. For this reason the oestrogen
receptor content of a tumour appears to act
as an independent prognostic guide, and when
used in combination with other prognostic
factors it allows clearer definition of the
likely outcome of local treatment.

Pre-menopausal patients were less likely to
have tumours which contained receptors for
oestrogen than patients who were past the
menopause. Despite this, the rate of recurrence of receptor positive and receptor
negative cancers was the same in both groups
and suggests that patients have either
"receptor positive or receptor negative
disease" irrespective of menopausal status.

In patients with axillary lymph node metastases, there was no significant difference,
as reported previously (2), between tumours
with or without receptors for oestrogen.
However, those patients with lymph node
involvement and receptor negative tumours
had the highest rate of recurrence of all
the groups studied. This finding is in agreement with that of Knight (4), who reported
that 50 per cent of a similar group of
patients had developed recurrence within
eighteen months.

In patients without axillary lymph node
metastases, a group usually thought to have
a good prognosis, the rate of recurrence
was unexpectedly high for those patients
whose tumours did not contain receptors for
oestrogen. For this group the rate of
recurrence was similar to that for all the
patients who had axillary node metastases.
The high rate of recurrence in patients
without lymph node involvement and without
receptors suggests that such patients should
be considered for inclusion in trials of
adjuvant chemotherapy.

Jenson et al. (8) has reported that in
patients with advanced carcinoma of the
breast there is a group of tumours which have
low levels of oestrogen receptor, and these
behave in the same way as receptor negative
cancers. In the present study no difference
was found in the levels of receptor protein
when oestrogen receptor positive tumours
with and without recurrence were compared.
However, the number of receptor positive
tumours which have recurred is low, and
longer follow-up is required.

This study confirms previous reports
that the presence or absence of oestrogen
receptors in primary cancer of the breast is
an independent guide to prognosis (3,4).
The combination of oestrogen receptor analysis and axillary lymph node histology allows
prognosis to be determined more precisely,
and this may be of benefit in the selection
of patients for adjuvant therapy (9).

REFERENCES

1. W. L. McGuire, P. P. Carbone, and E. P.
   Volmer, *Estrogen Receptors in Human
   Breast Cancer*. Raven Press, New York
   (1975).
2. T. Cooke, W. D. George, P. V. Maynard,
   K. Griffiths, and R. Shields, Oestrogen
   receptors and prognosis in early breast
   cancer. *Lancet* 1, 995 (1979).
3. P. V. Maynard, C. W. Blamey, C. W. Elston,
   J. L. Haybittle, and K. Griffiths,
   Estrogen receptor assay in primary breast
   cancer and early recurrence of the disease.
   Cancer Res. 38, 4292 (1978).
4. W. A. Knight, R. B. Livingston, E. J.
   Gregory, and W. L. McGuire, Estrogen
   receptor as an independent prognostic
   factor for early recurrence in breast
   cancer. *Cancer Res.* 37, 4669 (1977).
5. O. H. Lowry, N. R. Rosebrough, A. L. Farr,
   and R. J. Randall, Protein measurement
   with folin phenol reagent. *J. Biol. Chem.*
   193, 265 (1951).
6. H. A. Feldman, Mathematical theory of
   complex ligand-binding systems at equilibrium. *Anal Biochem.* 48, 317 (1972).
7. R. Peto, N. E. Armitage, D. R. Breslow,
   D. R. Cox, and S. V. Howard, Design and
   analysis of randomised clinical trials
   requiring prolonged observations of each
   patient. II. Analysis and Examples.
   Br. J. Cancer 35, 1 (1977).
8. E. V. Jensen, T. Z. Polley, S. Smith,
   E. Block, D. J. Ferguson, and E. R.
   DeSombre, Prediction of hormone depending

in human breast cancer. In *Estrogen
Receptors in Human Breast Cancer* (Edited
by W. L. McGuire, P. P. Carbone, and E. P.
Volmer) p. 37. Raven Press, New York
(1975).

9. S. K. Carter, Adjuvant chemotherapy in
breast cancer: critique and perspectives.
Cancer Chemother. Pharmacol. 1, 183
(1978).

The Relationship of Oestradiol Receptor (ER) and Histological Tumour Differentiation with Prognosis in Human Primary Breast Carcinoma

C. W. Elston*, R. W. Blamey*, J. Johnson*, H. M. Bishop*,
J. L. Haybittle** and K. Griffiths***

*Departments of Pathology and Surgery, City Hospital, Nottingham, U.K.
**Department of Physics, Addenbrooke's Hospital, Cambridge, U.K.
***Tenovus Institute for Cancer Research, Welsh National School of Medicine, Cardiff, U.K.

Correspondence to C. W. Elston, Departments of Pathology and Surgery, City
Hospital, Hucknall Road, Nottingham, U.K.

Abstract—In a series of 273 primary breast carcinomas oestradiol receptor
content (ER) has been measured by the dextran coated charcoal method, and
tumour differentiation assessed histologically. Fifty-two per cent of the
tumours were ER positive. There was a strong correlation between ER status
and histological grade, the better differentiated tumours tending to be ER
positive. This correlation was highly significant in post-menopausal women.
Both histological grade and ER status were related to prognosis, better
differentiated tumours and those which were ER positive giving a better
survival.

INTRODUCTION

The Nottingham Breast Cancer Study was established to examine the feasibility of producing a prognostic index so that future adjuvant therapy could be given in a more rational way. The approach has been multi-disciplinary, and a preliminary report has demonstrated the value of an index based on tumour size, pathological lymph node involvement and histological differentiation in identifying a group of patients with a poor prognosis (1). A further aspect of the study has been the assessment of oestradiol receptor (ER) status and its correlation with the other prognostic factors (2,3). This paper examines in particular the relationship between ER status and histological tumour differentiation, since previous reports have been at variance, one recording a positive correlation (4) but others suggesting that there is no significant relationship (5,6,7, 8). Preliminary aspects of the correlation of ER status and histological differentiation with prognosis will also be considered.

MATERIALS AND METHODS

1. Clinical Details

The study is based on a single surgical team and data are currently available on a consecutive series of 344 female patients (aged 27–70 years) with primary operable breast cancer. Clinically, tumours were less than 5 cm in diameter, freely mobile and there was no clinical evidence of metastatic spread (broad correlation with TNM Stage I and II breast cancer). A simple or subcutaneous mastectomy was performed in all cases,

with biopsy of lymph nodes from the low axilla, the apex of the axilla and the internal mammary chain via the second intercostal space. Details of follow-up procedure and definition of recurrence have been published elsewhere (1,2).

In brief, patients were seen at a post mastectomy clinic at three monthly intervals to 18 months and thereafter at six monthly intervals. Recurrence was defined as objective evidence of tumour deposits requiring a major change in treatment policy (e.g. major local recurrence in wound flaps or symptomatic axillary lymph nodes requiring radiotherapy, bone metastases seen on radiographs, enlarged liver with raised alkaline phosphatase).

2. Histopathology

In most cases specimens were examined in the fresh state immediately after operation, and representative portions of tumour tissue were immersed in liquid N_2 for subsequent assay. All mastectomy specimens were fixed in 10 per cent buffered formalin. Depending on tumour size, 1 to 4 tumour blocks were selected for histological examination, having regard to adequate sampling. Paraffin sections were cut at 4–6 μm and stained with Ehrlichs haematoxylin and eosin. Where necessary multiple sections were examined.

Histological tumour differentiation was assessed according to the method described by Bloom and Richardson (9). The degree of tubular differentiation, the variation in size and shape of tumour nuclei and the number of mitotic figures were each scored from 1 to 3, in ascending order of abnormality. Each tumour was therefore given a composite score of 3-9, which is arbitrarily divided as follows:

Grade I   (well differentiated) 3,4,5.
Grade II   (moderately differentiated) 6,7.
Grade III (poorly differentiated) 8,9.

The assessments were carried out by the two pathologists (C.W.E. and J.J.) independently, and without knowledge of clinical details or ER results. Agreement on the initial assessment was reached in 90 per cent of cases. The remaining 35 cases (10%) were re-examined independently and agreement was found in 30. In 5 cases final agreement was reached by consensus. In none of the cases did the original assessments differ by more than one subgroup.

3. Oestradiol Receptor Assay

Details of the assay used routinely have been published previously (2,10). Tumours were considered as positive only when they contained more than 15 fmol of specific oestradiol binding per mg. cytosol protein, and negative if they contained less than 5 fmol; results between 5 and 15 fmol were regarded as equivocal.

RESULTS

Of the 344 consecutive patients in the series ER assay was not carried out in 47 (in most of these cases tissue was not available for ER assay because the diagnosis of carcinoma had been established at prior excision biopsy). A further 20 patients were excluded from the analysis because the ER result was in the equivocal range, and in 5 patients the tumour was intraduct in type.

Table 1. Relationship between oestradiol receptor status and histological differentiation in 273 patients with primary breast carcinoma.

Histological Grade	Oestrogen receptor status Positive	Negative	Total
I	34	11	45
II	64	37	101
III	45	82	127
Total	143	130	273

$X^2 = 29.0$, 2 d.f., $p < 0.0005$.

Table 1 shows the relationship between ER status and histological differentiation in the 273 patients available for study. Fifty-two per cent of the tumours were ER positive. There is a significant correlation between ER status and histological grade, a greater percentage of ER positive tumours being well differentiated (Grade I, 76% positive, grade III, 35% positive).

It is of importance to establish the effect of menopausal status on these results, and this is shown in Tables 2 and 3.

Table 2. Relationship between oestradiol receptor status and histological differentiation in 92 premenopausal patients with primary breast carcinoma.

Histological Grade	Oestradiol receptor status Positive	Negative	Total
I	11	7	18
II	16	19	35
III	15	24	39
Total	42	50	92

$X^2 = 2.56$, 2 d.f., p 0.3 > p < 0.2.

Table 3. Relationship between oestradiol receptor status and histological differentiation in 179 post-menopausal patients with primary breast carcinoma.

Histological Grade	Oestradiol receptor status Positive	Negative	Total
I	22	4	26
II	47	18	65
III	30	58	88
Total	99	80	179

$X^2 = 32.9$, 2 d.f., $p < 0.0005$.

In one patient menopausal status could not be determined. In the premenopausal patients, the relationship does not reach significance, but in post-menopausal patients there is a highly significant correlation between ER status and histological differentiation.

Survival data are at a preliminary stage in this study, but there is a minimum follow-up of two years for the first 205 patients whose tumour ER status had been determined. Using life table analysis and the Mantel test (11) Fig. 1 shows that there is a significant relationship between the degree of histological differentiation and survival, patients with Grade I tumours having a better survival than those with Grade II and III tumours. Oestradiol receptor status also correlates with survival (Fig. 2) and post-menopausal women who are ER positive have a significantly more favourable prognosis.

DISCUSSION

Previous investigations into the relationship between histological tumour differentiation and ER status have yielded equivocal results. Although Heuson et al. (4) found

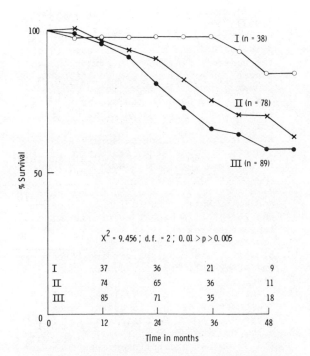

Fig. 1. Relationship between histological grade and survival in 205 patients with a minimum follow-up of two years.

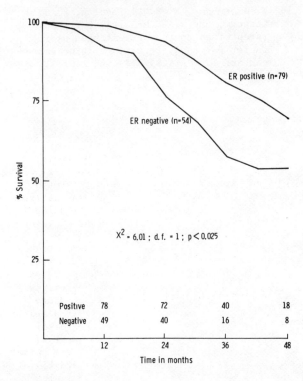

Fig. 2. Relationship between ER status and survival in 133 post-menopausal patients with a minimum follow-up of two years.

that poorly differentiated tumours were more likely to be ER negative, they graded only 85 tumours out of 214 studied for ER content.

Furthermore, a higher percentage of the graded tumours was ER positive than in the overall series (85 per cent compared with 73 per cent). Johansson et al. (5) could find no correlation between ER content and histological grade in a study of 31 breast cancers, and similar negative findings have been reported by Rosen et al. (6,7) in 120 and 177 primary breast carcinomas respectively, and in a Japanese series of 324 breast carcinomas (8).

The present study is thus the first large scale series in which an unequivocal correlation has been shown between histological grade and oestradiol receptor status. This relationship reaches a high level of significance in post-menopausal women, and the results suggest that ER status provides another measure of tumour differentiation, parallel to that which can be demonstrated histologically. This is in accord with recent dynamic studies (12) showing that when differentiation was measured by thymidine labelling, breast carcinomas with high rates of replication, and thus presumably less well differentiated, tended to be ER negative.

Assessment of tumour differentiation only assumes practical importance when it can be shown to correlate with prognosis. Histological grade has been shown by several authors to be of prognostic significance (9,13,14) and although follow-up data are at a preliminary stage this study has already confirmed this correlation between histological differentiation and prognosis, patients with Grade I tumours having a significantly better survival than those with Grade II or III tumours. This emphasises the potential usefulness of histological grade as a prognostic indicator.

Oestradiol receptor positive tumours have been shown to respond better to endocrine therapy than receptor negative patients (15), and it is therefore important to determine whether estimation of the ER status of primary tumours is of value in predicting prognosis. A report on a small number of patients stated that ER content of primary tumours is an independent prognostic factor, patients with ER negative tumours tending to suffer earlier recurrence than those with ER positive tumours (16). The present study confirms and extends this finding in a larger series of patients, for both recurrence-free interval (3), and survival are poorer in patients with ER negative tumours.

REFERENCES

1. R. W. Blamey, C. J. Davies, C. W. Elston, J. Johnson, J. L. Haybittle, and P. V. Maynard, Prognostic factors in breast cancer: the formation of a prognostic index. *Clinic. Oncology* (in press)(1979).
2. P. V. Maynard, C. J. Davies, R. W. Blamey, C. W. Elston, J. Johnson, and K. Griffiths, Relationship between oestrogen-receptor content and histological grade in human primary breast tumours. *Brit. J. Cancer* 38, 745 (1978).
3. P. V. Maynard, R. W. Blamey, C. W. Elston, J. L. Haybittle, and K. Griffiths, Estrogen receptor assay in primary breast

cancer and early recurrence of the disease. *Cancer Res.* 38, 4292 (1978).

4. J. C. Heuson, G. Leclercq, E. Longeval, M. C. Deboel, W. H. Mattheiem, and R. Heiman, Estrogen receptors: prognostic significance in breast cancer. In *Estrogen Receptors in Human Breast Cancer* (Edited by W. L. McGuire, P. P. Carbone and E. P. Vollmer) p. 57. Raven Press, New York (1975).

5. H. Johansson, L. Terenius, and L. Thorén, The binding of estradiol-17B to human breast cancers and other tissues in vitro. *Cancer Res.* 30, 692 (1970).

6. P. P. Rosen, C. J. Menendez-Botet, J.S. Nisselbaum, J. A. Urban, V. Miké, A. Fracchia, and M. K. Schwartz, Pathological review of breast lesions analysed for estrogen receptor protein. *Cancer Res.* 35, 3187 (1975).

7. P. P. Rosen, C. J. Menendez-Botet, R. T. Senie, M. K. Schwartz, D. Schottenfeld, and G. H. Farr, Estrogen receptor protein (E.R.P.) and the histopathology of human mammary carcinoma. In *Hormones, Receptors and Breast Cancer* (Edited by W. L. McGuire) p. 71. Raven Press, New York (1978).

8. H. Sugano, G. Sakamoto, A. Sakamoto, Y. Nomura, O. Takatani, and K. Matsumoto, Hormone receptors and histopathology in Japanese breast cancer. In *Hormones, Receptors and Breast Cancer* (Edited by W. L. McGuire) p. 59. Raven Press, New York (1978).

9. H. J. G. Bloom and W. W. Richardson, Histological grading and prognosis in breast cancer. *Brit. J. Cancer* 11, 359 (1957).

10. P. V. Maynard and K. Griffiths, Clinical, pathological and biochemical aspects of the oestrogen receptor in primary human breast cancer. In *Steroid Receptor Assays in Human Breast Tumours: Methodological and Clinical Aspects* (Edited by R. J. B. King) p. 86, Alpha Omega Alpha Publishing Co., Cardiff (1978).

11. N. Mantel, Evaluation of survival data and two new rank order statistics arising in its consideration. *Cancer Chemother. Rep.* 50, 163 (1966).

12. J. S. Meyer, B. R. Rao, S. C. Stevens, and W. L. White, Low incidence of estrogen receptor in breast carcinomas with rapid rates of cellular replication. *Cancer* 40, 2290 (1977).

13. B. Wolff, Histological grading in carcinoma of breast. *Brit. J. Cancer* 20, 36 (1966).

14. H. R. Champion, I. W. Wallace, and R. J. Prestcott, Histology in breast cancer prognosis. *Brit. J. Cancer* 26, 129 (1972).

15. W. L. McGuire, P. P. Carbone, M. E. Sears, and G. C. Escher, Estrogen receptors in human breast cancer: an overview. In *Estrogen Receptors in Human Breast Cancer* (Edited by W. L. McGuire, P. P. Carbone, and E. P. Vollmer) p. 1. Raven Press, New York (1975).

16. W. A. Knoght, R. B. Livingston, E. J. Gregory, and W. L. McGuire, Estrogen receptor as an independent prognostic factor for early recurrence in breast cancer. *Cancer Res.* 37, 4669 (1977).

Steroid Hormone Receptors in Mammary Carcinoma: the Effect of Tamoxifen

A. J. M. Koenders*, L. V. M. Beex**, J. Geurts-Moespot* and Th. J. Benraad*

*Department of Experimental Endocrinology, Medical Faculty, University of Nijmegen, Nijmegen, The Netherlands.
**Department of Medicine, Division of Endocrinology, University of Nijmegen, Nijmegen, The Netherlands.

Correspondence to A. J. M. Koenders

Abstract—*Estradiol receptor (ER) and progesterone receptors (PgR) were measured in biopsies of DMBA-induced mammary tumors before and during tamoxifen (200 µg/day) treatment. Regressing tumors during treatment had significantly higher pretreatment ER and PgR levels than non-regressing tumors. During tamoxifen administration cytoplasmic ER levels became undetectable, whereas PgR levels declined to 20% of the corresponding pretreatment levels. Also in human mammary carcinoma ER became undetectable during tamoxifen (40 mg/day) therapy. After tamoxifen discontinuation ER levels in sequential biopsies of patients with advanced breast cancer were consistently lower or occasionally ER-negative compared to the corresponding values obtained before therapy. There were 10 objective remissions in 20 ER-positive cases and none in 9 ER-negative cases. These results suggest that ER and PgR measurements may be useful in the selection of tamoxifen responsive tumors.*

INTRODUCTION

Antiestrogens are a class of compounds which prevent estrogens from expressing their full effect on estrogen target tissues. Although the mechanism of action of antiestrogens is not clearly defined, it is generally accepted that an interaction with the estradiol receptor is an essential step (1,2). Recently several studies have demonstrated a relation between growth response of DMBA-induced mammary tumors (3,4) or of human mammary carcinoma (5) to the antiestrogen tamoxifen and estradiol receptor levels (ER). However, currently no information is available with regard to the progesterone receptor (PgR).

In the present study the relation between pretreatment ER and PgR levels and DMBA-tumor response to tamoxifen administration was investigated. Furthermore the effect of this treatment on ER and PgR levels was studied. In addition ER levels were measured before, during and after tamoxifen administration in sequential biopsies of patients with metastatic breast cancer and were related to the clinical response of these patients.

MATERIALS AND METHODS

1. Measurement of Estradiol and Progesterone Receptor Binding Sites

Receptor binding sites were measured as published previously (6-8). Shortly, 50 µl cytosol samples were transferred into microtiterplates and incubated with six different concentrations of ^{3}H-E$_2$ (1-8 nM) or ^{3}H-R5020 (1-10 nM). The nonspecific binding was determined in the presence of 10^{-6} M nonradioactive E$_2$ or R5020 respectively. After incubation for 16-20 hr at 0-4°C the unbound steroid was removed by the addition of 100 µl dextran-coated charcoal suspension. The concentration of receptor binding sites and the equilibrium dissociation constant (K_d) were determined by Scatchard-analysis.

2. Treatment of the Animals and Classification of DMBA-induced Mammary Tumors.

Mammary tumors were induced in 50 day old female Sprague-Dawley rats (IFFA Creda, France) by a single intragastric feeding of 20 mg DMBA in 1.0 ml sesame oil in each animal. All tumor areas were calculated at least once every week by caliper measurements. Biopsies were taken before tamoxifen administration at random stages of the oestrus cycle, of tumors that reached an area of about 4 sq cm (length × width). When tumors regained prebiopsy size the animals received daily s.c. injections of 200 µg tamoxifen[x] in 0.1 ml sesame oil. After 3 weeks of tamoxifen treatment a second biopsy was taken 48 hr after the last injection from the same tumor already biopsied. Tumors, that had decreased at least 50% in size during these 3 weeks of treatment were

---

[x]Tamoxifen was kindly provided by ICI, Holland.

scored as regressing (33/47 = 70% of all
tumors), whereas tumors that remained static
or continued to grow (14/47 = 30% of all
tumors) were scored as non-regressing tumors.

3. Collection of Human Breast Tumor Specimens

Biopsies during tamoxifen treatment were
taken from non-responding patients (2-3
months after start of therapy) or from
relapsing tumors (10-20 months after therapy
was started).

RESULTS

1. ER and PgR Levels before Tamoxifen Treatment in Regressing and Non-Regressing DMBA-tumours (Fig. 1)

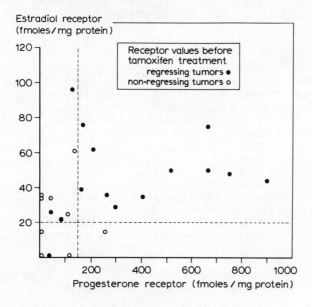

Fig. 1. Relation of pretreatment estradiol
and progesterone receptor levels of
regressing (o) and non-regressing
(o) DMBA-induced rat mammary tumors.
Broken lines indicate arbitrarily
chosen "critical levels".

ER and PgR were measured in 24 tumor biopsies (19 animals) taken before tamoxifen
200 µg/day treatment. Detectable amounts of
ER were found in 21 out of 24 tumors studied.
The mean of the ER levels, 46 ± 6 (range 0-95
fmoles/mg protein) in 15 regressing tumors
was significantly higher (p < 0.05, Wilcoxon
rank test) than the corresponding value,
25 ± 6 (range 0-60) of the 9 non-regressing
tumors. All 15 regressing tumors and 5 out
of the 9 non-regressing tumors revealed the
presence of PgR. Although there was overlap
of the lower values of the regressing tumors
(range 40-900 fmoles/mg protein) and the
higher values of the non-regressing tumors
(range 0-255), regressing tumors had significantly higher PgR levels than non-regressing
tumors (p < 0.01). No significant correlation
between individual ER and PgR levels was
observed in either group of tumors. Using
arbitrarily chosen "critical levels" of

20 fmoles/mg protein for ER and 150 for PgR,
it appears that all tumors (11/11) with
receptor levels above these "critical levels"
regressed during 3 weeks of 200 µg tamixifen
administration. In 2 tumors PgR activity
was present without detectable ER.

2. ER and PgR Levels in DMBA-tumors before and during Tamoxifen Administration (Fig. 2)

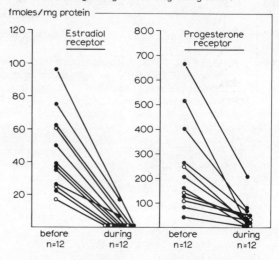

Fig. 2. Effect of 200 µg/day tamoxifen
treatment on estradiol and progesterone receptor levels of regressing
(o) and non-regressing (o) DMBA-
induced rat mammary tumors.

Fig. 2 compares ER and PgR levels of the
same tumor before and during tamoxifen treatment. During treatment ER levels were undetectable in 10 and another 2 tumors showed very
low ER levels. Tamoxifen treatment markedly
reduced PgR levels, but specific PgR binding
remained detectable in 9 out of 12 tumors
studied. The mean PgR level before treatment was 248 ± 55 and declined to 47 ± 17
fmoles/mg protein (80% reduction) after 3
weeks of 200 µg tamoxifen/day.

3. ER Levels before, during and after Tamoxifen Therapy in Sequential Biopsies of the same Patients (Fig. 3)

The ER levels before treatment ranged
between 20 and 480 fmoles/mg protein. During
tamoxifen administration no cytoplasmic ER
binding could be detected (n = 8). In 3 out
of 5 patients ER binding increased from
undetectable value during tamoxifen (40 mg
daily) to values that ranged between 30 and
145 after drug withdrawal. After tamoxifen
withdrawal the ER values appeared to be
consistently lower compared to the corresponding values measured before this treatment
was started. Two patients with ER-positive
metastases before therapy revealed ER-negative

tumors 6 and 8 weeks after termination of
this therapy. In 6 patients cytoplasmic ER
binding sites reappeared between 2 weeks and
3 months after cessation of treatment.

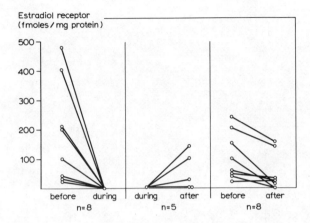

Fig. 3. Estradiol receptor levels before,
during and after tamoxifen (40 mg
daily) administration in sequential
biopsies of the same patients.

4. Relation between ER Activity and the
Clinical Response to Tamoxifen Therapy

Twenty-nine postmenopausal patients have
been treated with tamoxifen 40 mg daily.
All 9 patients with ER-negative tumors were
classified as non-responders, whereas in 10
out of the 20 patients with ER-positive
objective response to tamoxifen were recorded.

DISCUSSION

Several recent reports (3-5) have suggested
a relation between response of mammary tumors
to tamoxifen and quantitative estradiol receptor binding capacity. In the present study
it appears that tumors regressing during
administration of 200 μg tamoxifen/day have
significantly higher ER levels than non-
regressing tumors. However, there is no
definite separation between these tumors on
basis of ER levels, due to a considerable
overlap of ER levels from responding and non-
responding tumors.

Recently Horwitz et al. (9) suggested that
the progesterone receptor, being an ultimate
product of estrogen action, could serve as a
more reliable marker of endocrine responsiveness of breast tumors. As appears from the
results reported here, progesterone receptors
were detectable in all regressing and 5 out
of 9 non-regressing tumors. This observation
confirms that there is no absolute relation
between the presence or absence of PgR and
endocrine responsiveness of breast tumors
(10), but a higher rate of response to tamoxifen administration was observed when both

receptor levels were taken into account.
This indicates that measurement of PgR along
with ER provides additional although not
definitive information with regard to endocrine responsiveness of breast tumors.

During tamoxifen administration PgR levels
decreased in both regressing and non-regressing tumors confirming the observations by
Tsai and Katzenellenbogen (11), that the
effect of antiestrogens on tumor growth and
on PgR synthesis may be dissociated.

Two out of 8 patients with ER-positive
pretreatment tumors were measured ER-negative
6 and 8 weeks after tamoxifen withdrawal.
This observation suggests that a considerable
time may be required after discontinuation
of therapy before results of receptor assays
should form basis for therapy. In this study
no objective remission to tamoxifen administration was observed in ER-negative human
tumors.

REFERENCES

1. C. Burnett-Lunan and A. Klopper, Antiestrogens: A Review. *Clin. Endocr.*
   (Oxford) 4, 551 (1975).
2. B. S. Katzenellenbogen and E. R. Ferguson,
   Antiestrogen action in the uterus:
   biological ineffectiveness of nuclear
   bound estradiol after antiestrogen.
   Endocrinology 97, 1 (1975).
3. V. C. Jordan and T. Jaspan, Tamoxifen as
   an anti-tumour agent: oestrogen binding
   as a predictive test for tumour response.
   J. Endocr. 68, 453 (1976).
4. R. I. Nicholson, P. Davies and K.
   Griffiths, Nolvadex binding in mammary
   tumours in relation to response. In:
   Hormone Deprivation in Breast Cancer.
   Reviews on Endocrine-Related Cancer
   (Edited by M. Mayer, S. Saez and B. A.
   Stoll) p. 306. Supplement April, I.C.I.,
   Macclesfield, G.-B., (1978).
5. H. Westerberg, B. Nordenskjold, Ö. Wrange,
   J. A. Gustafsson, S. Humla, N. O. Theve,
   C. Silfverswärd and Per-Ola Granberg,
   Effect of antiestrogen therapy on human
   mammary carcinomas with different estrogen receptor contents. *Europ. J. Cancer*
   14, 619 (1978).
6. A. J. M. Koenders, A. Geurts-Moespot,
   S. Zolingen and Th. J. Benraad, Progesterone and estradiol receptors in DMBA-
   induced mammary tumors before and after
   ovariectomy and after subsequent estradiol
   administration. In: *Progesterone Receptors
   in Normal and Neoplastic Tissues* (Edited
   by W. L. McGuire, J. P. Raynaud and E. E.
   Baulieu) p. 71 Raven Press, New York
   (1977).
7. A. J. M. Koenders, J. Geurts-Moespot,
   K. H. Kho and Th. J. Benraad, Estradiol
   and progesterone receptor activities in
   stored lyophilised target tissue.
   J. Steroid Biochem. 9, 947 (1978).
8. A. J. M. Koenders. In *Steroid Hormone
   Receptors in Experimental and Human
   Mammary Carcinoma.* Dissertation, University of Nijmegen. Krips Repro, Meppel
   (1979).

9. K. B. Horwitz, W. L. McGuire, O. H. Pearson and A. Segaloff, Predicting response to endocrine therapy in human breast cancer: a hypothesis. *Science* 189, 726 (1975).

10. W. L. McGuire, Steroid receptors in human breast cancer. *Cancer Res.* 38, 4289 (1978).

11. T. L. S. Tsai and B. S. Katzenellenbogen, Antagonism of development and growth of 7,12-dimethylbenz (a) anthracene-induced rat mammary tumors by the antiestrogen U 23,469 and effects on estrogen and progesterone receptors. *Cancer Res.* 37, 1537 (1977).

Fine Needle Biopsy in Estrogen Receptor Determination in Breast Cancer

A. Lindgren*, J. Sällström* and H-O. Adami**

*Department of Pathology, Akademiska Sjukhuset, Uppsala, Sweden
**Department of Surgery, Akademiska Sjukhuset, Uppsala, Sweden

Correspondence to A. Lindgren, Department of Pathology, Akademiska Sjukhuset,
S-750 14 Uppsala, Sweden

Abstract—*Cytoplasmic estrogen receptors in mammary carcinoma was determined by iso-electric focusing in polyacrylamide gel using fine needle aspiration technique for tumor sampling. The method was compared with synchronous determination on homogenized tumor material and was found to give consistent results and to have advantages in sampling and analysis procedures such as need of minimal material, very little admixture of other cells or tissue and no need for homogenization. This technique also permits the receptor concentration to be expressed as number of cytoplasmic receptors per cell. Familiarity with the aspiration technique is necessary to extract the about 500,000 cells required for analysis. The fine needle biopsy would be especially suitable for analysis in recurrent breast cancer.*

INTRODUCTION

Determination of estrogen receptors (ER) in breast cancer has for some years been used to predict the response to endocrine treatment in recurrent disease (1). The introduction of an assay for iso-electric focusing in polyacrylamide gel (2) has enabled the analysis to be performed on very small amounts of tumor tissue and Silfverswärd et al. (3,4) have adopted this technique for analysis of fine needle aspiration biopsies. This technique has in our study been used for further clinical trial in patients with primary breast cancer. The aim of the study was to 1) compare pre-operative fine needle ER analysis to operation specimen fine needle and tissue homogenate analysis, 2) determine the minimal cell number necessary for adequate analysis and 3) develop a new method to quantify receptor content relative to tumor cell number.

MATERIAL AND METHODS

1. Patients

Aspiration was done through the skin, simulating in situ biopsy, on the breast tissue specimen from 29 patients. In another 11 patients, biopsies were taken both before surgery and after surgery on the breast tissue specimen. In all cases, a cube of tumor (size 1/2 cm) was taken for correlative studies. 31/40 patients were post-menopausal, defined as over 55 years of age.

Cell counting experiments on 29 patients include 7 of the 11 patients mentioned above.

2. Biopsies

Needle aspiration was done by the technique described by Franzén and Zajicek (5). Material from 2 aspirates with a 0.7 mm needle was ejected into 0,5 ml of hypo-tonic TRIS-EDTA buffer (20 mOsm) and immediately frozen to $-78^{o}C$ in a penthane-dry ice mixture. One drop of the cell suspension was smeared, air-dried and Giemsa-stained and checked for cellularity. The hypotonic buffer ruptures the cell membrane but leaves the nuclear membrane intact and cancer cells can easily be identified. Tissue specimens were taken from the cellular periferal parts of the tumor and frozen in the same way as the fine needle aspirates from 30-60 min after removal of the breast. This time has been found not to significantly influence the analysis (unpublished results). All fine needle biopsies and choice of tumor cube was done by an experienced pathologist.

3. Cell Counting

At the ER-analysis, the thawed suspension was thoroughly mixed by repeated pipetting through a Pasteur pipette in order to break up cell clusters. A 10 µl sample was diluted with an equal volume of 0.05% toluidine blue and the number of tumor cell nuclei per µl counted in a Bürker chamber. The total number of cells in the sample was calculated. Thus, the result of the ER-analysis could be related to the number of cells as either fmole receptor per cell or, using the Avogadro constant, as average number of receptor molecules per cell.

The minimal cell number necessary for analysis was studied by a stepwise dilution of the fine needle aspiration sample. The results were compared with the relative ^{3}H-estradiol binding in homogenized tissue specimens from the same cancer.

4. Cell Viability

Needle aspirate was ejected into phosphate buffered saline, pH 7.2 instead of into hypotonic TRIS-EDTA-buffer and very gently suspended. Small volumes of the cell suspension was mixed with equal volumes of either 0.05% toluidine blue or 0.2 μg/ml of fluoresceindiacetate and incubated at room temperature for 5 min and 15 min, respectively. The proportion of stained cells was determined in slide-coverslip preparations in which cell clusters were flattened, allowing all cells to be observed. For ER-analysis of such samples, the phosphate buffer was changed to the hypotonic TRIS-EDTA-buffer after 10 min centrifugation at 200 G at 4°C.

5. Estrogen Receptor Analysis

Samples were stored in a -70°C freezer for no longer than 3 weeks. The analysis of cytosol estradiol receptors was performed by isoelectric focusing in slabs of polyacrylamide gel (Ampholine[R] PAG-plates, pH-range 3.5-9.5, LKB Produkter, Bromma, Sweden) after mild trypsination, according to the method described by Wrange et al. (2). However, for hygienic reasons, addition of the isotope was done after the homogenization of the tissue and preparation of the cytosol. In a comparative study no significant difference could be demonstrated if the isotope was added before or after the preparation of cytosol. The radioactive steroid (2, 4, 6, 7, 16, 17-^{3}H) estradiol with a specific activity of 130-170 Ci/mmol (New England Nuclear Co) was added to the cytosol to a final concentration of 7 nM, and the sample was incubated for 45 min at 0°C.

Less than 0.1 fmol/μg DNA was considered ER-negative, 0.1-1 fmol/μg DNA weakly positive and more than 1 fmol/μg DNA as strongly positive.

RESULTS

Table 1. Comparison between ER-analysis of surgical and fine needle biopsies from the breast tissue specimen in 40 patients.

Cytology		Biopsy	
		ER-pos	ER-neg
	ER-pos	31	1
	ER-neg	2	6

Table 1 summarizes a comparison between cytologic and cold knife tissue specimen analysis. All but 3 cases were congruent in either presence or absence of ER. In ER-positive cases, tissue specimens varied from 0.1 to 7.2 fmol/μg DNA, cytology specimens from 0.1 to 9.3 fmol/μg DNA. In four cases, the tissue value for ER was strongly positive (≥ 1 fmol/μg DNA or more) while the cytology was weakly positive (less than 1 fmol/μg DNA), in 2 cases the opposite was true and in the remainder, values were equal.

By the stepwise dilution experiment, the minimal cell number for reliable analysis was found to be around 500,000 as exemplified by the experiment shown in Fig. 1.

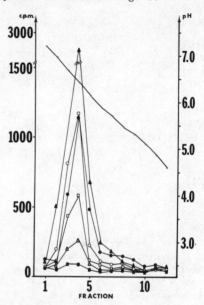

Fig. 1. Step-wise dilution of aspirate sample compared to tissue homogenate sample.

▲—▲   4 × 10[6] cells
○—○   2 × 10[6] cells
□—□   1 × 10[6] cells
△—△   0.5 × 10[6] cells
■—■   0.25 × 10[6] cells
●—●   homogenate
○—○   pH-gradient

The same experiment also demonstrated the difference in total ^{3}H-estradiol uptake relative to total DNA. The fine needle sample of 2 × 10[6] cells contained a total amount of 29 μg DNA while the corresponding tissue sample binding the same amount of ^{3}H-estradiol contained 115 μg giving a fmol/μg DNA of 4.1 for the cytologic sample, 1.0 for the tissue sample. This is due either to incomplete release of receptors to the cytosol or, more likely, to the amount of non-tumor DNA of the tissue specimen.

The 2 false negative needle biopsies showed inadequate material. The false negative surgical biopsy remains unexplained. 31 of

Table 2. 23 fine needle aspirate ER-analysis in primary breast
cancer.

Analysis	Range	Mean
Total DNA (µg)	10 - 131	38
Cell number	$0.4 - 9.0 \times 10^6$	2.8×10^6
DNA/cell (µg)	$0.4 - 2.9 \times 10^{-5}$	1.4×10^5
fmol/µg DNA	0.1 - 5.3	1.4
fmol/cell	$0.2 - 9.9 \times 10^{-5}$	2.0×10^{-5}
Receptors/cell	1,200-60,000	12,300

the patients were post-menopausal and 4 of these were ER negative.

Thus establishing the possibility to use fine needle aspirates for ER determination, further biopsies were taken pre- and post-operatively comprising 29 patients with primary breast cancer and cell counting was included in the analysis. 6 biopsies gave too little material. They were all pre-operative biopsies. Post-operative biopsies all conformed with the surgical biopsy control. ER-positivity was found in 17 (13 post-menopausal) and ER-negativity in 6 (4 post menopausal).

Table 2 lists the values obtained. It is concluded that the minimal amount of cells necessary for analysis is about 500,000 and that tumor cells contain an average of about 10.000 cytoplasmic receptors. 25-50% of the tumor cells are viable at the time of biopsy.

DISCUSSION

Determination of estrogen receptor content in breast cancer cells by ordinary techniques expresses the presence of ER in terms of fmole estradiol/µg DNA or µg protein of the sample. In such samples, the admixture of stromal connective tissue, vessels and inflammatory cells in the tumor cytosol influences the content of both DNA and protein. In this respect, fine needle aspirates are superior as only cancer cells and a small amount of inflammatory cells are withdrawn, as seen in the Giemsa-stained slides. By counting the amount of cancer cells in the specimen it is possible to express ER contents as number of receptors per cell, thus omitting the DNA analysis which requires a substantial amount of DNA in the specimen to give reliable results and includes irrelevant DNA content of non-tumor cells.

Cell viability varies considerably due to tumor size as well as histologic type. Another influencing factor is the site of sampling within the tumor. By correlating the ER value to the viable cells, this parameter is standardized. This would probably be a still better way of expressing the degree of receptor positivity and might improve the predictive value of ER analysis for response to endocrine therapy.

A minor advantage with the used technique is that it makes homogenization of the tumor unnecessary as the hypotonic buffer is enough

to ensure release of the cytoplasmic receptors to the medium.

Aspiration technique allows ER determination even in cases where the primary carcinoma is so small that otherwise all tumor tissue has to be used for histopathologic confirmation of the diagnosis.

A promising aspect of this new technique is the possibility to make ER-evaluation on recurrent cancer or metastases without the need for surgical intervention. Repeated analyses before, during and after endocrine and cytotoxic treatment might also improve our understanding of the tumor biology.

Preliminary results with biopsies taken routinely before surgery by the surgeon or in recurrent disease by the oncologist are promising but indicate the need for a well trained person to do the biopsies. Even so, a rather large percentage of failures to get enough material from cutaneous metastases is to be expected, considering the usual microscopic picture of these with few cancer cells in an abundant collagenous stroma. Investigations in progress will evaluate the usefulness of the described method for ER determination in clinical practice.

REFERENCES

1. W. L. McGuire, P. P. Carbone and E. P. Vollmer, Eds. *Estrogen receptors in human breast cancer*. Raven Press, New York (1975).
2. Ö. Wrange, B. Nordenskjöld and J-Å. Gustafsson, Cytosol estradiol receptor in human mammary carcinoma: an assay based on isoelectric focusing in poly-acrylamide gel. *Analyt. Biochem.* 85, 461 (1978).
3. J. Silfverswärd, *Estrogen receptors in human breast cancer*. Thesis, Stockholm (1979).
4. J. Silfverswärd and S. Humla, Estrogen receptor analysis on needle aspirates from human mammary carcinoma. *Acta Cytol.* In press (1979).
5. S. Franzén and J. Zajicek, Aspiration biopsy in diagnosis of palpable lesions of the breast. *Acta Radiol.* 7, 262 (1968).

Hormone Receptors in Breast Cancer

E. Engelsman

Antoni van Leeuwenhoek Ziekenhuis, Netherlands Cancer Institute, Plesmanlaan 121,
Amsterdam, The Netherlands

Correspondence to E. Engelsman

Abstract—*A short report is given of the results of the EORTC workshop on standardization of ER assay, held in March 1979 in Amsterdam. A practical method to decide on an effective cut-off point between ER "positive" and "negative" will be demonstrated; a division between positive and negative can be chosen so that this distinction has optimal predictive value for clinical hormone sensitivity.*

EORTC WORKSHOP ON ESTROGEN ASSAY STANDARDIZATION

In March 1979 a Workshop on Estrogen Receptor assay standardization was held in the Netherlands Cancer Institute, organised by the EORTC Breast Cancer Group, under chairmanship of Prof. P. Jungblut. Full agreement was reached on a standard procedure for the assay of both estrogen and progesterone receptors in breast cancer tissue. This standard assay will be used by all centres taking part in EORTC Breast Cancer Group clinical trials.

An organization for quality control was set up: the first samples of tissue powder have already been sent round by Dr. Benraad, in Nijmegen, Holland.

The protocol for the standard assays will be published as soon as possible. With this standard ER assay it will be feasible to stratify patients according to ER status in future clinical trials.

A CUT-OFF POINT FOR ER NEGATIVE AND POSITIVE WITH MAXIMUM PREDICTIVE POWER

In the Netherlands Cancer Institute we wanted to find the cut-off point for ER positivity that should give maximum prediction of response to endocrine therapy in advanced breast cancer.

We collected responses and failures to endocrine treatment, and made cumulative frequency curves of both, in relation to the ER quantities measured in the tumours (Fig. 1).

From Fig. 1 it is clear that any of the values a, b and c should have some predictive value if used as the cut-off between ER- and ER+: most of the responses with ER+ tumours, most of the failures with ER-tumours. If the line should be shifted to the right, no failures would be seen with ER+ tumours, but most responses with ER- tumours. Shifting the line to the left should mean many ER+

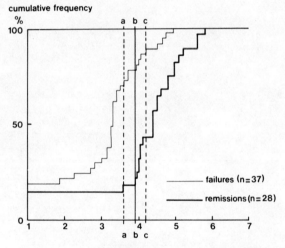

Fig. 1. Relation between cumulative frequency of failures/remissions and ER-level.

tumours, and many failures with ER+ tumours.

It seems that the maximum vertical distance between the curves indicates the ER value that could best be used as the cut-off value. A curve can be constructed illustrating the vertical distance between the two curves at all the measured ER values (Fig. 2).

The value which had been used arbitrarily as the border between ER- and ER+ (b in Fig. 1 and Fig. 2) seems to have been chosen very efficiently (10 fmol/mg tissue protein).

Table 1 shows the remission rates obtained with ER+ tumours if two different cut-off points are used.

The predictive value of the ER determination is slightly better if b is chosen as the cut-off value.

From these data one can calculate the

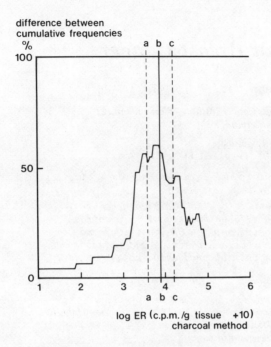

Fig. 2. Difference between cummulative
         frequencies of failures and
         responses in relation to ER- level.

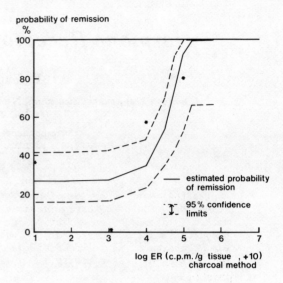

Fig. 3. Relation between probablity of
        remission and ER- level.

Table 1. Remission rates by endocrine therapy, if different
         cut-off points are chosen between ER+ and ER-
         (a, b: see Fig. 1 and Fig. 2).

Cut-off point	ER	Number tumours	Remissions	Remissions %
a	+	34	23	.68
	–	31	5	.16
b	+	31	23	.74
	–	34	5	.15

relation betwen the probability of obtaining
a remission by endocrine therapy and the ER
values measured (linear logit model).

Figure 3 shows that in our material the
probability of achieving a remission by
endocrine therapy increases with higher ER
values. Our data indicate that 10 fmol/mg
tissue protein is a good cut-off value for
ER, to predict hormone responsiveness by
ER positivity. The higher ER values seem to
predict a better chance that the tumour
will respond to hormone therapy.

Use of Blue Sepharose for the Purification of Cytoplasmic Estrogen Receptors from DMBA-Induced Rat Mammary Tumors

G. Leclercq*, A. Tenenbaum** and A. Hepburn*

**Clinique et Laboratoire de Cancerologie Mammaire, Service de Medecine,
Institut Jules Bordet, 1000 Bruxelles, Belgium*
***Laboratoire d'Endocrinologie, Service de Medecine, Institut Jules Bordet, 1000
Bruxelles, Belgium*

Correspondence to G. Leclercq

Abstract—*Free and estradiol-complexed forms of the estrogen receptor from
DMBA-induced rat mammary tumors were shown to display a different chromatographic behaviour on Blue Sepharose. At $4^{o}C$ the complexed form was not
retained on the column whereas the free was tightly adsorbed. At $18^{o}C$
adsorbed ER might be extracted from the Blue Sepharose matrix with ^3H-estradiol.
This process was relatively slow and required several hours. At the end of
the extraction period no protein could be detected in the medium; protein
still being detectable in 100-times diluted cytosol it seems that ER was
purified at least by a factor of 100. Sieving of extracted ER on Sephadex
G 200 Superfine gave a single and sharp peak suggesting that the macromolecular
structure of the purified receptor corresponds to a single estrogen-binding
unit.*

*These properties define a rapid method for obtaining highly purified ER
from rat mammary tumors. However, recovery of ER from the Blue Sepharose
matrix was found to vary from one cytosol to another. Therefore, search is
still required to improve the yield of the extraction procedure.*

Purification of uterine cytoplasmic estrogen receptors (ER) has attracted attention
over the last decade, but successful purifi-
cations of ER from mammary tumors are still
scarce, although they might produce pro-
gresses in the study and treatment of hormone-
dependent breast cancer. This technique may
improve the clinical relevance and understanding of the cellular action of estrogen
receptors.

The difficulty of obtaining large amounts
of breast cancer tissue and the relatively
low content of cytoplasmic ER in the majority
of tumors imposes very efficient purification
processes. The use of specific adsorbents,
recently developed (1,2), appears therefore
the most appropriate approach for this task.
Among these adsorbents, Heparine-conjugated
Sepharose was shown to be highly effective
in the isolation of cytoplasmic ER from
uterus (2) and mammary gland (3,4). In our
laboratory, attempts using such a matrix
with cytosol preparations from DMBA-induced
rat mammary tumors were disappointing in view
of the low adsorption property of ER from a
large proportion of tumors (unpublished
data).

On the other hand, we observed a major
difference between the free and estradiol-
complexed forms of ER from DMBA-induced rat
mammary tumors in respect to their chromatographic behaviour on Blue Sepharose
columns (5). At $4^{o}C$ the complexed form was

not retained on the column whereas the free
one was tightly adsorbed. Additional experiments demonstrated that washing the column
with Cibacron Blue (0.5 mg/ml) yielded a
fraction that bound ^3H-estradiol (^3H-E_2).
The suppression of this labeling by 100-fold
excess of cold estradiol indicated the presence of ER in the fraction. Finally, it
was found that adsorbed receptors might
also be extracted with labeled estrogens
(^3H-estradiol or ^3H-diethylstilbestrol) from
the Blue Sepharose matrix at $18^{o}C$. We are
presently evaluating whether or not these
properties might be used for the purification
of ER from rat mammary tumor ER. The data
reported here summarize our preliminary
results in this regard.

1. Kinetics of the Extraction Process

Fig. 1 analyses the kinetics of the extraction of ER from the Blue Sepharose matrix at
$18^{o}C$ in a typical experiment (experimental
procedures in the legend of the figure). It
shows that the process is relatively slow
and requires several hours. As in all
extraction processes, the present one progressively slows down. Thus, after 10 hours
the amount of receptors released from the
matrix was about 70% of the amount released
after 50 hours.

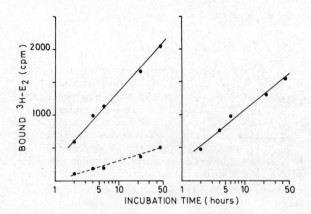

Fig. 1. Kinetics of extraction from Blue
Sepharose of adsorbed cytoplasmic
ER from DMBA-induced rat mammary
tumors. In the left panel, the
full line refers to the extraction
by ^{3}H-E$_2$ alone; the dotted line, to
the extraction by ^{3}H-E$_2$ in presence
of an excess of unlabeled E$_2$. In
the right panel, the line refers
to the specific extraction $\left(\left(^3\text{H-E}_2\right)\right.$
$\left.- \left(^3\text{H-E}_2 + \text{excess E}_2\right)\right)$.

Experimental procedure
Cytosol from DMBA-induced rat mammary tumors was prepared as previously described (6) and stored
in liquid nitrogen until chromatography (1 week). Two and a half
g of Blue Sepharose CL-6 B (Phar-
macia, Uppsala, Sweden) was equili-
brated with 8 ml of 10 mM Tris-1.5
M EDTA buffer pH 7.8 containing
6 mM/ß-mercaptoethanol (TEM buffer)
in a chromatographic column at 4°C
($\sim$ 11 g of packed gel).

Adsorption of ER:
Two ml of cytosol were applied to
the top of the Blue Sepharose
column and eluted with TEM buffer
to remove all non-binding proteins.
Elution was pursued with 1.5 M KCl
in TEM buffer until collection of a
second protein fraction. The column
was then washed with TEM buffer to
remove KCl. None of these elution
fractions contained detectable ER
(5).

Extraction of ER:
Blue Sepharose was removed from the
column and suspended in 10 ml of
TEM buffer added with 10^{-8}M ^{3}H-E$_2$
(86 Ci/mM, Radiochemical Center,
Amersham, UK) at 18°C to extract
ER. The specificity of the extraction was assessed by a parallel
incubation of ^{3}H-E$_2$ plus a 1000-
fold excess of unlabeled E$_2$. Aliquots of 500 µl were taken at
various times and centrifuged (5
min; 2,000 × g). Bound ^{3}H-E$_2$ was
then estimated in aliquots of 250 µl

of supernatant by a dextran-coated
charcoal procedure (6). For each
experimental value, the remaining
radioactivity at time zero (blank)
was subtracted.

2. Efficiency of the Extraction Procedure

Five cytosol samples were adsorbed on Blue Sepharose and
extracted by ^{3}H-E$_2$ at 18°C.
Recovery of ER varied from one cytosol
to another. The reason of this variability
remains unknown. However, in two experiments
a very good yield (80%) was obtained after a
long extraction period. At the end of the
extraction procedure no protein could be
detected in the medium by the Bio-Rad assay
(Bio-Rad, Richmond, California) as well as
by U.V. spectrophotometry (λ 280 mµ). Protein being still detectable in 100-times
diluted cytosol seems to indicate that ER was
purified at least by a factor of 100.

Finally, sieving of extracted ER on Sephadex G 200 superfine gave a single and sharp
peak of bound ^{3}H-E$_2$ (Fig. 2). This pattern
suggests that the macromolecular structure
of the purified ER corresponds to a single
estrogen-binding unit.

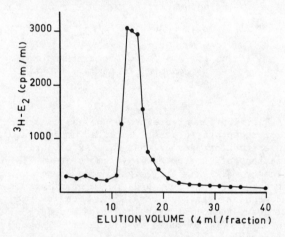

Fig. 2. Elution on Sephadex G 200 superfine
of ER extracted from Blue Sepharose. Before elution, extracted
receptors were $\sim$ 20 times concentrated by the aquacide technique
to allow the application of a fine
band on the top of the Sephadex
column.

The experiments described here define a
rapid method for obtaining highly purified
cytoplasmic ER from DMBA-induced rat mammary
tumors. However, recovery of the receptors
varied from one cytosol to another. Therefore, search is still required to find the
origin of the variability and improve the
yield of the extraction procedure (extraction
at various ^{3}H-E$_2$ concentrations, temperatures,
pH, ionic strengths...).

ACKNOWLEDGEMENT

This work was supported by a grant from
the "Fonds Cancérologique de la Caisse
Générale d'Epargne et de Retraite", Belgium
and by contract n°1-CM-53840 from the National
Cancer Institute, Bethesda, Maryland.

REFERENCES

1. V. Sica, I. Parikh, E. Nola, G. A. Puca
   and P. Cuatrecasas, Affinity chromatography and the purification of estrogen
   receptors. *J. Biol. Chem.* 248, 6543
   (1973).
2. A. M. Molinari, N. Medici, B. Moncharmont
   and G. A. Puca, Estradiol receptor from
   calf uterus: Interaction with heparine-
   agarose and purification. *Proc. Natl.
   Acad. Sci. (US)* 74, 4886 (1977).
3. F. Aurichio, A. Rotondi, P. Sampaolo
   and E. Schiavone, Cytosol oestrogen
   receptor of lactating mammary gland.
   Effect of heparine on the aggregation
   of the receptor and interaction of the
   receptor with heparine sepharose.
   Biochem. J. 171, 137 (1978).
4. A. Rotondi and F. Auirichio, Oestrogen
   receptor of calf mammary gland. Purification by use of sodium bromide and
   Heparine-Sepharose. *Biochem. J.* 178,
   581 (1978).
5. A. Tenebaum and G. Leclercq, Different
   chromatographic behaviour on Blue
   Sepharose CL-6 B of free and estradiol
   complexed forms of the estrogen receptor
   from DMBA-induced rat mammary tumors,
   submitted for publication.
6. G. Leclercq and J. C. Heuson, Specific
   estrogen receptor of the DMBA-induced
   mammary carcinoma and its estrogen-requir-
   ing molecular transformation. *Europ. J.
   Cancer* 9, 675 (1973).

New Aspects of Endocrine Treatment
of Advanced Disease

Recent Developments in the Endocrine Treatment of Breast Cancer

B. A. Stoll

Departments of Oncology, St. Thomas' Hospital and Royal Free Hospital, London, U.K.

Correspondence to B. A. Stoll, Department of Oncology, St. Thomas' Hospital, London SE1 7EH, U.K.

Abstract—*In the last 30 years we have improved our ability to select those patients more likely to benefit from endocrine therapy, and also the method more likely to help the individual patient. We have also developed new endocrine modalities with less morbidity, yet with the same objective response rate. Since cytokinetic factors dictate the maximum proportion of patients who will show significant tumour regression under either endocrine or cytotoxic therapy, we have reached a plateau in the regression rate possible from these treatments unless limiting factors in the individual tumours can be overcome.*

One method is to take advantage of the heterogeneity of the majority of breast cancers. A combination of endocrine and cytotoxic therapies should yield a higher response rate than either alone, and this has indeed been shown in early trials of oophorectomy and polychemotherapy in premenopausal patients, and a combination of tamoxifen and polychemotherapy in postmenopausal patients. Whether the modalities should be given concurrently or consecutively, and in which order, depends on both tumour and host factors and needs further investigation.

The last 30 years have produced a large number of methods for changing the endocrine environment of the tumour in the patient with advanced breast cancer. However, the evidence suggests that there is a plateau in the regression rate which depends on the cell kinetic characteristics of breast cancer, and we cannot get beyond it with our present methods.

Effective progestins lead to an overall regression rate of 30%, whatever the agent and whether low or high dosage is used. Recent reports on the use of aminoglutethimide show a similar overall response rate. The regression rate reported from the effective new androgens is the same 30% as for the older androgen and the results of transsphenoidal hypophysectomy or Yttrium ablation of the pituitary are similar. Anti-oestrogens such as clomiphene or nafoxidine yield a regression rate of 30% and the same figure applies to tamoxifen.

The magic 30% overall regression rate from all methods is not merely a coincidence. Nor does it necessarily mean that all endocrine methods have the same mechanism of action on breast cancer. The figure of 30% represents the proportion of tumours which show at least 50% decrease in their diameter and this necessitates a 90% decrease in their volume. Proliferating cells represent only a part of the tumour mass and even if 99% of them die, tumour shrinkage will occur only if the other cytokinetic characteristics of the tumour are favourable. The conclusion is that we cannot

improve the overall regression rate to be expected from endocrine therapy unless we are able to change certain limiting factors in many of the tumours. These include poor vascularity, heterogeneity of the tissue, low proportion of proliferating cells, site factors which diminish response or a prolonged cell cycle which delays response.

A similar plateau has been reached in the regression rate from cytotoxic therapy in breast cancer, and this also is due to cell kinetic factors. But the plateau for cytotoxic therapy is set at 50% compared to a 30% plateau for endocrine therapy. The reason for this is suggested by the recent finding that both ER+ and ER- tumours show a 50% likelihood of response to cytotoxic therapy, whereas ER- tumours show only a 10% likelihood of response to endocrine therapy. This explains the difference in overall regression rate between the two methods. Apart from this, there is little difference between cytotoxic and endocrine therapy either in the proportion of patients with complete remission or in the average duration of remission. This has been shown in a randomised comparison of the two methods. Most large series confirm that the proportion of complete responders and the mean duration of response is remarkably similar for tamoxifen therapy as for polychemotherapy.

Is there any way we can extend the duration of response to endocrine therapy? There are several possible explanations as to why a breast cancer finally loses its sensitivity

to endocrine therapy. After endocrine ablation, homeostatic adjustment occurs in hormonal secretion, while after administration
of a hormonal agent, changes in its metabolic
disposal may change its effectiveness. Many
explain the development of autonomy on the
basis that the tumour is multiclonal and that
hormone resistant cells gradually replace
the destroyed sensitive cells, while others
suggest that all tumours progress naturally
to autonomy, possibly as a result of changes
in receptor activity. Most of the evidence
points to the likelihood that breast cancer
is a multiclonal tumour.

This suggests that one way of breaking
through the present plateau in regression
rate, degree of regression and duration of
regression, may lie in combining endocrine
with cytotoxic therapy. The evidence from
clinical trials is so far not statistically
significant, but it does suggest that a
combination of oophorectomy and cytotoxic
therapy for the premenopausal patient may
lead to better results than either method
alone. Similarly, a combination of tamoxifen
and cytotoxic therapy in the postmenopausal
patient may lead to better results than
either alone. The benefit from a combination
of stilboestrol and cytotoxic agents is more
doubtful.

What progress then have we made in endo-
crinal therapy in the past 30 years? We have
developed new methods associated with much
less morbidity, yet with the same overall
response rate. This means that the patient's
quality of life during the remission is
considerably improved. We have also improved
our ability to select those patients who are
most likely to benefit from endocrine therapy
and also for selecting the method most likely
to help the individual patient.

Tamoxifen is associated with a much greater
patient compliance rate than the oestrogens
and androgens used previously. A withdrawal
rate from treatment of less than 3% in about
1000 patients, proves tamoxifen to be a well
tolerated agent.

The use of the ER assay for selecting
patients for endocrine treatment is well
established and the measurement of progesterone receptor in addition, may further
improve our ability to predict the response.
The recent finding of low tumour ER levels
in breast cancer patients within the first
few years after the menopause provides an
explanation for what clinicians have observed
for many years - a poor response rate in that
age group to endocrine therapy of any type.

What then is the present guide to the
selection of endocrine therapy in late breast
cancer? In a collected series of premenopausal patients treated by tamoxifen, an
overall regression rate of 30% has been shown.
Tamoxifen may therefore be an alternative to
castration, particularly for the ER+ tumour
involving soft tissue rather than bone. In
the postmenopausal patient, ER+ soft tissue
tumour is certainly an indication for a trial
of tamoxifen while bone metastases may respond
better to androgens such as fluoxymesterone.
For the ER- tumour on the other hand,
polychemotherapy is preferred in both age
groups.

In the case of the rapidly growing tumour
however, there is no time to wait for the
results of what may turn out to be unsuccess-
ful therapy, and it may be better to ignore
the results of ER assay in such cases. A
combination of endocrine and cytotoxic
therapy is more likely to be effective than
either alone, and the addition of cortico-
steroid will help to achieve a more immediate
response.

How do I see future developments in the
selection of systemic therapy for advanced
breast cancer? Selective treatment based on
receptor assay is inadequate. This is suggested by the better and more prolonged
remissions achieved from the combinations of
endocrine and cytotoxic therapy. We will
need to develop direct methods of testing
tumour sensitivity to combinations of agents,
either in vitro or on transplants growing in
nude mice. We also need to investigate the
potential of conjugated compounds of hormones
and cytotoxic agents, which will enable the
antimitotic effect to be exerted selectively
at the target tissue.

The Changing Role of Endocrine Therapy in the Management of Advanced Breast Cancer

J. L. Hayward

Guy's Hospital, London SE1 9RT, U.K.

Correspondence to J. L. Hayward

Abstract—*The past few years have witnessed significant changes of emphasis in the endocrine treatment of advanced breast cancer. Firstly, receptor site assays have proved effective in predicting response to therapy. Secondly, compounds are now available which, although giving the same response rate as androgens or oestrogens, lack almost all the unpleasant side effects. Thirdly, medical treatments are now available which have a similar effect as the major ablative procedures. It is likely that within a short time the operations of oophorectomy, adrenalectomy and hypophysectomy may become obsolete.*

In the early 1950's, the introduction of adrenalectomy and hypophysectomy as practical measures for the treatment of patients with advanced breast cancer fundamentally changed attitudes on the management of this disease. Previously, ovarian ablation had been used in the treatment of premenopausal patients, and androgens and oestrogens had been available for postmenopausal women, but the duration of benefit was short and, certainly in terms of the additive compounds, side-effects were severe. It had been appreciated for some time that after the failure of these measures, further benefit might accrue if the secretions of the adrenal or pituitary glands could be abolished, but surgical ablation of these glands was impossible because patients died in Addisonian crisis and, for the same reason, attempts at partial adrenalectomy proved too hazardous for routine use.

Then, with the synthesis of cortisone, the whole situation changed. Adrenalectomy and hypophysectomy became practicable procedures and initial reports of series of patients treated in this way engendered enormous enthusiasm for a treatment which, when successful, gave a greater degree of benefit for a longer duration than had ever been reported before. Subsequently, cases were described where patients had had a remission of 10 or more years and who had been living a more or less normal life for that period. Research efforts were centered partly on attempting to find methods of predicting which patients would respond and partly trying to determine why failure occurred. An accepted pattern of management developed. Premenopausal patients were treated initially by oophorectomy, menopausal patients by androgen therapy and postmenopausal patients by oestrogen therapy. When these treatments failed, adrenalectomy or hypophysectomy was carried out. The decision to use the operations was based partly on the history of

success or failure of previous treatment and partly on the use of urinary steroid estimations which gave a somewhat imprecise measure of the likelihood of success. There has been considerable change since this relatively stable situation, and a number of factors have been responsible.

First has been the development of assays of hormone receptor proteins in the cytosol of the cancer cell. Measurement of these proteins has proved more accurate than urinary steroid measurements in predicting the response of patients to ablative endocrine therapy and, moreover, it has enabled the response of patients to additive therapy also to be predicted. Possibly more important, it has directed attention away from the function of the endocrine glands and towards the cancer cell itself. Furthermore, the identification of these receptor proteins has provided a more logical explanation of the mechanism of endocrine response.

Second, antioestrogens have been developed. Tamoxifen, the best of these compounds, has provided an effective substitute for both androgens and oestrogens and, most importantly, has proved to have almost none of their unpleasant side effects.

Third, and possibly predictably, medical methods of inhibiting the secretion of the adrenal and to some extent the pituitary gland, are being developed. Aminoglutethimide can effectively inhibit the secretion of the adrenals, and prednisone partly achieves the same effect. Regarding the pituitary, prolactin secretion can be effectively inhibited by bromoergocryptine and, in the case of the ovary, although not by the same sort of mechanism, the anti-tumour effect of ablation can be achieved by the prescription of tamoxifen.

Fourth, there has been a major improvement in the efficacy of chemotherapy. Not only have new and more effective compounds been developed, but the use of combination treatment has given a further impetus to this method of treatment. Possibly more important than the development of chemotherapy has been the emergence of expert chemotherapists. The appearance of trained specialists in this field has meant not only that the treatment is given more effectively, but often preferentially over more traditional methods of therapy.

These developments are continuing and are having a profound effect on the management of the patient and on the direction of research. The use of receptor site assays has resulted in greater emphasis being placed on detailed analysis of the primary tumour. Although these assays can be carried out on material biopsied from secondary deposits, it is not always possible to obtain such tissue if metastases are present only in such sites as brain, lung or bone. Also, because tamoxifen is easy to prescribe and has so few side effects, it is often more practicable to try the drug rather than subject the patient to an additional biopsy. It is becoming almost as important to do these assays on the primary tumour as it is to carry out the usual histological examination.

The demonstration of the presence of these receptor proteins has directed attention back to the cancer cell and to its biochemistry.

Not only will assays of receptors become more precise and carried out on fixed material, but more specific typing of these proteins may enable more accurate predictions of tumour behaviour to be made. With this information will come the stimulus for more effective blocking agents to be synthesised, and the availability of these agents should enable the endocrine glands to be left undisturbed in the majority of patients.

If more specific medical measures for inhibiting natural hormone production becomes available, there will be demand for their use, but only in patients shown to have endocrine sensitive tumours. Those patients who have endocrine insensitive tumours will be referred for chemotherapy at an early stage. It is also likely that there will be earlier recourse to chemotherapy in those with sensitive tumours who are failing to respond to endocrine treatment. Still largely unexplored is the use of a combination of endocrine and chemotherapy.

The use of the major ablative operations is already waning and fewer are being carried out each year. It can be predicted with a fair degree of certainty that, within the next decade, the role of surgical adrenalectomy and hypophysectomy in the management of patients with advanced breast cancer will become largely historical.

The Tamoxifen Trial - A Double-Blind Comparison with Stilboestrol in Post-Menopausal Women with Advanced Breast Cancer

H. J. Stewart*, A. P. M. Forrest**, J. M. Gunn*, T. Hamilton**, A. O. Langlands*, I. J. McFadyen** and M. M. Roberts**

*Department of Radiation Oncology, University of Edinburgh
**Department of Clinical Surgery, University of Edinburgh

Correspondence to H. J. Stewart, Department of Radiation Oncology, Western General
Hospital, Crewe Road, Edinburgh EH4 2XU, U.K.

Abstract—The results of a double-blind randomly controlled crossover trial, comparing tamoxifen with stilboestrol as first palliation in postmenopausal women under the age of 80 with advanced and metastatic breast carcinoma, are described. Patients were stratified and randomised to receive coded drugs from the hospital pharmacy. Treatment was continued until disease was deemed progressive, when the alternative preparation was prescribed. Seventytwo postmenopausal women were entered, of whom 39 received the two drugs in sequence. Response to treatment was assessed according to British Breast Group criteria and was subject to external review. The drug code was not broken until one year after closure. Our results indicate that the two drugs appear to act independently, that the greater frequency of intolerance to stilboestrol is a significant disadvantage, and that tamoxifen should be the first hormone drug of choice for postmenopausal patients with advanced breast cancer.

INTRODUCTION

Previous reports by Cole et al. (1) and Ward (2) indicated that benefit from tamoxifen therapy could occur in 30%-40% of women with advanced breast carcinoma. The drug was described as an antioestrogen and the recorded incidence of side effects was low. In August 1973 in the combined breast clinic in Edinburgh a randomly controlled trial to assess the place of tamoxifen therapy in the management of patients with advanced and metastatic breast carcinoma was commenced with the support of ICI Pharmaceuticals UK. At its commencement the trial was designed in two parts to allow inclusion of patients in whom initial treatment included prophylactic oophorectomy. In each part of the trial tamoxifen was to be compared with oestrogen therapy in postmenopausal patients (LMP more than 5 years previously) and androgen therapy in menopausal patients (LMP from 2 to 5 years previously). Those patients who had failed to respond to a previous therapeutic oophorectomy were to be included in the postmenopausal group.

MATERIALS AND METHODS

1. Protocol

A description of the protocol including subsequent modification has been published elsewhere (3).

All patients with proven advanced breast carcinoma attending the Edinburgh combined breast clinic were considered for inclusion providing they were under the age of 80 and had not received previous systemic therapy for their breast carcinoma other than prophylactic or failed therapeutic oophorectomy. Patients were excluded by a previous history of malignant disease of another site and if they had had an unrelated hysterectomy or bilateral oophorectomy.

The hormones under study were supplied in a double-blind fashion and given consecutively with a 4 week gap between drugs when evidence of relapse or failure to respond was obtained.

Stratification into sub-groups according to disease type (local or systemic), disease-free interval and menstrual status was carried out and allocation to treatment within these stratification sub-groups was by a system of random cards prepared by the statistician.

2. Treatment

The hospital pharmacy was supplied with the three coded hormone preparations similarly prepared and packaged, namely tamoxifen 10 mgs, diethy-stilboestrol 5 mgs and fluoxymesterone 5 mgs. On submission of their selection card, patients received the appropriate package from the pharmacist with instructions to take 3 tablets daily.

3. Conduct of the Trial

Clinical examination findings, with measurements and clinical photographs where applicable, were recorded together with the results of a full radiological survey on entry. Biochemical tests of liver function, serum calcium and haematologic levels were performed on entry and repeated at 1 month and 3 months subsequently. At 3 months a preliminary clinical and radiological assessment was made of known disease and at 6 months after entry full assessment was repeated and the patient's response grade recorded.

4. Progress

A preliminary review of the first 60 patients entered showed that there was little point in continuing with the tamoxifen/fluoxymesterone arm of the study into which only 4 patients had been entered after $2\frac{1}{2}$ years. This comparison was therefore abandoned. The last patient was selected in April 1977, making a total of 76 patients in all, 72 of whom are available for analysis. Sixtyfour are now dead, and of the remaining 8 only 2 remain on a trial drug.

5. External Review

In May 1976 the clinical and trial records of over 40 patients for whom internal assessment had been made were externally reviewed and response to treatment defined according to BBG criteria (4). For this assessment the drug codes were not broken. Although some internal assessments were downgraded, the most striking effect of this external review was the exposure of minor errors of inclusion and selection. In all 38 protocol infringements in 30 of the 72 trial patients occurred. The majority of these infringements have been ignored for this analysis as they are not considered to be relevant to the drug comparisons. Two patients who were over age had only just passed their 80th birthday: of 4 given previous systemic therapy, 2 received short-term prednisone for lung disease prior to entry to the trial and 2 had received intermittent adjuvant 5-fluorouracil as part of their initial treatment. The original reason for excluding patients with a previous hysterectomy was in order to be able to define the natural menopause: of 6 incorrectly included because of a previous hysterectomy, 5 were over 60 years at the time of entry and have therefore been deemed postmenopausal. Although no allowance in the protocol was made for breaking the drug code, 8 in whom the knowledge of the drug prescribed was considered important for subsequent management have not been withdrawn since the correct second drug was eventually given. The remaining patient was prescribed the incorrect drug by her general practitioner before the trial package was supplied and has been included in the analysis according to this prescription. The reason for defining a withdrawal period between drugs was in order to test for withdrawal response, but as this is only likely to follow a response to treatment, the 12 patients in whom the withdrawal period was less than 4 weeks when it followed either toxicity or continued progression of disease, have been included. Five patients were randomised within the wrong subgroup but have been analysed according to their true grouping. Incorrect disease classification resulted from inconsistent handling of those patients who had contralateral as well as local disease. For this analysis they have been included in the local only group despite the selection of some of them within the systemic disease category.

Following a second external review session, 79 out of the 111 drug treatments given within the trial have been externally reviewed. This means that for this analysis 32 internal assessments have been included without subsequent external confirmation.

6. Withdrawals (Table 1)

Of the 72 patients for assessment, 16 have been termed not assessable, mostly by our external reviewers. Included in this group are 8 patients in whom drug toxicity was such that treatment had to be discontinued before an assessment could be made. Two patients have been excluded because of inadequate duration of therapy and death shortly after entry to the trial.

RESULTS

Shortly before closing the trial an analysis of the blood results of 34 patients was carried out by the clinical research department of ICI. No significant differences were detected on comparison of the biochemical parameters at 0, 1, 3, 6 and 12 months but WBC levels became significantly higher after stilboestrol therapy. Details of the actual drugs prescribed were sent to the research department for this analysis but the trial codes were not officially broken until 1 year after entry to the trial closed.

Those patients classified as having clear-cut objective remissions, those with remissions lasting less than 6 months (temporary response) and those accepted as having failed to progress as a result of the drug treatment (static response) have been added together. In the 56 patients available for analysis, comparison of the two drugs given either as the first treatment or the second treatment, shows no significant difference in the rate of response, as defined above (Table 2). For tamoxifen the response rate is similar whether administered first or second.

Median duration of remission in those deemed to have responded to tamoxifen was greater whether the drug was given as first or second treatment but the difference does not reach significance. It is noticeable, however, that of the 9 patients deemed to have had a clear-cut objective remission, 6 had this to tamoxifen therapy and 1 patient remains in remission (first drug).

Table 1. Reasons for withdrawal from the analysis of 16 og the
72 patients selected within the trial.

	Tamoxifen	Stilboestrol
Inadequate trial (< 7 days therapy)	2	0
No assessable disease or inadequate recording	2	2
No follow-up after entry	2	0
Intolerance	1	7
Total	7	9

Table 2. The response to 90 assessable treatments in 56 patients.
* denotes clear-cut objective remissions according to
BBG criteria. x denotes significant difference at 10%
level by Wilcoxon's rank Sum test.

Randomised Treatment	Number	Remissions	Median Duration (Week)	Range
Tamoxifen				
1st drug	29	9 ****	38	15 - 221 +
2nd drug	17	5 **	51	23 - 129
Total	46	14	44.5	15 - 221 +
Stilboestrol				
1st drug	27	6 ***	32.5	25 - 48
2nd drug	17	4	27.5	25 - 45
Total	44	10	27.5 x	25 - 48

Responses to both drugs were more frequent in those with widespread metastatic disease compared to those with only local or contralateral disease. The distribution of the disease types is not significantly different nor is the response rate when the two drugs are compared.

More than half the patients who were entered into the trial presented with inoperable stage III or stage IV disease (Table 3).

The distribution between the two drug treatments is similar and although there would appear to be a trend in favour of tamoxifen for inoperable disease, this difference is not significant. The disease-free interval defined according to the stratification requirements has not influenced the response to either drug nor is there a difference between the drug responses (Table 3).

The absence of side effects has not always

Table 3. The response to 90 assessable treatments according to
whether or not a previous mastectomy had been performed
and according to disease-free interval. * denotes
patients with inoperable primary disease controlled by
radiation therapy prior to entry to trial.

	Tamoxifen		Stilboestrol	
	No.	No. with remission	No.	No. with remission
Mastectomy	20	5	22	5
No mastectomy	26	9	22	5
F I < 1 year	30	8	21	7
F I 1 -5 years	12***	5	14**	2
F I > 5 years	4	1	5	1
Total	46	14	44	10

been recorded but assuming that no comment means no serious toxicity, then a breakdown of the information available on all 72 patients (that is including those deemed non-assessable) shows a significant increase in toxicity in the patients given stilboestrol (Table 4).

In almost half of them this led to discontinuation of the drug, despite the fact that its nature was not known at the time. Toxicity from tamoxifen was at no time severe.

In 28 of the patients included in the trial, tumour was available for oestrogen receptor protein estimation and done by the method previously described by Hawkins et al. (5). In most the tissue was obtained at the time of diagnostic biopsy of an inoperable primary lesion. The association of positive receptors and response to drug treatment is confirmed in this small group of patients but no difference has been found when the two drugs are compared (Table 5).

Of the 23 patients in whom oestrogen receptors were detected, only 13 received both drugs. Of the 10 of them who have had both drugs assessed, 1 patient had a double remission while 4 failed to respond to either drug.

The original aim of this trial was to give all patients both drugs in sequence. Inevitably in practice this was not possible and was achieved in only 39 out of the 72 patients. In 12 of these 39 patients one drug was not assessable (Table 6).

When the drug given was stilboestrol the reason for this was toxicity while with tamoxifen the reasons were similar to those detailed previously (Table 1) with the one addition of inadequate withdrawal.

Of the 27 patients in whom the effects of both drugs have been assessed, 16 or 59% responded to neither. However, as can be seen from Table 7, 3 patients responded to both drugs independently. All 3 patients had systemic disease and all 6 remissions

Table 4. Side-effects in 72 patients given either tamoxifen or stilboestrol. The paired numbers refer to those with side-effects following first and second treatments.

	Tamoxifen - 56	Stilboestrol - 55
Nausea	5 + 0 (5)	12 + 4* (16)
Jaundice	-	1
C.C.F.	-	1
Hypercalcaemia	3	4
No. who stopped drug	2	7 + 2 (9)
Death on drug	2 + 3 (5)	6 + 2 (8)

$\chi^2 = 4.3$, p < .05

Table 5. Drug response related to oestrogen receptor assay in 28 patients.

Eostrogen receptors	Tamoxifen assessments		Stilboestrol assessments	
	total	remissions	total	remissions
Positive 23	18	7	15	5
Negative 5	5	0	2	0

Table 6. Reasons for one drug being termed non-assessable in 12 patients in whom both drugs were given.

	Tamoxifen	Stilboestrol
Intolerance	1	7
Inadequate duration	2	0
Nil to assess	1	0
No withdrawal after response to first drug	1	0
	5	7

Table 7. Results of double-assessed treatments in 27 patients
expressed as duration of remissions in weeks according
to whether this occurred to first or second drug given.
* denotes clear-cut remissions (BBG criteria).

First drug given	First remission	Second remission
Tamoxifen	72 weeks	27 weeks
	16 weeks	25 weeks
	94 weeks*	none
	38 weeks*	none
	27 weeks	none
	none	28 weeks
Stilboestrol	39 weeks	23 weeks
	39 weeks*	none
	26 weeks*	none
	25 weeks	none
	none	51 weeks

were of the intermediate category. In 1 the
second remission lasted longer than the first.
Of the 8 patients who responded to one drug
only, the response was to the first drug
given in 6 but in 2 the response followed
previous failure.

When these results are combined with the
single assessments to give a total of 39
patients who were given both drugs within
the trial a patient remission of 44% is
obtained (17 of 39) with a treatment remission
of 26% (20 of 78). This compares reasonably
well with previous reports of the effect on
metastatic breast carcinoma of hormone therapy
in general.

DISCUSSION

The biggest disappointment in the conduct
of this trial was the rapid fall-off in rate
of entry. Although initially uncertain as
to the comparative values of the two drugs
studied, experience gained from the use of
tamoxifen in non-trial patients and its relative lack of side effects led to a preference
for it in the clinic.

The lessons learned from the first external
review were notable. The number of protocol
infringements initially detected were mostly
unexpected and stressed the importance of
good protocol design. They were considered
due largely to the number of doctors involved
in the conduct of the trial and their failure
to refer at regular intervals to the protocol.
In particular the importance of having
specially designed trial records and one
individual totally responsible for their
availability and continuous updating was
made apparent. This is especially important
in trials dealing with metastatic breast
cancer when many departments, and even several
hospitals, may be involved with the management
of the patients. All who were involved with
the external review benefitted from it, as
did the subsequent running of the trial. We
now believe that no trial should be reported
without at least some external review of the
records and response assessments. When
expected, this discipline can only lead to
greater attention to detail and greater
accuracy of recording by the trial staff,
and therefore in the long run, more reliable
conclusions.

Under the conditions of our study, no
significant difference in the duration or
rate of response between the two drugs has
been found. There is a suggestion however
that when response to tamoxifen occurs it is
not only more effective but also longer.
The fact that in two patients benefit was
recorded from the second drug following a
lack of response to the first, suggests that
the drugs do not necessarily act in the same
way. This supports the previous report by
Ward (6). The greater frequency of intolerance to stilboestrol was confirmed in this
trial and is considered a definite significant
disadvantage in its use in postmenopausal
women. Tamoxifen does have side effects
but these are less often troublesome and
often only mentioned by the patient in retro-
spect when the drug is stopped. From this
trial, under the circumstances of the present
analysis we conclude that as far as hormone
therapy for postmenopausal patients with
advanced or metastatic breast carcinoma is
concerned, tamoxifen should be the first
hormone drug of choice.

ACKNOWLEDGEMENT

Many clinicians from the Departments of
Clinical Surgery and Radiation Oncology in
Edinburgh have been involved with the running
of this trial as well as with the care and
assessment of patients included in it. We
acknowledge the part that all have played.

H. J. Stewart *et al.*

REFERENCES

1. M. P. Cole, C. T. A. Jones, and I. D. H. Todd, A new anti-oestrogen agent in late breast cancer. An early appraisal of ICI 46474. *Br. J. Cancer* 25, 270 (1971).
2. H. W. C. Ward, Anti-oestrogen therapy for breast cancer: a trial of tamoxifen at two dose levels. *Br. Med. J.* 1, 13 (1973).
3. M. M. Roberts, A. P. M. Forrest, T. Hamilton, A. O. Langlands, W. Lutz, Ida J. McFadyen, and Helen J. Stewart, Preliminary Report of a Controlled Trial in Advanced Breast Cancer comparing a Tamoxifen with Conventional Hormone Therapy. *Cancer Treatm. Rep.* 60, 1461 (1976).
4. British Breast Group. Assessment of response to treatment in advanced breast cancer. *Lancet* 2, 38 (1974).
5. R. A. Hawkins, R. Hill, and B. Freedman, A simple method of the determination of oestrogen receptor concentrations in breast tumours and other tissues. *Clin. Chim. Acta* 64, 203 (1975).
6. H. Ward, Clinical Experience with Anti-Hormone Therapy. Proceedings of a symposium on the Hormonal Control of Breast Cancer, September 1975. Imperial Chemical Industries Ltd., Pharmaceuticals Division, Alderley House, Alderley Park, Macclesfield, Cheshire.

Serum Concentrations of Tamoxifen and Major Metabolite during Long-term Nolvadex Therapy, Correlated with Clinical Response

J. S. Patterson*, R. S. Settatree**, H. K. Adam* and J. V. Kemp*

*I.C.I. Pharmaceuticals Division, Macclesfield, Cheshire, U.K.
**Birmingham & Midland Hospital for Women, Birmingham, U.K.

Correspondence to J. S. Patterson

Abstract—*Serum levels of tamoxifen and N-desmethyltamoxifen (DMN) were measured during a study of tamoxifen (Nolvadex)* and bromocriptine (Parlodel) in postmenopausal women with advanced breast cancer. Steady state serum levels of tamoxifen were achieved after 4 weeks therapy with 20mg twice daily indicating an elimination half life of approximately 7 days. The N-desmethyl-tamoxifen reached maximal serum levels after 8 weeks suggesting an elimination half life of 14 days. Concomitant bromocriptine therapy caused a significant elevation of serum tamoxifen. There was no correlation between steady state serum drug levels and response in this small study, nor was response correlated to the serum oestradiol level.*

INTRODUCTION

The antioestrogen tamoxifen has gained wide acceptance in the treatment of advanced breast cancer (1). Previous pharmacokinetic and metabolic studies were limited to the use of radio labelled drug (2) due to the lack of a suitable assay technique. Adam et al. (3) has now described a reliable assay for serum tamoxifen and has also determined that the major human serum metabolite is N-desmethyltamoxifen (DMN) (4).

Tamoxifen is thought to act by competing with endogenous oestrogens for a high affinity cytoplasmic binding protein (5). It is said to bind with considerably less affinity than 17-β-Oestradiol (6) and therefore an excess of circulating drug is required to inhibit hormone sensitive cells. The advent of a method for the measurement of circulating drug allows us the opportunity to compare steady state serum levels with response to therapy and with endogenous oestrogen concentrations. Furthermore, information on the pharmacokinetics and metabolism of tamoxifen may facilitate the design and interpretation of future clinical studies as, unlike cyto-toxic chemotherapy, monitoring of circulating drug levels has not previously been possible with endocrine therapy.

MATERIALS AND METHODS

64 post menopausal women with advanced, measurable breast cancer were entered into a study in which they received either tamoxifen 20 mg bd or tamoxifen 20 mg bd plus bromo-criptine 2.5 mg tds. 39 patients, of whom 22 received tamoxifen alone, were assessable both for response - according to the U.I.C.C. criteria (7) - and for steady state tamoxifen and metabolite levels. Responses were confirmed by an external independant clinical assessor.

Blood samples were taken by vene puncture prior to therapy and at 2, 6, 12, 19 and 26 weeks on therapy. Patients were all seen, bled and assessed by one worker (RS) at a special clinic where the exact timing of each sample was recorded. Samples were allowed to clot, spun, separated and the serum stored frozen. Analysis, in batches, was by the following methods:

Serum tamoxifen by the thin-layer densito-metry procedure of Adam et al (3).

Serum oestrogens by the method of Kandeel (8).

Serum cortisol by the method of Morris (9).

Tamoxifen was administered as Nolvadex tablets containing the citrate salt, equiva-lent to 10 mg tamoxifen base per tablet.

Bromocriptine 2.5mg tablets were a gift of the Sandoz company who supported, in part, the clinical aspects of this study.

Approximate elimination half lives were calculated by the methods of Ballard and Menczel (10) and van Rossum (11). The statis-tical significance of our results was tested using "student's" two tailed t-test. Results are given as Mean (± S.E.M.).

RESULTS

We assessed the effect of bromocriptine

---

*Nolvadex is a registered trade mark property of ICI Ltd.

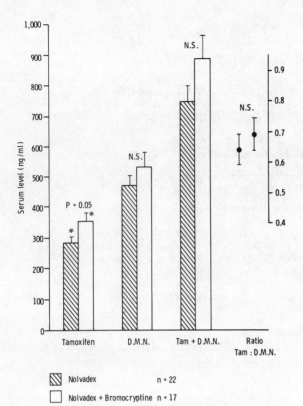

Fig. 1. Effect of Bromocriptine on steady
state serum levels of tamoxifen,
DMN, tamoxifen + DMN and the ratio
tamoxifen: DMN.

tamoxifen Alone

tamoxifen + Bromocriptine

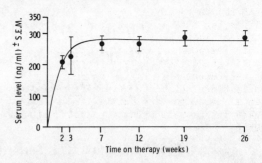

Fig. 2. Mean Serum levels of tamoxifen
(± SEM) in ng/ml versus time after
Commencement of Chronic therapy
with 20mg b.i.d.

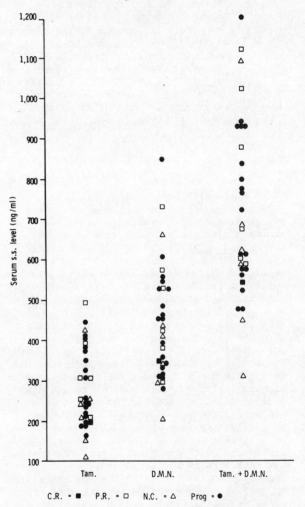

C.R. = ■   P.R. = □   N.C. = △   Prog = ●

Fig. 3. Clinical response in relation to
S.S. serum levels of tamoxifen
(ng/ml) DMN and DMN + tamoxifen.

■ – Complete Response

□ – Partial Response

△ – No Change

● – Progression

upon serum tamoxifen and DMN levels (Fig. 1).
Bromocriptine was associated with higher
mean serum steady state (S.S.) tamoxifen
levels viz 358 ± 31 ng/ml versus 285 ± 19
ng/ml (P = 0.05), with a similar but non
significant trend for DMN. As a result of
this finding, all pharmacokinetic evaluation
is based upon results generated from the
22 women who received tamoxifen alone.

Patients receiving tamoxifen 20 mg twice
daily achieved steady state levels of 285 ±
19 ng/ml tamoxifen (range 153–494). These
levels were achieved after 4 weeks on therapy
(Fig. 2) and from this graph, it can be
seen that the women achieved 74% and 80% of
the steady state levels after 2 and 3 weeks
respectively. In contrast, DMN reached steady
state levels of 477 ± 35 ng/ml (range 189–802)
after 8 weeks on therapy. Patients had
achieved only 43% of the steady state level
at 2 weeks, 69% at 3 weeks and 92% after
7 weeks. These results yield approximate
biological half lives

$$\left(\frac{\text{Time to (9)\% S.S.}}{3.3} \right)$$

of 7 and 14 days for tamoxifen and DMN
respectively.

There was no correlation between the steady
state concentrations of tamoxifen or DMN
or the sum or ratio of these values and the
clinical response (complete plus partial

response) to tamoxifen therapy (Fig. 3).
This is not a function of serum oestrogen
levels as Table 1 shows all levels to be
within the post menopausal range and no
significant difference between responders and
non responders. Tamoxifen did not significantly alter the circulating oestradiol level
over 12 weeks therapy but Table 2 shows a
marked increase in serum cortisol during
therapy.

over the 100 fold excess required for compe-
titive binding. As this study gives data
upon neither the protein binding in serum
nor the tissue concentrations achieved,
conclusions concerning the significance of
this high anti oestrogen: oestrogen ratio
must be drawn cautiously.

The long elimination half life of tamoxifen
and DMN in this chronic study confirms the
findings of Wilkinson (14) and Fabian (15)

Table 1. Serum oestradiol levels (pg/ml).

	Responders (mean ± S.E.M.)	Non responders (mean ± S.E.M.)	Sig.
Pre treatment	24.36 ± 2.54	23.85 ± 2.3	N.S.
12 weeks	24.35 ± 2.42	24.46 ± 2.4	N.S.
Sig.	N.S.	N.S.	

Table 2. Serum cortisol levels (ng/ml).

	Responders (mean ± S.E.M.)	Non responders (mean ± S.E.M.)	Sig.
Pre treatment 0	194 ± 22	173 ± 24	N.S.
2	290 ± 27	217 ± 39	N.S.
6	324 ± 32	310 ± 20	N.S.
12	313 ± 23	298 ± 13	N.S.
12 week mean increase	119	125	

DISCUSSION

This study has established the chronic
pharmacokinetic behaviour of tamoxifen and
its major serum metabolite during long term
therapy in advanced breast cancer. The
finding that serum steady state levels do
not correlate with the clinical response is
interesting. However, subtle variations due
to differences in serum concentrations may
be submerged by other prognostic variables,
such as oestrogen receptor status, in this
limited study. We have shown that one such
variable, the endogenous oestrogen level, is
not responsible for this negative finding.
Furthermore, Willis has reported that oestrogen levels rise in non responders to
tamoxifen therapy (12). Our study has failed
to confirm this observation.

Our finding of a significant rise in circulating cortisol levels, during tamoxifen
therapy, in both responders and non responders
may be due, in part, to a rise in cortisol
binding globulin as described by Sakai (13).
The relevance of this finding is unclear. It
is possible that such a change may effect
the protein binding of tamoxifen and therefore
the ability of the drug to diffuse out of the
circulation.

In vitro tamoxifen binds to the oestrogen
receptor with an affinity that is between
1% and 10% of that of oestrodiol dependent
upon the conditions used. Total serum anti
oestrogen levels were considerably in excess
of the total circulating oestrogen with well

in acute and sub acute studies. This prolonged elimination phase leads to two pharmacokinetic conclusions. Firstly, the final
steady state should be (and is) achieved
relatively slowly. Secondly, the consequent
high serum levels magnify numerically, the
inter subject variation that always occurs
due to the normal biological and genetic
differences between patients. The presence
of such a wide inter subject spread in serum
steady state levels of tamoxifen and DMN
should facilitate the search for a correlation
between serum concentrations and clinical
response.

Several corollaries emerge from this study.
In pharmacokinetic terms, the serum levels
achieved by dosing at 20mg twice daily are
almost identical to those projected for
once daily dosing with the same quantity of
drug (40 mg daily). However, in the absence
of a clear "therapeutic concentration" any
change of the dosage regimen must await a
clinical comparison of once versus twice
daily dosing.

It is tempting to associate the slow
build up of tamoxifen in serum with the
delayed onset of response that is seen with
tamoxifen compared to that of cytotoxic
therapy. This may just be due to the more
slowly growing tumours being those which
respond to endocrine therapy. This concept
may now be tested as, in kinetic terms, it
is possible to use loading doses as suggested
by Fabian (15) to attain the final steady
state value more rapidly. However, Ward (16)

has suggested that the higher doses of tamoxifen are less well tolerated by the patient. The place of a loading and/or once daily dosage scheme must be examined clinically as the theoretical advantages may be outweighed by its decreased acceptability.

Significant levels of DMN are achieved on chronic administration of tamoxifen. This metabolite has an almost identical pharmacological profile in laboratory studies to that of the parent compound (17). It follows, therefore, that its clinical effect is likely to be additive to that of the parent compound. Thus, even greater total "anti oestrogen" levels are achieved than was previously considered. The significance of this finding requires resolution but the fact that the major serum metabolite is an anti oestrogen of considerable activity and a prolonged elimination phase suggests that measurement of tumour oestrogen receptor protein should be delayed for at least 4 half lives of DMN (8 weeks) after cessation of chronic tamoxifen therapy if a true result is to be seen. If tissue retention is prolonged beyond the serum elimination, an even greater wash out period must be envisaged.

ACKNOWLEDGEMENTS

We are grateful to Professor W R Butt and his staff for their assistance and for undertaking the oestrogen and cortisol assays.

REFERENCES

1. H. Mouridsen, T. Palshof, J. Patterson and L. Battersby, Tamoxifen in advanced breast cancer. *Cancer Treat. Reviews* 5, 131 (1978).

2. J. M. Fromson, S. Pearson and S. Bramah, The metabolism of tamoxifen (ICI 46,474) Part II: In Female Patients *Xenobiotica* 3, 711 (1973).

3. H. K. Adam, M. A. Gay and R. H. Moore, Quantification of tamoxifen and metabolites in biological samples by thin layer densitometry. *J. Endocr.* (in press).

4. H. K. Adam, E. J. Douglas and J. V. Kemp, The metabolism of tamoxifen in humans. *Biochem Pharmacol* 27, 145 (1979).

5. V. C. Jordan and L. J. Dowse, Tamoxifen as an anti-tumour agent: effect on oestrogen binding. *J. Endocr.* 68, 297 (1976).

6. R. I. Nicholson, C. P. Daniel, P. Davies and K. Griffiths, (^{3}H) Tamoxifen binding studies in dimethylbenzanthracene-induced mammary carcinomata. *J. Endocr.* 75, 26P (1977).

7. J. L. Hayward, P. P. Carbone, J. C. Heuson, S. Kumaoka, A. Segaloff and R. D. Rubens, Assessment of response to therapy in advanced breast cancer. *Europ. J. Cancer* 13, 89 (1977).

8. F. R. Kandeel, W. R. Butt, D. R. London, S. S. Lynch, R. Logan Edwards, B. T. Rudd. Oestrogen amplification of LH-RH response in the polycystic ovary syndrome and response to clomiphene. *Clin. Endocrinol.* 9, 429 (1978).

9. R. Morris, A simple and economical method for the radioimmunoassay of cortisol in serum. *Ann. Clin. Biochem.* 15, 178 (1978).

10. B. E. Ballard and E. Menczel, Multiple-dosing drug kinetics. *J. Pharm. Sci.* 60, 406 (1971).

11. J. M. van Rossum, Pharmacokinetics of accumulation. *J. Pharm. Sci.* 57, 2162 (1968).

12. K. J. Willis, D. R. London, H. W. C. Ward, W. R. Butt, S. S. Lynch and B. T. Rudd, Recurrent breast cancer treated with the anti oestrogen tamoxifen: correlation between hormonal changes and clinical course. *Brit. Med. J.* i Feb. 12th, 425 (1977).

13. F. Sakai, F. Cheix, M. Clavel, J. Colon, M. Mager, E. Pommateau and S. Saez. Increases in steroid binding globulins induced by tamoxifen in patients with carcinoma of the breast. *J. Endocr.* 76, p. 219 (1978).

14. P. Wilkinson, G. Ribeiro, H. K. Adam, J. Kemp and J. S. Patterson, Tamoxifen citrate pharmacokinetics in patients with metastatic breast cancer. XV Annual Meeting of the American Society of Clinical Oncology 20, p. 309, Abstr. C-71 (1979).

15. C. Fabian and L. Sternson, Tamoxifen (TAM) Blood levels following initial and chronic dosing in patients with breast cancer: correlation with clinical data. XV Annual Meeting of the American Society of Clinical Oncology 20, p. 326, Abstr. C-145 (1979).

16. H. W. C. Ward, Clinical experience with anti-hormone therapy. Proceedings of a Symposium of 'The Hormonal Control of Breast Cancer,' Alderley Park September 1975, p. 53, ICI Ltd., Pharmaceuticals Division, Alderley Park, Macclesfield, Cheshire (1976).

17. S. R. Slater and A. E. Wakeline (personal communication).

Hormone Therapy in Advanced Breast Cancer: High Dose Medroxyprogesterone Acetate (MAP) vs Tamoxifen (TMX). Preliminary Results

F. Pannuti, A. Martoni, F. Fruet, E. Strocchi and A. R. Di Marco

Oncology Division, M. Malpighi Hospital, Bologna, Italy

Correspondence to F. Pannuti

Abstract—*Preliminary results of a prospective, randomized clinical trial comparing high dose Medroxyprogesterone Acetate (MAP) orally (2000 mg/day) versus Tamoxifen (TMX) (20 mg/day) in advanced breast cancer are reported. The study is still in progress. Up to this time 9/21 (43%) patients with MAP and 5/20 (25%) patients with TMX presented partial objective remission for a median duration of 5+ months and 13+ months respectively.*

The differences are not statistically significant. The only statistically significant difference between the two treatments concerns pain remission (83%) with MAP, 22% with TMX).

A further widening of the study is necessary before drawing any conclusion.

INTRODUCTION

In 1973 we proposed the use of high doses of Medroxyprogesterone Acetate (MAP) in oncology (1). A MAP dose of 1500 mg/day/ i.m. for 30 days induced objective remissions (RC+RP) in 43% (19/44) of patients suffering from advanced breast carcinoma (2).

Apart from objective remission, this treatment induced a significant analgic effect (92%, 37/40) and a considerable improvement in performance status (average from 49.31 to 65.00, S.E. 2.084, P < 0.001, in 29 patients one month from the beginning of treatment) on which we reported elsewhere (3). A successive randomized and perspective controlled study comparing the 30 days MAP regimen of 1500 mg/day/i.m. with a 30 days MAP regimen of 500 mg/day/i.m., confirmed previous results and proved that, with the same objective remission rate (CR+PR) and median remission duration, patients suffering from advanced breast carcinoma treated with the higher dosage regimen showed a better survival rate (4). Other authors employing high i.m. doses of MAP (> 500 mg/day) and using the same assessment criteria used by us, obtained an objective remission in more than 40% of cases, thus confirming our results (5,6).

We moreover proved the following:
1) in treating metastatic breast cancer, it is possible to use even higher i.m. doses of MAP (2000 mg/day for 30 days) without increasing toxic effects (7);
2) these high doses (2000 mg/day for 30 days) can also be administered orally obtaining a significant anabolizing effect in a group of patients suffering from various types of solid tumors, and an antalgic effect as well as a reduction in local toxic effects in a lower percentage of cases with the same

systemic effects as before (8).

Another hormone agent which proved active in treating advanced breast carcinoma (32% of objective remission on average (9)) is the Tamoxifen antiestrogen (TMX), which has been clinically employed for some time.

The purpose of this study is the following:
1) to verify whether MAP, administered orally in high doses, is active in treating advanced breast carcinoma;
2) to verify this activity in randomized and perspective comparison with TMX and in historical comparison with MAP i.m. administered in the same doses;
3) to compare tolerance of the above treatments;
4) to verify further effectiveness of the two drugs after cross-over.

MATERIAL AND METHODS

At the present time 23 patients have been randomized in order to receive MAP 2000 mg/day/orally for 30 days and later on, continuously for 15 days a month (primary treatment: MAP/1); 27 patients have been randomized in order to receive TMX 10 mg b.i.d. (primary treatment: TMX/1).

These treatments were carried out up to progression/relapse of the disease or drug intolerance; in these cases patients treated with MAP/1 passed to TMX/2 and those treated with TMX/1 passed to MAP/2 (secondary treatment was carried out as stated above).

Clinical analysis of the 41 female patients, who can be assessed at present in terms of objective response (follow-up longer than 3 months), is shown in Table 1.

Patients eligible for this study had to have the following characteristics: a histological diagnosis of advanced breast carcinoma;

F. Pannuti *et al.*

Table 1. Clinical characteristics (41 pts.).

	MAP/1	TMX/1
Patients Randomized	23	27
Patients Evaluable	21	20
Time from Menopause (years)		
1 - 5	5	4
> 5	12	12
Castrated *	4	4
Age (years)		
< 50	5	5
50 - 60	7	7
61 - 70	7	7
> 70	2	1
Free Interval (years)		
0 - 2	6	7
> 2	15	13
Previous Systemic Treatment *		
None	20§	19
Chemotherapy	1	1
Performance Status (%)		
30 - 50	5	5
60 - 70	9	5
80 - 100	7	10
Dominant Metastatic Sites		
ST	7	4
O	11	10
V	3	6
§§ C.I. $= \dfrac{V}{ST + O}$	0.18	0.43

Legenda: * = Prophylactic castration
          ** = Previous systemic treatment for advanced disease
          § = 2 patients had received adjuvant polychemotherapy
     §§ C.I. = Comparative index (4)

a state of physiological menopause for at least 1 year or to have undergone castration; tumoral lesions which could be measured or assessed in progress; no prior treatment with the drugs tested in this study; no andineoplastic treatment for at least one month; "quoad vitam" prognosis longer than 2 months; performance status $\geq$ 30%; normal heart, renal and hepatic functions. Patients with hepatic or CNS metastases were excluded.

The following elements were considered for randomization: dominant metastatic site (soft tissues—ST—, osseous metastases—O— and viscera—V—), age, free interval and systemic treatments previously carried out for disseminated disease.

The assessment of the response was carried out after a month of treatment and, if there is not progression, it was repeated in the occasion of following clinical control. Clinical control was carried out at 1-2 month

intervals and radiological examinations every 3-6 months. Patients who had followed at least 20 days of therapy and had passed on to another treatment, owing to a rapid progression of the disease, were also considered for assessment. Assessment of objective response was made according to the following criteria: complete remission (CR) was defined as the disappearance of all signs of the disease for at lease 6 months; partial remission (PR) was defined as > 50% decrease in the surface of all measurable lesions and/or a considerable improvement in lesions which could be assessed but not measured, for at least one month, or, in the case of bone lesions, a stationary condition for more than 3 months with remission of pain and, at the same time, remission of the tumor in other sites; minimal remission was defined as $\geq$ 25%-< 50% decrease in the surface of measurable lesions; no change (NC) was defined as the stationary condition of lesions or < 25% decrease in measurable lesions; progression (P) was defined as a surface increase of even one lesion > 25%, or the appearance of a new lesion; relapse was defined as > 25% expansion of the surface of a lesion or the appearance of a new lesion after a period of remission or a stationary condition.

Subjective response was assessed by recording changes in performance status and a considerable reduction or disappearance of the following signal-symptoms : pain, dyspnoea, asthenia, anorexia, walking impairment.

Before and after a month of treatment patients received hematologic tests (wbcs, rbcs, hemoglobin, platelets, total protein, SGOT, bilirubin, total cholesterol, alkaline phosphatase, glucose, BUN, creatinine, uric acid, Na, K, Ca, P); radiological data were reassessed by extramural radiologists. The statistical analysis was carried out using X^2 test and Student's "t" tests.

RESULTS

9/21 (43%) of patients treated with MAP/1 and 5/20 (25%) of patients treated with TMX/1 presented objective remission (RC+RP) (Table 2).

Table 2. Primary Treatment: Objective response.

	MAP/1 *	TMX/1 *
CR	-	1 (5%)
PR	9 (43%)	4 (20%)
MR	1	1
NC	4	3
P	7	11
Total	21	20

* No significant difference between the two treatments (χ^2)

Median remission duration is 5+ months (range 4+-10+) for MAP/1 and 13+ months (range 7+-10+) for TMX/1. The analysis of results on the basis of the dominant metastatic site shows that, among patients classified ST, remission occurred in 3/7 for MAP/1 and 1/4 for TMX/1; among patients classified 0 objective remission occurred in 6/11 and 4/10 respectively, while none of patients classified V had objective remission.

Table 3. Primary treatment: Subjective remission.

	MAP/1	TMX/1
Pain	10/12 (83%)*	2/9 (22%)*
Dyspnoea	2/7 (29%)°	3/5 (60%)°
Asthenia	5/8 (63%)°	2/9 (22%)°
Anorexia	4/4 (100%)°	3/5 (60%)°
Walking impairment	6/9 (67%)°	0/4 -
Performance status	8/21 (38%)°	4/20 (20%)°

*P < 0.01
°no significant difference (χ^2)

Table 4. Secondary treatment: Objective response.

	TMX/2	MAP/2
CR	-	-
PR	2 (22%)	4 (29%)*
MR	-	1
NC	2	4
P	5	5
Total	9	14

*One patient had received inadequate primary treatment (TMX).

Table 3 shows the analysis of subjective remission after a month treatment. The pain remission rate is significantly higher after MAP ($P < 0.01$). The other parameters considered also show that response to MAP/1 is more favourable with the exception of dyspnoea. After a month of treatment patients that were given MAP/1 showed a significant weight increase (from 63.68 to 65.12 Kg, S.E. 3.125, $P < 0.01$, average increase of 2.19 Kg), while patients treated with TMX/1 did not show significant changes (from 69.17 to 68.32 Kg, S.E. 3.532, average decrease of 0.85 Kg).

At present 5 patients are still on MAP/1 and 7 patients are on TMX/1. After progression 7 patients have not started the secondary treatment; 31 patients have undergone a secondary treatment. Up to now, 9/13 patients treated with TMX/2 and 14/18 treated with MAP/2 can be assessed for the purpose of objective response. Secondary treatment induced objective remission in 2/9 (22%) of patients treated with TMX/2 and in 4/14 (29%) of patients treated with MAP/2 (Table 4).

Remission duration was 5 and 6 months for TMX/2 and 5, 5, 5+, 6+ months for MAP/2. The two patients responsive to TMX/2 had presented PR and P respectively after MAP and the four patients responsive to MAP/2 had presented MR (1 patient) and P (2 patients) to TMX, while the 4th was not assessable as regards TMX since she underwent an insufficient period of treatment (15 days) deriving from protocol violation (when MAP/2 treatment was started, patient was undoubtedly in progression).

It should be pointed out that 3 patients presented PR in cutaneous lesions while the disease progressed in the bones: these patients were given TMX/1, TMX/2 and MAP/2 respectively.

Median survival calculated from the beginning of primary treatment is 11+ months (range 2-18+) for MAP/1 and 11+ months (range 2-19+) for TMX/1.

At a toxicologic level, the statistical comparison of blood tests carried out before and after one month of primary treatment showed that MAP/1 causes a significant increase in leucocyes ($P < 0.02$) and a decrease in glucose ($P < 0.01$), while no significant change was induced by TMX/1 (Table 5).

Table 6 reports the overall side-effects noted during primary and secondary treatment. Secondary side-effects to MAP never prevented the treatment from being carried out. One patient suffered from bleedings after the first month of treatment. A cavity revision revealed the presence of simple endometrium hyperplasia: in this case maintenance therapy was not carried out. As for other cases vaginal spotting was very limited and temporary. TMX/2 treatment was suspended after 8 days in one case, owing to persistent vomiting and severe vulvar itching. Hypercalcemia appeared in 2 patients with bone metastases after 6 and 17 days respectively: after temporary withdrawal of treatment when calcium levels had returned to normal, TMX was resumed without the reappearance of hypercalcemia. 2 cases on TMX/1 showed moderate leucopenia (WBC 3.800/mmc after 125 days and 3.400/mmc after 17 days) which disappeared after discontinuation of treatment and treatment was resumed in one case after 15 days (in the other case progression of the

Table 5. Toxicology - Blood data.

	MAP/1			TMX/1		
	$\bar{X}$ Before	$\bar{X}$ After	P*	$\bar{X}$ Before	$\bar{X}$ After	P*
WBC	5.96	7.41	< 0.02	6.14	5.97	ns
RBC	4.19	4.24	ns	4.38	4.28	ns
Hemoglobin	12.30	12.50	ns	13.18	12.62	ns
Platelets	240.54	264.36	ns	185.18	207.82	ns
Alkaline Phos.	66.83	63.78	ns	61.53	78.47	ns
SGOT	14.41	11.0	ns	13.28	13.78	ns
Bilirubin	0.50	0.53	ns	0.51	0.52	ns
BUN	19.45	20.2	ns	21.0	20.3	ns
Creatinine	0.83	0.80	ns	1.01	0.97	ns
Uric acid	4.35	4.48	ns	6.29	5.22	ns
Glucose	91.85	80.65	< 0.01	94.0	92.5	ns
Cholesterol	204.47	205.06	ns	215.64	204.5	ns
Total protein	6.89	6.92	ns	6.75	6.93	ns
Ca	9.61	9.35	ns	10.34	9.89	ns
P	3.64	3.65	ns	3.78	3.66	ns

*Student's "t" test.

Table 6. Toxicology: Side-effects. (Primary + secondary
treatment).

MAP (41 PTS)*			TMX (40 PTS)**	
Sweating	9 (22%)	Nausea	7	(17.5%)
Cramps	8 (20%)	Vomiting	3	(7.5%)
Vaginal spotting	8 (20%)	Hot flushes	3	(7.5%)
Fine tremors	7 (17%)	Hypercalcaemia	2	(5%)
Constipation	3 (7%)	Leukopenia	2	(5%)
Headache	2 (5%)	Diarrhoea	2	(5%)
Vulvar itching	1 (2%)	Ichthyosis	2	(5%)
Insomnia	1 (2%)	Anorexia	2	(5%)
Thrombophlebitis	1 (2%)	Sweating	2	(5%)
		Pain	2	(5%)
		Thrombocytopenia	1	(2.5%)
		Urinary incontinence	1	(2.5%)
		Headache	1	(2.5%)
		Thrombophlebitis	1	(2.5%)

*MAP/1:23 pts + MAP/2:18 pts = 41 pts
**TMX/1:27 pts + TMX/2:13 pts = 40 pts

disease occurred). Finally as regards one
patient on TMX/1, several brief interruptions
occurred due to severe perspiration, hot
flushes and nausea.

DISCUSSION

This study is still under way and results
reported here are preliminary and do not make
it possible to draw final conclusions.

It should be noted that the caution with
which the results should be interpreted is
further confirmed by the fact that the number
of patients with visceral lesions is slightly
higher for TMX and as a result the two groups
of patients are not perfectly balanced.

At present high doses of MAP administered
orally seem able to induce an objective
remission rate similar to those obtained
when MAP was administered by way of i.m.
(2,4,7): this rate is higher than that
obtained with TMX; however a statistical
comparison does not show any significant
difference. Our objective results obtained
with Tamoxifen are consistent with results
reported by other authors (9). Up to now
objective remission duration obtained with
TMX is higher than that obtained with MAP.
Previously, high doses of MAP at i.m. for
only one month induced remissions lasting
an average of 7 months (2). Should a wider
study confirm a decrease in remission duration, a possible explanation could be that
the MAP maintenance therapy employed here
is not the optimum therapy and research
should be made into other forms of treatment.

However kinetic studies on the drug, which
are under way in our department, may be useful in order to solve this problem.

On a subjective level, it should be noted
that MAP proved to be more effective.

The results of secondary treatment are
also of some importance, even though very few
patients can be assessed at present. On the
basis of these initial data it is possible
for us to present the combination of the two
drugs as a feasible and useful hypothesis,
and our studies also have this end in view.

ACKNOWLEDGEMENTS

We are grateful to Dott. Nino Monetti and
Dott. Vittorio Morselli for having assessed
the radiological data.

REFERENCES

1. F. Pannuti, A. Martoni, E. Pollutri,
   P. Camera, F. Losinno and H. Giusti,
   Massive doses progestational therapy in
   oncology (medroxyprogesterone). Preliminary results. *Panminerva Med.* 18, 129
   (1976).
2. F. Pannuti, A. Martoni, G. R. Lenaz,
   E. Piana, and P. Nanni, A possible new
   approach to the treatment of metastatic
   breast cancer: massive doses of medroxyprogesterone acetate (MAP). *Cancer Treat.
   Rep.* 62, 499 (1978).
3. F. Pannuti, A. Martoni, A. P. Rossi, and
   E. Piana, The role of endocrine therapy
   for relief of pain due to advanced cancer,
   in *Advances in Pain Research and Therapy,*
   Vol. 2; International Symposium on Pain of
   Advanced Cancer. (Edited by J. J. Bonica
   and V. Ventafridda) p. 145, Raven Press,
   New York (1979).

4. F. Pannuti, A. Martoni, A. R. Di Marco,
   E. Piana, F. Saccani, G. Becchi,
   G. Mattioli, F. Barbanti, G. A. Marra,
   W. Persiani, L. Cacciari, F. Spagnolo,
   D. Palenzona and G. Rocchetta, Prospective,
   randomized clinical trial of two different
   high dosages of medroxyprogesterone acetate
   (MAP) in the treatment of metastatic
   breast cancer. *Europ. J. Cancer* 15, 593
   (1979).

5. D. Amadori, A. Ravaioli and F. Barbanti,
   L'impiego del medrossiprogesterone acetato
   ad alti dosaggi nella terapia palliativa
   del carcinoma mammario in fase avanzata.
   Minerva Med. 67, 1 (1976).

6. G. Robustelli Della Cuna, A. Calciati,
   M. R. Bernardo Strada, C. Bumma and
   L. Campio, High dose of medroxyprogesterone
   acetate (MPA) treatment in metastatic
   carcinoma of the breast: a dose-response
   evaluation. *Tumori* 64, 143 (1978).

7. F. Pannuti, A. Martoni, G. R. Lenaz,
   E. Piana and P. Nanni, Management of
   advanced breast cancer with medroxy-
   progesterone acetate (MAP, F.I. 7401,
   NSC - 26-386) in high doses. In *Functional
   Explorations in Senology*. (Edited by
   C. Colin, P. Franchimont and W. Gordenne)
   p. 253, European Press, Ghent (1976).

8. F. Pannuti, F. Fruet, E. Piana, E. Strocchi
   and A. Cricca, The anabolic effect induced
   by high doses of medroxyprogesterone
   acetate (MAP) orally in cancer patients.
   IRCS Med. Sci. 6, 118 (1978).

9. H. Mouridsen, T. Palshof, J. Patterson
   and L. Batterby, Tamoxifen in advanced
   breast cancer. *Cancer Treat. Rev.* 5, 131
   (1978).

Aminoglutethimide in the Management of Advanced Breast Cancer

I. E. Smith*, R. C. Coombes***, H. T. Ford*, J-C. Gazet*,
C. Harmer**, M. Jones**, J. A. McKinna** and T. J. Powles*

*The Royal Marsden Hospital, London and Surrey
**The Combined Breast Clinic, St. Georges' Hospital, London
***The Institute of Cancer Research, London and Surrey

Correspondence to I. E. Smith, The Royal Marsden Hospital, London and Surrey, U.K.

Abstract—One hundred and five patients with advanced breast cancer were
treated with aminoglutethimide, a drug which inhibits the synthesis of adrenal
steroids, and the conversion of androgens to oestrogens in peripheral tissues.
Eighty-eight patients are so far assessable for response: 24 (27%) achieved an
objective response. A further 19 patients achieved significant bone pain
relief but without objective evidence of response. Responses were most
commonly seen in soft tissue and bone metastases, but were rarely seen in
patients with metastases in lung or liver. The median duration of response
has not yet been reached, but the predicted median is in excess of one year.
Survival in responding patients was significantly longer than in non-responders,
and the median duration of survival has not yet been reached in responding
patients. Side effects were mild and transient in the majority of patients;
the most important were an initial period of drowsiness and sleepiness in
47% of patients, and a transient self-limiting rash in 20%. Aminoglutethimide
appears to be a useful agent in the endocrine management of advanced breast
cancer, and particularly in the control of painful bone metastases.

INTRODUCTION

Aminoglutethimide suppresses the synthesis
of all adrenal steroid hormones by inhibiting
the enzymic conversion of cholesterol to
pregnenolone (1). More recently, it has also
been shown to inhibit the conversion of
androgens to oestrogens in peripheral tissues
(2). The drug has therefore been used as an
alternative to surgical adrenalectomy in the
treatment of advanced breast cancer, with
similar response rates reported (3,4).

We have used aminoglutethimide in the treatment of 105 patients with advanced breast
cancer during the last 2 years. Eighty-eight
of these are so far assessable and we report
our findings here.

MATERIALS AND METHODS

Eighty-eight patients with clinical or
radiological evidence of metastases from
histologically proven breast cancer were
included in the study. All were postmenopausal or had previously undergone
oophorectomy. Forty-five had been treated
with previous assessable endocrine therapy,
and 22 of these had responded.

Aminoglutethimide was given orally in a
dose of 250 mg. 4 times a day, with cortisone
acetate orally 25 mg. 2 times daily and
fludrocortisone 0.1 mg on alternate days.
Overall objective response to therapy was
defined according to the UICC criteria for
advanced breast cancer (5).

Response for each involved site of disease
was also involved independently.

RESULTS

Eighty-eight patients are so far assessable
for response to therapy and of these 24 (27%)
achieved an objective response; 12 showed no
change on therapy for at least a three month
period, and the remaining 52 showed progressive disease on treatment. One of the most
striking features of this drug was bone pain
relief: 28 out of 68 patients with painful
bone metastases achieved marked relief for a
period of at least two months (41%), although
only 9 (13%) showed objective evidence of
re-sclerosis on X-ray.

Response by site is shown in Table 1:
responses were most commonly seen in soft
tissue and bone metastases; responses were
rare in lung, and only 1 out of 13 patients
with liver metastases achieved a partial
response.

Responses were more common in patients who
had achieved a response to previous endocrine
therapy (41%) than in those who had not
responded to previous endocrine therapy (17%).
Details of response after previous endocrine
therapy are shown in Table 2.

The median duration of response has not
yet been reached. One patient has so far
relapsed after three months and two after
six months, but several remain in remission

Table 1. Response by site to aminoglutethimide.

		Responders	
	Total	n	%
Soft tissue	26	8	31%
Nodes	12	4	33%
Bone	68	9 (28)*	13% (41%)*
Lung	21	2	10%
Pleura	15	2	13%
Liver	13	1	8%

*Includes relief of bone pain

Table 2. Response to aminoglutethimide after previous endocrine therapy.

		Responders	
Previous endocrine therapy	Total	n	%
Responders	22	9 (7)*	41 (73)*
Non-responders	23	4 (7)	17 (30)
Not given or not assessable	43	11 (20)	26 (47)

*Includes relief of bone pain

at periods of 18 months or more, and the predicted median duration is in excess of one year. Survival in responding patients is significantly longer than that in non-responders (P less than 0.01) (Fig. 1).

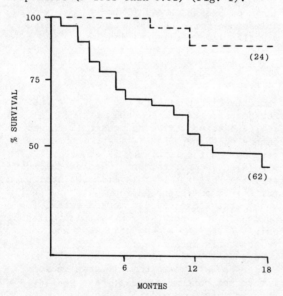

Fig. 1. Survival after aminoglutethimide: responders, 24 patients (- - -); non-responders, 62 patients (——).

Serious side effects were rare with aminoglutethimide. The most common problem was transient sleepiness and lethargy which occurred to some extent in 41 patients (47%). Usually this settled spontaneously within 2 or 3 weeks of starting treatment; in the minority of patients this was more severe,

and in 7 (8%) was associated with significant ataxia. These symptoms were dose related, and usually settled on a temporary dose reduction to 750 mg. daily. The symptoms were also age related, and were more common in the elderly, and were particularly severe in patients over 70. 18 patients (20%) developed an itchy erythematous maculo-papular rash over the trunk and limbs 8 to 10 days after the start of treatment. The severity of this varied considerably between different patients, but was occasionally associated with general malaise and pyrexia. In the first 3 patients, treatment was discontinued, but subsequently we discovered that in all patients the rash settled spontaneously within 4 days, and never returned. In the first 6 months of the study, 4 patients developed clinical features resembling adrenal insufficiency while on treatment, with malaise, prostration, hypotension, nausea and vomiting. All responded rapidly to parenteral hydrocortisone. Subsequently all patients were given fludrocortisone 0.1 mg on alternate days in addition to cortisone acetate supplements, and since then we have not seen this problem. Twelve patients had transient initial nausea, but in only 2 of these was this a serious problem.

DISCUSSION

These results confirm our preliminary experience (5) and that of others, that aminoglutethimide is an effective agent in the management of advanced breast cancer. The response rate of 27% in 88 patients has fallen compared with the response rate of 37.5% in the initial 42 patients on whom we

reported; this does not surprise us, since
patients entering the study latterly were
largely unselected, whereas those entering
initially tended to have shown evidence of
previous endocrine response. This response
rate, in association with a response rate of
38% in 50 patients reported by Santen's group
(4) suggests that aminoglutethimide is as
effective as surgical adrenalectomy in
achieving responses in patients with metastatic breast cancer. It is not yet possible
for us to say whether the median duration of
response will be as good as that achieved by
surgical adrenalectomy, but we predict that
our median duration will be in excess of one
year, and Santen's group report a mean
duration of 18 months.

The agent seems particularly effective in
achieving rapid relief of bone pain, confirming previous experience with adrenalectomy
(6). We feel this is of particular importance in view of the relative ineffectiveness
of additive hormone therapy and chemotherapy
against bone metastases (7,8). It is important to note however that only the minority
of patients achieving significant bone pain
relief subsequently showed evidence of
re-sclerosis on X-ray. This raises the
question of how response in bone metastases
from breast cancer may be best assessed,
and we are at present looking into this
problem further.

As might be expected, responses were most
commonly seen in patients previously
responding to other forms of endocrine
therapy. Nevertheless the fact that
responses were also seen in 17% of patients
who had failed to respond to previous endocrine therapy suggests that aminoglutethimide
may still be worth trying in such patients.

Although aminoglutethimide is usually well
tolerated in the dosage described here,
problems can occasionally arise in the early
stages of treatment. The drowsiness and
lethargy experienced by many patients
initially is usually mild and disappears
within two to three weeks. Nevertheless
because of the association of this symptom
with both dosage and age, it is now our
practice to start older patients on a reduced
dose of 750 mg daily, and to instruct other
patients to make a similar dose reduction
themselves if their symptoms become severe.
All patients are warned of the risk of
developing a rash around a week after
starting treatment; although this is always
self-limiting, the associated itchiness and
general malaise occasionally require a
temporary hospital admission. In the last
15 months, no one has had to discontinue
therapy permanently because of this side
effect.

The ease of administration of aminoglutethimide, and its rapid reversibility if
ineffective, encourage us to believe that
this agent may have significant advantages
over surgical adrenalectomy in the treatment
of advanced breast cancer. A control trial
comparing the two types of therapy is currently
underway in the U.S.A., to answer this question more fully. Likewise, the relative
merits of aminoglutethimide and the anti-

oestrogen tamoxifen are not yet established,
and we are currently investigating this.

ACKNOWLEDGEMENTS

We wish to thank the nursing staff of the
Royal Marsden Hospital for their help and
care in the management of the patients described in this study. We also thank Miss
T. K. Berry for her skill and efficiency in
the preparation of the manuscript.

REFERENCES

1. R. Cash, A. J. Brough, M. N. P. Cohen and
   P. S. Satoh, Aminoglutethimide as an
   inhibitor of adrenal steroidgenesis
   mechanism of action and therapeutic trial.
   J. Clin. Endocr. 27, 1239 (1967).
2. R. J. Santen, J. D. Veldhuis, E. Samojlik,
   A. Lipton, H. Harvey and S. A. Wells.
   Mechanism of action of aminoglutethimide
   in breast cancer. *Lancet* 1, 44 (1979).
3. H. H. Newsome, P. W. Brown, J. J. Terz
   and W. Lawrence. Medical and surgical
   adrenalectomy in patients with advanced
   breast carcinoma. *Cancer* 39, 542 (1977).
4. S. A. Wells, R. J. Santen, A. Lipton,
   D. E. Haagensen, E. J. Ruby, H. Harvey
   and W. G. Dilley. Medical adrenalectomy
   with aminoglutethimide: Clinical studies
   in post-menopausal patients with metastatic breast carcinoma. *Ann. Surg.* 187,
   475 (1978).
5. I. E. Smith, B. M. Fitzharris, J. A.
   McKinna, D. R. Fahmy, A. G. Nash, A. M.
   Neville, J-C. Gazet, H. T. Ford and T. J.
   Powles. Aminoglutethimide in the treatment
   of metastatic breast carcinoma. *Lancet* 2,
   646 (1978).
6. A. A. Fracchia, H. T. Randall, and J. H.
   Farrow. The results of adrenalectomy in
   advanced breast cancer in 500 consecutive
   patients. *Surg. Gynecol. Obstet.* 125, 747
   (1967).
7. B. A. Stoll, *Hormonal management in breast
   cancer* p. 38, London (1969).
8. G. P. Canellos, V. T. de Vita, G. L. Gold,
   B. A. Chabuer, P. S. Schein and R. C.
   Young, Cyclical combination chemotherapy
   for advanced breast cancer. *Brit. Med. J.*
   1, 218 (1974).

Medical Adrenalectomy with Aminoglutethimide-Cortisol in the Treatment of Metastatic Breast Carcinoma

R. Paridaens, C. Van Haelen and J. C. Heuson

Service de Médecine, Laboratoire d'Investigation Clinique, Institut J. Bordet,
1, rue Héger-Bordet, 1000 Brussels, Belgium

Correspondence to R. Paridaens

Abstract—*Twenty-eight post-menopausal patients with generalized breast cancer were treated in a phase II trial with Aminoglutethimide (1,0 g/day) plus low dose cortisol replacement therapy (40 mg/day). Treatment was rapidly stopped because of severe toxicity in 6 patients. Eighteen of the 22 remaining patients were found evaluable and were assessed according to the U.I.C.C. criteria. Five patients (28%) had an objective partial response lasting from 3 to 17 months and are still in remission. An additional patient showed a mixed response lasting 10 months and another showed stabilization of her lesions for 13 months. Treatment failed in 11 patients (61%). Our results are comparable to those reported by other groups which used higher doses of corticosteroids. Objective responses appear to be merely due to aminoglutethimide rather than to replacement doses of glucocorticoïds. Side effects occurred in 15/28 patients (54%) and consisted mainly of skin rashes and drowsiness appearing early in the course of therapy. A reduction of the initial dosage of AG is recommended in order to prevent CNS side effects. Orthostatic hypotension was observed in 3 cases and this complication was controlled in two by mineralocorticoïds. Liver toxicity was suspected in two cases. Blood cholesterol levels increased frequently. A gain in body weight was often noted but a mild Cushing's syndrom was rarely observed.*

INTRODUCTION

Griffiths et al. (1) have shown that Aminoglutethimide (AG), when given together with corticosteroïds produces remissions in post menopausal patients with advanced breast cancer. The effectiveness of this association has recently been confirmed in several trials (2-5). In these studies, however, glucocorticoïds have been given in pharmacological rather than replacement doses. It is therefore difficult to assess the respective roles of AG and glucocorticoïds in the induction of remissions.

Two years ago, we started a clinical phase II trial in post-menopausal patients with advanced breast cancer treated with AG plus low doses of hydrocortisone replacement therapy. We report here the results of this study.

MATERIAL AND METHODS

Patients selection: twenty eight patients with advanced histologically proven breast cancer were treated at the Institut Jules Bordet. All were postmenopausal or had undergone oophorectomy (11 patients). All had evolutive disease and measurable or evaluable lesions. Patients with CNS metastic involvement or with severe or rapidly progressive visceral metastases were excluded.

To be included in the study, patients had to have a performance status of at least 40% according to the Karnofsky's scale and expected survival of at least 3 months. Twenty patients (71%) had been treated previously for their disease with hormones (16 patients) and/or chemotherapy (12 patients). These treatments were interrupted at least one month before starting AG and this delay was increased to two months for those who received long acting hormone preparations.

Treatment: AG 1 gram daily per os was given in four divided doses. Hydrocortisone was given by mouth in three divided doses: 10 mg at 8 am and 5 pm and 20 mg at bedtime.

Follow-up evaluation: all patients but one were ambulatory. Physical examination, recording of side effects and biological controls were performed before therapy, after 15 and 45 days, and thereafter at monthly intervals. Immediately before treatment, the following investigations were also performed: chest X ray, liver and bone scans, radiological skeletal survey and bone marrow biopsy. Except for the latter, these investigations were repeated after 3 months. All cases were reviewed by two independent clinicians in order to assess the response according to the U.I.C.C. criteria (6).

RESULTS

Of the 28 patients included in the study, 2 were found inevaluable for lack of assessable lesions. Two were also judged ineligible because of insufficient delay after stopping previous hormonal therapy (1 pt) and poor general condition (1 pt). Six of the 24 remaining patients rapidly interrupted the treatment for unacceptable side effects. Eighteen patients were found evaluable for treatment efficacy. Fifteen completed a course of 3 months of therapy while 3 others showed earlier evidence of progressive disease requiring another treatment.

patients and were sufficiently severe in 6 (21%) to require withdrawal of AG. Toxicity was judged to be severe in 4 (14%) and mild in 5 (18%) others. Three patients exhibited untractable somnolence that led to the interruption of the treatment while 4 had milder symptoms which subsided after 1 month of therapy. Cutaneous toxicity occurred in 8 patients (29%). Among these, six had a transient pruritic skin rash, while two others had to stop therapy for a severe purpuric eruption (1 case) and erythema nodosum (1 case). Mineralocorticoïd insufficiency occurred in 3 patients with abrupt unpredictable hypotension. Additional fludrocortisone administration controlled

Table 1. Responses related to sites of metastases and sites of dominant lesions.

	No. patients	Partial response (PR)	No change (NC)	Failure (F)
Metastatic site				
· Soft tissue	10	4		6
· Bone	10	3		7
· Lung	3	1	1	1
· Marrow with myelophtysic anemia	2	2		
Dominant site				
· Soft tissue	5	1		4
· Bone	9	2		7
· Viscera	4	2	1	1

Five patients had an objective sustained partial regression of their lesions (Table 1). All five responders are still in remission for periods longer than 17, 13, 10, 7 and 3 months respectively. Among these, only one had undergone prior castration which was followed by stabilization of the disease for 1 year.

Two others had been treated previously and had responded to cytostatics (1) or to Tamoxifen (1). An additional patient had a mixed response with regression of cutaneous lesions and correction of myelophtysic anemia lasting 10 months while she exhibited simultaneous slow progression of bone lesions.

Among 10 patients with bone metastases, 2 showed recalcification of lytic lesins and experienced early relief of severe pain. A third patient presented, after 3 months of treatment, distinct densification of osseous areas which showed increased isotopic uptake on the bone scan and normal radiological appearance prior to treatment; this patient was interpreted as having PR because of the regression of cutaneous and pulmonary lesions.

Subjective improvement and especially reduction of bone pain were only noted in patients who experienced an objective response.

Side effects were recorded in 15/28 (54%)

this problem in two but not in the third patient, whose treatment had to be withdrawn.

No electrolyte changes were recorded in any case but circulating aldosterone levels dropped, sometimes below detectable limits in most patients.

One patient presented a marked jaundice with cytolysis after 6 weeks of therapy, which vanished 3 weeks after stopping AG. A definite diagnosis of toxic as opposed to viral hepatitis could not be made but reinstitution of AG was uneventful. Another patient had a transient mild increase in transaminases after 3 months. No hematological changes were noted in any patient except in two who had correction of their myelophtysic anemia (1 PR; 1 MR). Serum cholesterol levels increased frequently, especially after long term courses of treatment. Fasting glucose levels and TSH values did not increase. A weight gain of 2 to 6 kg was noted in about half the patients who were treated for 3 to 6 months. Mild clinical features of Cushing's syndrome (moon face) were observed in only 2 patients after prolonged therapy.

DISCUSSION

Surgical adrenalectomy produces objective

tumor regression in approximately one third
of postmenopausal patients with advanced
breast cancer. Corticosteroîds were then
used in an attempt to achieve "medical
adrenalectomy" in these patients. Replacement doses of cortisone were however unable
to induce true objective responses (7,8).
Larger supraphysiological doses of glucocorticoîds induce a low rate, always below
20%, of short lived objective remissions (9).
These disappointing results could be
explained by a poor control of the production
of adrenal androgens, and furthermore by a
lack of control of ovarian androgens secretion in non castrated postmenopausal women.
Aminoglutethimide, a drug formerly used as
an anticonvulsant, was shown to be able to
block the whole adrenal steroidogenesis by
inhibiting the enzymic conversion of cholesterol to pregnenolone (10). This drug exerts
also an extra adrenal action for it inhibits
the enzymic conversion of androgens into
estrogens. This was demonstrated in in vitro
experiments (11-12) and recently confirmed
in vivo in patients with advanced breast
cancer (13). When given to patients, AG
had however to be associated with a corticosteroid in order both to prevent a rebound
ACTH rise and the appearance of clinical
symptoms of adrenal insufficiency.

After the initial clinical report of
Griffiths et al. (1), other groups (2-5)
confirmed that this drug combination could
induce a good response rate in postmenopausal
women with advanced breast cancer. In these
studies, the reported objective remission
rates ranged from 22 to 38%. Treatment
regimens used in these series were however
very different from each other. Because of
the limiting CNS toxicity (drowsiness) of
AG at higher doses (1,2), most of the authors
administered one gram per day as we did in
the present study.

Large supraphysiological doses of dexamethasone were needed to achieve a sustained
adrenal suppression (2,14). Santen could
subsequently explain this phenomenon, and
showed that under AG therapy the metabolism
of dexamethasone was accelerated. He advocated the use of cortisol in combination
with AG since the near physiological dose
of 40 mg per day of this steroid efficiently
prevented a rebound ACTH rise (14). More
recently, Smith et al. (5) using AG in
combination with cortisone at slightly higher
doses (50-75 mg per day) reported very favourable results.

Because of the use of larger than replacement doses in all previous studies, the
respective roles of steroids and AG in the
induction of remissions remained to be clarified. In the present study, drug dosage and
schedule of administration were those recommended by Santen et al. (14,15). The low
daily dose of 40 mg hydrocortisone seems very
unlikely to have a role in the induction of
objective remissions, as mentioned above.
Larger doses of corticosteroîds used in other
studies did not seem to produce distinctly
higher response rate than ours (28%) and
appear therefore unjustified. This also

suggests that these favourable results were
merely due to the action of AG rather than
to the action of glucocorticoîds. Unlike
others, however, we did not find any improvement or reduction of metastatic bone pain in
patients who did not experience an objective
response. This antalgic effect reported
elsewhere (1-2,4-5) was probably the result
of a non specific anti-inflammatory action
of higher doses of steroîds.

Finally, in the present study, side effects
of AG, especially drowsiness and skin rashes,
were quite severe and imposed discontinuation
of therapy in about 20% of the cases.
Attempts are currently made to improve drug
tolerance. As others (5,16) we observed
that CNS side effects tended to vanish after
several weeks of therapy.

In order to avoid this complication, we
are now starting with low daily doses of AG
(250 to 500 mg) which are gradually increased
until full dosage is reached. The lower
proportion of severe skin rashes observed in
other series (2,4,5,15) could be due to a
concealment of this reaction by the larger
doses of corticosteroids used. Three of
our patients, aged 63, 75 and 77 years
respectively, had orthostatic hypotension.
This complication, which had also been
mentioned by others (2,5) seemed to occur
especially in elderly patients, as previously
suggested by Smith et al. (5). It is likely
to be a consequence of the drop in blood
aldosterone levels observed here. Fishman
et al. (17) has also shown that larger doses
of AG (2 gram per day) decreased aldosterone
production in normal subjects. In order to
prevent hypotension, we recommend to give
fludrocortisone in addition to cortisol,
especially in elderly patients. Incidentally,
since there is no readily available method
to assay blood levels of AG, measurement of
blood aldosterone level could be used as a
control of patient compliance.

REFERENCES

1. C. T. Griffiths, T. C. Hall, Z. Saba,
   J. J. Barlow and H. B. Nevinny, Preliminary trial of Aminoglutethimide in breast
   cancer. *Cancer* 32, 31 (1973).
2. R. J. Santen, A. Lipton and J. Kendall,
   Successful medical adrenalectomy and
   Aminoglutethimide. *J.A.M.A.* 230, 1661
   (1974).
3. K. E. Gale, P. R. Sheehe, L. V. Gould,
   R. Rohner, Treatment of advanced breast
   cancer with Aminoglutethimide: an 8
   year experience. *Clin. Res.* 24, 376A
   (1976).
4. H. H. Newsome, P. W. Brown, J. J. Terz
   and W. Lauwrence Jr, Medical and surgical
   adrenalectomy in patients with advanced
   breast carcinoma. *Cancer* 39, 542 (1977).
5. I. E. Smith, B. M. Fitzharris, J. A.
   McKinna, D. R. Fahmy, A. G. Nash, A. M.
   Neville, J. C. Gazet, H. T. Ford and
   T. J. Powles, Aminoglutethimide in treatment of metastatic breast carcinoma.
   The Lancet 2, 646 (1978).

6. J. L. Hayward, P. P. Carbone, J. C.
Heuson, S. Kumaoka, A. Segaloff and
R. D. Rubens, Assessment of response to
therapy in advanced breast cancer.
Europ. J. Cancer 13, 89 (1977).

7. A. Segaloff, R. Carabasi, B. N. Horwitt,
J. V. Schlosser and P. J. Murison,
Hormonal therapy of cancer of the breast.
VI. Effect of ACTH and cortisone on
clinical course and hormonal excretion.
Cancer 7, 331 (1954).

8. T. L. Dao, E. Tan and V. Brooks, A
comparative evaluation of adrenalectomy
and cortisone in the treatment of
advanced mammary carcinoma. *Cancer* 14,
1259 (1961).

9. J. C. Heuson, Hormones by administration.
In *The Treatment of Breast Cancer*.
(Edited by Professor Sir Hedley Atkins
K.B.E.) p. 113, Medical and Technical
Publishing Co. Ltd. Lancaster (1974).

10. R. N. Dexter, L. M. Fishman, R. C. Ney
and G. W. Liddle, Inhibition of adrenal
corticosteroid synthesis by aminoglutethimide: Studies on the mechanism
of action. *J. Clin. Endocrinol. Metab.*
27, 473 (1967).

11. E. A. Thompson, S. B. Bolton and P. K.
Siiteri, Kinetic studies of placental
steroid aromatase. *Fed. Proc.* 30,
1160 (1971).

12. J. Chakraborty, R. Hopkins and D. V.
Parke, Inhibition studies on the aroma-
tization of Androst-4-ene-3, 17 dione
by human placental microsome preparations.
Biochem. Journ. 130, 19 (1972).

13. R. J. Santen, S. Santner, B. Davis,
J. Veldhuis, E. Samojlik and E. Ruby,
Aminoglutethimide inhibits extraglandular
estrogen production in postmenopausal
women with breast carcinoma. *J. Clin.
Endocrinol. Metab.* 47, 1257 (1978).

14. R. J. Santen, S. A. Wells, S. Runic,
C. Gupta, J. Kendall, E. B. Ruby and
E. Samojlik, Adrenal Suppression with
Aminoglutethimide. I. Differential
effects of aminoglutethimide on glucocorticoid metabolism as a rationale for
use of hydrocortisone. *J. Clin. Endocrinol. Metab.* 45, 469 (1977).

15. R. J. Santen, E. Samojlik, A. Lipton,
H. Harvey, E. B. Ruby, S. A. Wells and
J. Kendall, Kinetic, hormonal and
clinical studies with aminoglutethimide
in breast cancer. *Cancer* 39, 2948 (1977).

16. R. J. Santen, J. D. Veldhuis, E. Samojlik,
A. Lipton, H. Harvey and S. A. Wells,
Mechanism of action of aminoglutethimide
in breast cancer. *Lancet* 1, 44 (1979).

17. L. M. Fishman, G. W. Liddle, D. P. Island,
N. Fleischer and O. Kuchel, Effects of
aminoglutethimide on adrenal function in
man. *J. Clin. Endocrinol. Metab.* 27, 481
(1967).

Therapeutic Effect of Tamoxifen versus combined Tamoxifen and Diethylstilboestrol in Advanced Breast Cancer in Postmenopausal Women*

H. T. Mouridsen*, M. Salimtschik, P. Dombernowsky***,
K. Gelshoj**, T. Palshof****, M. Rorth*,
J. L. Daehnfeldt**** and C. Rose******

*Department R II - R V, Finseninstitute, Copenhagen
**Department A, Finseninstitute, Copenhagen
***Medical Department C/T, Bispebjerg Hospital, Copenhagen
****The Fibiger Laboratory, Copenhagen

Correspondence to H. T. Mouridsen, M.D., Department R II - R V, Finseninstitute,
49, Strandboulevarden, 2100 Copenhagen 0, Denmark

Abstract—This study was undertaken to compare the therapeutic efficacy of
tamoxifen (TAM) with tamoxifen plus diethylstilboestrol (TAM + DES). One
hundred and twenty two postmenopausal patients with advanced breast cancer,
those less than 68 years of age resistant to previous chemotherapy, and
those more than 68 years of age with or without resistance to chemotherapy,
entered the trial. Sixty five were randomized to treatment with TAM 10 mg
× 3 daily and 57 to treatment with TAM 10 mg × 3 daily plus DES 1 mg × 3
daily. Remission (partial and complete) was obtained in 39% of the
patients with TAM compared to 37% with TAM + DES (p > 0.7), no change in
31% versus 33% and progressive disease in 31% versus 30%. Median duration
of remission was 11+ months with TAM and 9+ months with TAM + DES and
median duration of no change was 9 months versus 7½ months. Toxicity was
significantly more pronounced with the combination. Thus the addition of
DES to TAM does not increase the therapeutic effect but increases
toxicity.

INTRODUCTION

Estrogens have until recently been the most
widely used agents when additive endocrine
treatment is indicated in patients with
advanced mammary carcinoma. Some 20-30% of
the patients will respond to treatment (1)
and the response rate is increasing with
daily dose from 1.5 mg to 1500 mg however
at the expence of increasing toxicity (2).

Since the antiestrogenic compound tamoxifen
seems to have the same efficacy and milder
side effects this drug has now replaced
estrogen in additive endocrine therapy (3).

However, the major part of patients still
fail to respond to estrogens and antiestrogens. The lack of a full understanding of
steroid hormone action and the absence of a
good experimental animal model for combined
endocrine treatment makes it reasonable -
on entirely imperical basis - to combine
different kinds of additive and/or ablative
procedures.

The aim of the present study has been to
compare the therapeutic effect of tamoxifen
alone with the effect of tamoxifen plus
diethylstilboestrol in postmenopausal
patients with advanced breast cancer.

MATERIAL AND METHODS

The material include consecutive patients
admitted to the departments R II - R V and
R/A, Finseninstitute and Medical Department
C/T, Bispebjerg Hospital between September 1,
1977 and August 1, 1978.

Eligibility requirements for the study
were:

1) The patients must be postmenopausal
defined as at least 6 months spontaneous
menostasia. Patients previously hysterectomized must be more than 50 years of age.
Patients previously oophorectomized
could enter the study 3 months after
surgical or 6 months after actinic castration.

2) Patients less than 68 years of age must
be clinical resistant to at least one
cytotoxic combination regimen. Patients
more than 68 years of age could enter the
study despite clinical resistance to
cytostatic treatment.

3) There must be measurable and/or evaluable
disease.

4) The performance status must be ≤ 3.

5) Previous additive endocrine treatment
must not have been given.

6) The patients should have given their
verbal informed consent.

The patients were randomly allocated
(using a stochastic array of numbers, closed
envelope system) to one of two treatment
groups. Treatment with tamoxifen 10 mg 3
times daily or treatment with tamoxifen 10 mg
3 times daily + diethylstilboestrol 1 mg

*Supported by a grant from the Danish Cancer Society.

3 times daily.

The treatment should, if possible, be maintained for at least 3 months when the response to treatment was assessed. If at 3 months there still was progressive disease the patient was taken off study. If at 3 months there was no change or a remission the patient continued on study until progression or relapse. Pretreatment examinations included physical examination, chest roentgenogram, skeleton survey, laboratory tests (blood cell counts, serum-calcium and liver function tests) and estimations of performance status. All visible and palpable lesions were measured to provide a baseline for subsequent examinations. These were repeated at 1-3 months intervals.

Further, when ever possible, prior to therapy biopsies from tumor tissue were taken for analyses of estrogen receptor protein using the dextran charcoal method (4).

Response to treatment was defined according to the UICC-criteria (5).

RESULTS

One hundred and twenty two patients entered the trial (Table 1). Four patients in each group were inevaluable. In the TAM-group 2 patients due to early death and 2 due to toxicity requiring early discontinuation of treatment. In the combination group 1 due to early death and 3 due to toxicity with early discontinuation of treatment.

rank sum test of unpaired data).

Nor were the duration of response different in the two treatment groups (see Table 3).

Only few data is available concerning the relation between frequency of response and estrogen receptor contents (Table 4) but in agreement with other studies the major part of the responders are found among the estrogen receptor positive tumors.

Side effects occurred most frequently and were most pronounced with the combined treatment (Table 5).

Two patients receiving TAM and 3 patients receiving TAM + DES discontinued treatment due to nausea after 1-2 months of treatment. Vaginal bleeding occurred in 8 patients on treatment with TAM + DES. In one case after 1 month of treatment. At that time this patient had rapidly progressive disease and died 1 week later. In one case the bleeding stopped spontaneously and treatment was continued. Among the other 6 cases 3 occurred after 3 months of treatment, 1 after 4 months, and 2 after 5 months. In all these cases a curettage demonstrated the endometrium to be hyperplastic and the patients continued on TAM only without any further episodes.

DISCUSSION

The result from the present study shows that treatment with TAM is equally good as the combination of tamoxifen and diethylstilboestrol.

Because an assay for tamoxifen is not at

Table 1. Tamoxifen (TAM) versus tamoxifen plus diethylstilboestrol (TAM + DES) in advanced breast cancer. Material.

	TAM	TAM + DES
Patients entered, no.	65	57
Patients evaluable, no.	61	53
Age, median (range), years	69 (34-83)	69 (46-82)
Disease-free interval, median (range), years	$2\frac{1}{2}$ (0-17)	$2\frac{1}{4}$ (0-22)
Performance status, median (range)	1 (0-3)	1 (0-3)
Previous chemotherapy, %	40	41
Dominant disease site,		
% in soft tissue	51	50
% in bone	20	21
% in viscera	29	29

Among the other 114 patients 61 were randomized to treatment with TAM and 53 to treatment with TAM + DES. As appears from Table 1 the two groups of patients were comparable with respect to age, disease-free interval, performance status, previous chemotherapy and localization of the dominant site of disease.

The response to treatment appears from Table 2.

No difference was observed when comparing rate of PR + CR (p > 0.7) or when comparing the overall results (p > 0.9) (Man-Whitney

our disposal the possibility of pharmacokinetic interactions between tamoxifen and diethylstilboestrol cannot be ruled out. Experimental results from the rat uterus (6) and DMBA induced rat mammary tumors (7) support the idea that tamoxifen exhibits its effect by opposing the replenishment of the cytoplasmic estrogen receptor.

The mode of action of pharmacologic doses of estrogens remains largely unknown. Using the rat uterus as an experimental model it seems that high doses of estrogens deplete

Table 2. Tamoxifen (TAM) versus tamoxifen plus diethylstilboestrol (TAM + DES) in advanced breast cancer.
Results.

	TAM	TAM + DES
PD[x]	20/65 = 31%	17/57 = 30%
NC	20/65 = 31%	19/57 = 33%
PR	14/65 = 22%	13/57 = 23%
CR	11/65 = 17%	8/57 = 14%
PR + CR	25/65 = 39%	21/57 = 37%

[x]Includes 4 patients in each group with early death or early discontinuation
of treatment due to toxicity.

Table 3. Tamoxifen (TAM) versus tamoxifen plus diethylstilboestrol (TAM + DES) in advanced breast cancer.
Duration of response (months).

	TAM	TAM + DES
NC	9 (2-20)	7½ (3-15)
PR + CR	11+ (4-18+)	9+ (2-16+)

Table 4. Tamoxifen (TAM) versus tamoxifen plus diethylstilboestrol (TAM + DES) in advanced breast cancer.
Relation between response (PR + CR) and ER content.

	TAM	TAM + DES	Total
ER positive[x]	6/12	5/8	11/20 ∿ 55%
ER negative	1/9	1/8	2/17 ∿ 12%

[x]ER positive is defined as an ER protein concentration of $\geq$ 20 fmols/mg of
protein.

Table 5. Tamoxifen (TAM) versus tamoxifen plus diethylstilboestrol (TAM + DES) in advanced breast cancer.
No. of patients with side effects.

	TAM	TAM + DES
nausea, vomiting	5	10
vaginal bleeding	0	8
pain in breast	0	6
tumor pain	2	0
restless legs	0	2
flushing	1	0
oedema	0	1
thrombophlebitis	0	1
Total	8/65	28/57

the cytoplasma for estrogen receptors (8) and
thereby rendering the tissue irresponsive to
continued estrogen stimulation. For theoretical reasons therefore there is no evidence of
pharmacodynamic interference at the receptor
level.

Data from the human mammary cell line MCF-7
indicates that the effect of high doses of
estrogen is in part non-specific and not
entirely mediated through the estrogen
receptor (9).

However, in the present clinical study
any difference as regards mode of action
has not resulted in any additive effect from

treatment with the combination of estrogen
and antiestrogen.

REFERENCES

1. J. L. Hayward, *Hormones and human breast cancer*. Springer-Verlag, Berlin Heidelberg New York (1970).
2. A. C. Carter, N. Sedransk, R. M. Kelley, F. J. Ansfild, R. G. Ravdin, R. W. Talley and N. R. Potter, Diethylstilboestrol: Recommended dosages for different categories of breast cancer patients. *JAMA* 237, 2079 (1977).
3. H. T. Mouridsen, T. Palshof, J. Patterson and L. Battersby, Tamoxifen in advanced breast cancer. *Cancer Treatm. Rev.* 5, 131 (1978).
4. J. L. Daehnfeldt and P. Briand, Determination of high affinity gestagen receptors in hormone responsive and hormone-independant GR mouse mammary tumors by an exchange assay. In *Progesterone Receptors in Normal and Neoplastic Tissues*. (Edited by W. L. McGuire, J.-P. Raynaud and E. E. Baulieu) p. 59, New York, Raven Press (1977).
5. J. L. Hayward, P. P. Carbone, J.-C. Heuson, S. Kumaoka, A. Segaloff and R. D. Rubens, Assessment of response to therapy in advanced breast cancer. *Europ. J. Cancer* 13, 89 (1977).
6. V. C. Jordan, C. J. Dix, K. E. Naylor, G. Prestwich and L. Rowsby, Non steroidal antiestrogens: Their biological effects and potential mechanisms of action. *Jr. of Toxicol. and Environ. Health* 4, 363 (1978).
7. R. I. Nicholson, M. P. Golder, P. Davies and K. Griffiths, Effects of estradiol-17 and tamoxifen on total and accessible cytoplasmic estradiol-17 receptors in DMBA-induced rat mammary tumors. *Europ. J. Cancer* 12, 711 (1976).
8. A. J. W. Hsueh, E. J. Peek and I. H. Clark, Progesterone antagaonism of the estrogen receptor and estrogen-induced uterine growth. *Nature* 254, 337 (1975).
9. M. Lippman, Hormone-responsive human breast cancer in continuous tissue culture. In *Breast Cancer:* Trends in research and treatment. (Edited by J.-C. Heuson, W. H. Mattheiem and M. Rozencweig), p. 111. New York, Raven Press (1976).

New Aspects of Chemotherapy of Advanced Disease

Alternating Cyclical Hormonal-Cytotoxic Combination Chemotherapy in Postmenopausal Patients with Breast Cancer. An EORTC Trial*

J.-C. Heuson*, R. Sylvester** and E. Engelsman***

*Clinique et Laboratoire de Cancérologie Mammaire, Service de Médecine, and
**EORTC Data Center, Institut J. Bordet, Brussels, Belgium
***Antoni van Leeuwenhoek Ziekenhuis, Amsterdam, The Netherlands

Correspondence to J.-C. Heuson, Institut Jules Bordet, rue Héger-Bordet,
1000 Brussels, Belgium

Abstract—Based upon concepts derived from estrogen receptor studies and theoretical considerations on drug resistance, a phase II exploratory trial was conducted where tamoxifen was administrated concomitantly with cytotoxic chemotherapy in postmenopausal patients with advanced breast cancer. Chemotherapy was composed of two 28-day cycles given alternatively. Cycle A consisted of adriamycin and vincristine (AV), and cycle B of cyclophosphamide, methotrexate and 5-fluoronracil (CMF). Of 95 patients who were found eligible and reviewed, 74 were fully evaluable. In this group, complete remissions (CR) were obtained in 16 patients (22%) and partial remissions (PR) in 37 patients (50%). The overall response rate (CR + PR) was 72%. The CR rate was significantly higher when the site of the dominant lesion was soft tissue (60%) as compared to bone or viscera (10%, 12%). In contrast, the overall response rate (CR + PR) by site did not show significant differences. When response rates were computed from the whole series of 95 eligible patients, including 74 fully evaluable cases, 3 toxic deaths, 9 cases of premature interruption of therapy, 4 early deaths and 5 cases lost to follow up, the rate of CR + PR was 56%. The median duration of response was 16 months. The median duration of survival was 30 months in responders and 7 months in the combined group of non-responders and non-evaluable cases.

INTRODUCTION

The basic programme of this study involved:
1. the concomitant use of hormonal and cytotoxic chemotherapy, and
2. the alternation of two non-cross resistant cyclical cytotoxic combinations.

This programme was devised with the aim of hopefully increasing the response rate, the duration of response and the survival of postmenopausal women with advanced breast cancer over those achieved by existing treatment modalities.

The rationale of this programme was threefold. First, it was assumed that the concomitant use of hormonal and cytotoxic chemotherapy might have additive effects. Endocrine responsiveness is often conceived as a all- or- nothing property of breast cancer. An alternative view has recently been proposed according to which most breast cancers are in fact hormone dependent to some degree (1). As a consequence, most patients would derive benefit from endocrine treatments even though only about 30% will experience a clear-cut, objectively recognizable remission. Secondly, it was hypothesized that alternating non-cross-resistant cytotoxic drug combinations might increase therapeutic efficacy. This was based on the assumption that relapse after remission was due to resistance to a given treatment and that perhaps failure to obtain a remission was due to early resistance in such a manner that reduction of tumor size could never be clinically recognized. By starting a second treatment at the

*Supported in part by Grant 5R10 CA 11488-07 awarded by the National Cancer Institute, DHEW (U.S.A.). This work was done by the E.O.R.T.C. Breast Cancer Cooperative Group with as chairman, J. C. Heuson; secretary, W. H. Mattheiem; statistician, R. Sylvester; EORTC Coordinator, M. Staquet; and EORTC representative, H. J. Tagnon; present chairman, E. Englesman. The following institutions participated in the study: Antoni van Leeuwenhoek Ziekenhuis, Amsterdam, The Netherlands (E. Engelsman); Institut J. Bordet, Brussels, Belgium (J. C. Heuson); Universitätskliniken, Ulm, West-Germany (W. Schreml); Universitäts-Krankenhaus-Eppendorf, Hamburg, West-Germany (H. Maass); Institut Médical des Mutualités Socialistes, La Hestre, Belgium (J. Michel); Kliniek Minnewater, Brugge, Belgium (A. Clarysse); Rotterdamsch Radiotherapeutisch Instituut, Rotterdam, The Netherlands (D. Blonk-Van Der Wijst); Finseninstitutet, Copenhagen, Denmark (H. Mouridsen); Centre Henri Becquerel, Rouen, France (J. P. Julien); St Radboud Ziekenhuis, Nijmegem, The Netherlands (L. Beex). The study protocol was elaborated by J. C. Heuson, chairman, J. S. Williams and G. J. Flowerdew, statisticians, and W. H. Mattheiem, secretary, with the collaboration of Y. Kenis and M. Rozencweig.

time of either recurrence or recognition of
failure, the problem of resistance may be
overcome but the tumors will have returned
to their original size or have grown. If
one supposes that alternating treatments in
a schedule such as ABAB ... avoids or delays
resistance, then each cycle will act on
tumors of scalewise decreasing volume until
regression is clinically recognized. On the
basis of these theoretical assumptions, one
may hope to obtain a higher rate and a longer
duration of remission. Thirdly, alternating
cycles A and B may hopefully have the advantage of decreasing the cumulative toxicity
of such drugs as adriamycin or vincristine
thereby delaying the occurrence of toxicity
and increasing the maximum tolerated total
doses.

Tamoxifen was selected as the endocrine
part of the treatment. It is a typical antiestrogenic compound which, like nafoxidine
(2,3), was shown to induce remissions in
postmenopausal patients with advanced breast
cancer (4,5,6). Non-cross resistant cytotoxic cyclical combinations were those
reported by Brambilla et al. (7,8) namely
cyclophosphamide, methotrexate, and fluorouracil (CMF), and adriamycin plus vincristine (AV).

The trial was devided into two sequential
phases. The initial phase was meant to be
an exploratory trial involving a large
enough sample of patients so as to provide
a fairly accurate assessment of the results.
A decision was then to be taken according to
predetermined criteria whether to extend the
trial into a fully randomized comparative
trial for more definitive results. The
purpose of the present communication is to
report the results of the initial exploratory
phase, which is now complete. An interim
report has appeared earlier (9).

PATIENTS AND METHODS

Patients were admitted into the study when
they had advanced breast cancer and were at
least 1 year postmenopausal. Six premenopausal patients were also admitted when they
had progressive disease after surgical castration. No patient received prior cytotoxic

therapy but five had been treated with short
courses of hormones.

To be admitted into the study, patients
had to meet the criteria of eligibility of
the EORTC Breast Cancer Cooperative Group
(3). One departure from this protocol was
that patients with massive liver involvement
were accepted provided their performance
status was $\geq$ 60 (Karnofsky index). Not
accepted were those having extensive radiological bone involvement, myelophthistic
anemia or hypercalcemia, a record of previous
massive X-irradiation of the bones,
leukopenia (WBC < 4,000), thrombocytopenia
(platelets < 120,000), or altered kidney
function (creatinine > 1.1 mg .).

Drug doses, schedule and route of administration for treatments A and B are given in
Table 1.

In patients above age 68, the doses of
cytotoxic drugs were reduced by one third.
During treatment, a reduced dose schedule
was also used, especially when there was
myelosuppression. If at initiation of either
cycle A or B, WBC were below 4,000 and/or
platelets below 100,000, treatment was
delayed 1 or at most 2 weeks. At the time
of drug administration, if the leukocyte
count was between 3,000 and 4,000 per mm^3,
half of the calculated dose of each drug
(except vincristine and tamoxifen) was given.
If the leucocyte count was between 2,000 and
3,000 and/or the platelet count was between
50,000 and 100,000 per mm^3, 25% of the calculated dose (except vincristine and tamoxifen)
were given. Below these levels, drug administration (except tamoxifen) was discontinued
until leucocytes and platelets were above
the upper threshold levels.

Patients were stratified according to
presence or absence of a free interval, site
of dominant lesion and the presence of
massive liver involvement, previous endocrine therapy, or age > 68 years. They were
randomized to either sequence ABAB... or
BABA... in order to detect a possible
although unexpected difference between them.
Treatments were alternated every 28 days for
the first year then every 56 days for the
second year. A few patients (about 10%)
received only CMF during the second year.
During the third year and thereafter, the

Table 1. Treatment and dose schedules.

Therapy	Drug	Dose	Schedule	Route
A	Adriamycin	75 mg/m^2	Day 1	i.v.
	Vincristine	1.4 mg/m^2	days 1 & 8	i.v.
	Tamoxifen	20 mg	twice/day	p.o.
B	Cyclophosphamide	100 mg/m^2	days 1 to 14	p.o.
	Methotrexate	60 mg/m^2	days 1 & 8	i.v.
	Fluorouracil	600 mg/m^2	days 1 & 8	i.v.
	Tamoxifen	20 mg	twice/day	p.o.

Note: For the patients from 68 to 75 years of age, the dose of the cytotoxic
drugs was reduced by one third.

treatment in responders was usually withheld although some patients received various types of unrecorded therapy.

The criteria of objective remission were those of the EORTC Breast Cancer Cooperative Group (3). Assessment was performed 4 months after initiation of therapy. One important provision was that all cases were subjected to extramural review by two independent investigators. Duration of remission and of survival was measured from the start of therapy and calculated by the actuarial method.

RESULTS

A total of 95 patients entered during the period July 1974-March 1976 were found to be eligible and were assessed by extramural reviewers. Seventy-four were fully evaluable while 21 were not for the reasons given in Table 2.

cases (Table 2), was 56%. The difference in response rates by site (soft tissue: 61%, bone: 33%, viscera: 61%) is not statistically significant (P = .10).

Table 4 presents the duration of response and of survival according to whether or not the patients responded. In the 74 evaluable patients, the responders who represented 72% of the group had a median duration of response of 16 months and a median survival time of 30 months. Three patients are known to still be in CR and three in PR beyond 3 years. In the group of non-responders, the median duration of survival was 10 months. If one considers the whole series of 95 eligible cases, the responders, namely those having a long survival, represented only 56% of the group. The remainder had a duration of survival close to that of the non-responders in the group of evaluable cases.

The toxic side effects ranged from mild to severe. The most significant were nausea and

Table 2. Distribution of patients entered July 1974-March 1976.

Total eligible and reviewed	95
Total evaluable	74
Toxic death	3
Toxicity/refused treatment	9
Early death	4
Lost to follow up	5

Table 3. Therapeutic results. May 1979.

Dominant site of lesions	Evaluable cases					All cases		
	No cases	CR No	CR %	CR+PR No	CR+PR %	No cases	CR+PR No	CR+PR %
Soft tissue	15	9	60%	11	73%	18	11	61%
Bone	10	1	10%	6	60%	18	6	33%
Viscera	49	6	12%	36	73%	59	36	61%
Total	74	16	22%	53	72%	95	53	56%

CR = complete response; PR = partial response.

The therapeutic results are presented in Table 3. Since the rate of response was nearly identical whether the patients were treated with sequence ABAB... or BABA..., the results for the two groups were pooled. It is seen from the Table that in the 74 fully evaluable cases, complete responses (CR) were obtained in 16 patients (22%) and partial responses (PR) in 37 patients (50%). The overall response rate was 72%. The difference in complete response rates by the dominant site of lesions (soft tissue: 60%, bone: 10%, viscera: 12%) is statistically significant (P < 001). When one looks at the combined CR + PR rates by site, the difference is no longer statistically significant. The overall response rate for all 95 eligible cases, including the non-evaluable

vomiting which occurred to some extent in most patients, weakness and pain, of which two thirds of the patients complained, and hematologic changes, which were recorded in half of the patients. Alopecia occurred in all cases.

There were three toxic deaths from leukopenia and infection, one due to accidental overdosage. Nine patients had their treatment stopped (4 cases) or refused to continue their treatment (5 cases) prior to 16 weeks due to toxicity. There were 4 early deaths (2 to 9 weeks), one being due to infection, not related to treatment, and three to unknown causes.

Table 4. Duration of response and survival in this trial as
compared to other treatment modalities.

| Treatment | No cases | % | Responders | | Non-responders |
			Median duration (months)	Median survival (months)	Median survival (months)
Androgens*	521	21%	10	26	6
Estrogens†	357	37%		21	7
Adrenalectomy‡	583	36%		25	8
CMF/AV sequential[X]	105	54%	9	23	10-14
CMF/AV alternating†	110	56%	12		
This trial					
evaluable cases	74	72%	16	30	10
all cases	95	56%	16	30	7

*C.B.C.G., 1964 (10); †A.M.A., 1960 (11); ‡Silverstein et al., 1975 (12);
[X]Brambilla et al., 1976 (8); †Brambilla et al., 1978 (13).

DISCUSSION

The present trial, based on concepts derived from estrogen receptor studies and theoretical considerations on drug resistance, associated endocrine and cytotoxic therapies. It gave satisfactory results with respect to therapeutic efficacy. A complete remission rate of 22% and an overall (CR + PR) remission rate of 72% have rarely been reported for combination chemotherapy in studies involving strict criteria for assessment of response. Treatment A (AV) alone was reported to achieve CR in 8% of the patients and CR + PR in 52%, the corresponding figures being 10% and 47% for treatment B (CMF) (8). Of special interest is the duration of response and of survival obtained with the present treatment regimen. In this regard, Table 4 compares our results with those of five large reported series. Three are concerned with the classical endocrine treatment modalities, androgen or estrogen administration, and adrenalectomy, and the remaining two with the same cytotoxic combinations as here but given without hormone, and used either sequentially or in an alternating schedule. In all series, as expected, responders had a much longer survival than non-responders. In this trial, the median duration of response and the median survival of responders were longer than with endocrine or cytotoxic chemotherapy alone. The most striking difference however was in the higher proportion of patients experiencing a response and thereby having a prolonged survival. It is fully acknowledged that these comparisons are made between patient samples that are not necessarily alike, and that any conclusion should therefore be drawn with great caution.

A definite weakness of the present trial lies in the rather large proportion of non-evaluable cases (21/95 = 22%; see Table 2). Since the cause of early death or loss to follow up (9 cases) may well in fact be tumor progression, it may be wise to include the corresponding cases in the calculations of response rates. The same holds true for patients who died from toxicity or had their treatment prematurely stopped due to toxicity. Inclusion of these cases in the analysis lowers the calculated response rates as shown in Tables 3 and 4 but does not substantially affect the duration of response or of survival (Table 4). However, with regard to toxic deaths (3 cases) and premature interruption of therapy (9 cases), their number could probably be reduced by a better skill on behalf of the physician in conducting this difficult treatment modality. Improved schedules of administration and more appropriate adjustment of drug dosages should be worked out.

If one tentatively admits that the apparent therapeutic superiority of the present regimen over conventional chemotherapy alone actually exists, it remains to be determined whether the difference is due to the concomitant administration of tamoxifen and chemotherapy, or to the use of two alternating cycles or both. An ongoing clinical trial of the EORTC comparing CMF with or without tamoxifen will be reported by Dr. H. Mouridsen later on at this Conference and may answer part of these questions. On the other hand, the concept of alternating two non-cross-resistant combinations in the treatment of solid tumors has been tried in Hodgkin's disease (14), in small cell bronchogenic carcinoma (15) and in breast cancer (13). This approach led to a high response rate in the first study and to an increased rate in the second although in neither one is it established whether a benefit is obtained in terms of duration of response or survival. In the third study, the authors conclusion is that the alternating scheme is in no way better than the sequential use of the same combinations. We think that the evidence presently available neither proves nor disproves the potential value of alternating non-cross-resistant combinations in the

treatment of advanced (or early) breast
cancer and that this approach is worthy of
further exploration.

REFERENCES

1. J. C. Heuson, E. Longeval, W. H.
   Mattheiem, M. C. Deboel, R. J. Sylvester
   and G. Leclercq, Significance of quantitative assessment of estrogen receptors
   for endocrine therapy in advanced breast
   cancer. *Cancer* 39, 1971 (1977).
2. J. C. Heuson, A. Coune and M. Staquet,
   Clinical trial of nafoxidine, an oestrogen antagonist in advanced breast cancer.
   Europ. J. Cancer 8, 387 (1972).
3. J. C. Heuson, E. Engelsman, J. Blonk-van
   der Wijst, H. Maass, A. Drochmans,
   J. Michel, H. Nowakowski and A. Gorins,
   Comparative trial of nafoxidine and
   ethinyl-oestradiol in advanced breast
   cancer. An E.O.R.T.C. Breast Cancer
   Cooperative Group Study. *Br. Med. J.* 2,
   711 (1975).
4. M. P. Cole, C. T. A. Jones and I. D. H.
   Todd, A new anti-oestrogenic agent in
   late breast cancer. An early clinical
   appraisal of ICI 46474. *Br. J. Cancer* 25,
   270 (1971).
5. H. W. C. Ward, Anti-oestrogen therapy
   for breast cancer: a trial of tamoxifen
   at two dose levels. *Br. Med. J.* 1, 13
   (1973).
6. R. C. Heel, R. N. Brogden, T. M. Speight
   and G. S. Avery, Tamoxifen: a review of
   its pharmacological properties and
   therapeutic use in the treatment of
   breast cancer. *Drugs* 16, 1 (1978).
7. G. Bonadonna, Symposium on Cytotoxic
   Chemotherapy for Mammary Cancer, Padova
   (1974).
8. C. Brambilla, M. de Lena, A. Rossi,
   A. Valagussa and G. Bonadonna, Response
   and survival in advanced breast cancer
   after two non-cross-resistant combinations. *Br. Med. J.* 1, 801 (1976).
9. J. C. Heuson, Current overview of
   E.O.R.T.C. clinical trials with tamoxifen.
   Cancer Tr. Rep. 60, 1463 (1976).
10. I. S. Goldenberg, Testosterone propionate
    therapy in breast cancer. *J. Am. Med. Ass.*
    188, 1069 (1964).
11. AMA Council on Drugs, Androgens and
    estrogens in the treatment of disseminated
    mammary carcinoma. Retrospective study
    on nine hundred fourty-four patients.
    J. Am. Med. Ass. 172, 1271 (1960).
12. M. J. Silverstein, R. L. Byron, Jr.,
    R. M. Yonemoto, D. U. Riihimaki and
    G. Schuster, Bilateral adrenalectomy for
    advanced breast cancer: a 21 year
    experience. *Surgery* 77, 825 (1975).
13. C. Brambilla, P. Valagussa and
    G. Bonadonna, Sequential combination
    chemotherapy in advanced breast cancer.
    Cancer Chemother. Pharmacol. 1, 35
    (1978).
14. D. C. Case, C. W. Young, L. Nisce, B. J.
    Lee III and B. D. Clarkson, Eight-drug
    combination chemotherapy (MOPP and ABDV)
    and local radiotherapy for advanced
    Hodgkin's disease. *Cancer Tr. Rep.* 60,
    1217 (1976).
15. M. H. Cohen, D. C. Ihde, P. A. Bunn,
    B. E. Fossieck, M. J. Matthews, S. E.
    Shackney, A. Johnston-Early, R. Makuch
    and J. D. Minna, Cyclic alternating
    combination chemotherapy for small cell
    bronchogenic carcinoma. *Cancer Tr. Rep.*
    63, 163 (1979).

CMF versus CMF Plus Tamoxifen in Advanced Breast Cancer in Post-menopausal Women. An EORTC* Trial

H. T. Mouridsen*, T. Palshof*, E. Engelsman** and R. Sylvester***

*Finseninstitute, Copenhagen, Denmark
**Antoni van Leeuwenhoek Ziekenhuis, Amsterdam, The Netherlands
***EORTC Data Center, Institut Jules Bordet, Bruxelles, Belgium

Correspondence to H. T. Mouridsen, M.D., Department R II, Finseninstitute,
49, Strandboulevarden, 2100 Copenhagen 0, Denmark

Abstract—263 patients were randomized to treatment with CMF or CMF plus tamoxifen. At the time of this preliminary analysis the response to therapy could be evaluated in 150 cases. In 50 of them the assessment by the local investigator was reviewed extramurally and agreement was observed in only 56% of the cases. In 12% the review committee increased the responserate and in 32% it was decreased. Among the 150 evaluable cases (the evaluation of the review committee if available and if not the evaluation of the local investigator) the rate of response (partial + complete remission) was 45% with CMF compared to 70% with CMF plus TAM, no change was observed in 26% versus 17% and progressive disease in 29% versus 13%. These differences are significant in favour of the combined treatment but it must be emphasized that only 33% of the patients have been reviewed extramurally. On the other hand analysis of the time to progression which depends less on the disagreement between the evaluations of the local investigator and the extramural review committee also shows that the addition of TAM to CMF significantly improves the treatment results.

INTRODUCTION

Systemic treatment of advanced breast cancer in postmenopausal subjects includes chemotherapy and endocrine therapy. With combination chemotherapy response is achieved in 50-60% of the cases (1,2). Concerning endocrine therapy the drug of choice today is tamoxifen. The response rate obtained is 20-40%, increasing slightly with age (3).

In premenopausal subjects the combination of oophorectomy plus chemotherapy has been demonstrated to be slightly superior to either of the two treatments alone (4,5,6). Similarly in postmenopausal subjects the addition of androgen (7) or estrogen (8) to combination chemotherapy increased the efficacy of the treatment but not significantly so.

The present study was undertaken to compare in a randomized trial CMF with CMF plus TAM with respect to rate and duration of response, toxicity and survival.

MATERIAL AND METHODS

The study included those patients admitted consecutively to the participating centers from March 1977 to March 1979. Eligibility requirements for the study were as follows:

1. Histological evidence of breast cancer.
2. Postmenopausal status (at least 1 year after last menstrual period) but age less than 68.
3. Progressive disease with measurable and/or evaluable lesions.
4. UICC performance status grade 2 or below.

*EORTC Breast Cancer Cooperative Group.
Participating members:
J. C. Heuson, W. L. Mattheiem, Institut Jules Bordet, Brussels, Belgium.
J. Michel, Centre Hospitalier de Tivoli, La Louviere, Belgium.
E. Engelsman, Antoni van Leeuwenhoek Ziekenhuis, Amsterdam, The Netherlands.
T. Blonk - van der Wijst, Rotterdamsch Radiotherapeutisch Institut, Rotterdam, The Netherlands.
L. Beex, St. Radboud Ziekenhuis, Nitmegen, The Netherlands.
K. Rosendaal, Onze Lieve Vrouwe Gasthuis, Amsterdam, The Netherlands.
E. Engelsman, Binnen Gasthuis, Amsterdam, The Netherlands.
H. T. Mouridsen + T. Palshof, Finsen Institute, Copenhagen, Denmark.
W. Schreml, Universitats Kliniken, Ulm, West Germany.
R. Sylvester + B. Wessen + M. van Glabbeke, EORTC Data Center, Institut Jules Bordet, Brussels, Belgium.

Supported in part by grant SR 10 CA 11488-07 awarded by the National Cancer Institute, U.S.A.

5. Normal hematological values.

6. Normal creatinine and calcium levels.

Criteria of ineligibility were the following:

1. UICC performance grade 3 or 4.

2. Previous treatment with the agents used in the study.

3. Treatment for the present disease by endocrine ablative procedures.

4. Less than 4 weeks of cessation of additive endocrine treatment. This delay must be increased accordingly for long acting or depot hormones.

5. Previous or concomitant malignancies with the exception of excisional biopsy of in situ carcinoma of the cervix uteri and adequately treated basal or squamous cell carcinoma of the skin.

6. Sarcoma of the breast.

7. Patients in whom pleural effusion, ascites, metastases in the central nervous system or osteoblastic bone lesions are the sole manifestation of the disease.

The patients were stratified by institution and according to the dominant site of the disease and randomized to one of two treatment groups: Group A, treatment with CMF (oral cyclophosphamide 100 mg pr m^2 d 1–14, i.v. methotrexate 40 mg per m^2 d 1 and 8, i.v. 5-fluoro-uracil 600 mg per m^2 d 1 and 8, cycle repeated every 4 weeks). Group B, treatment with CMF as in group A plus tamoxifen 20 mg twice daily. The treatment was if possible continued for at least 2 months at which time the response was assessed. If at 2 months there was progressive disease the patient was taken off study. If at two month there was no change or a remission the patient continued on study until progressive disease or relapse. In case of complete remission treatment was usually discontinued after 1 years duration of complete remission.

The relative dose of CMF was adjusted according to platelet and white blood cell counts according to the following scheme: Platelets ($\times 10^3$ per µl) > 100 and WBC ($\times 10^3$ per µl) > 4: 100% of dose; platelets > 100 and WBC 3–4: 50% of dose; platelets 50–100 and/or WBC 2–3: 25% of dose; platelets < 50 and/or WBC < 2: no drug. If, at the beginning of a 28-day cycle the platelet count was < 100 and/or WBC was < 4 the cycle was delayed one or two weeks.

Pretreatment examinations, follow up studies and assessment of response were defined according to the UICC criteria (9).

RESULTS

A total of 263 patients entered the trial and at present the response to treatment could be evaluated in 150 cases. The reasons for inevaluability are: too early, 81; incomplete data, 9; refusal of treatment, 5; early death, 3; protocol violation, 3 and other, 12.

Currently the response to treatment has been assessed by extramural reviewers in 33% of the evaluable patients entered on trial.

The results from the extramural review appears in Table 1 which shows the relation between the assessment by the review committee and the local investigator.

As can be seen, agreement was present in only 56% of the cases. In 12% the response was increased by the review committee and in 32% it was decreased. As also appears from Table 1 the percentage of patients for whom the response was decreased was equal in the two treatment groups whereas the review committee increased the response in only 1 of the patients treated with CMF as compared to 5 of the patients treated with CMF plus TAM.

The overall treatment results are shown in Table 2. It must be emphasized that the results in Tables 2–5 are preliminary as only 33% of the cases have been reviewed

Table 1. Comparison of response to treatment by review committee and local investigator.

	Total	CMF	CMF + TAM
Review committee agreed in	56% (28/50)	63% (17/27)	48% (11/23)
Increased response in	12% (6/50)	4% (1/27)	22% (5/23)
Decreased response in	32% (16/50)	33% (9/27)	30% (7/23)

Table 2. Overall treatment results. (Review committee/local investigator).

	CMF	CMF + TAM
PD	21 (29%)	10 (13%)
NC	19 (26%)	13 (17%)
PR	26 (36%)	38 (49%)
CR	7 (10%)	16 (21%)
PR + CR	33 (45%)	54 (70%) p = 0.003
Total	73	77

Table 3. Treatment results in patients with soft tissue as the
dominant site of disease. (Review committee/local
investigator).

	CMF	CMF + TAM
PD	5 (18%)	1 (4%)
NC	5 (18%)	6 (22%)
PR	13 (46%)	12 (44%)
CR	5 (18%)	8 (30%)
PR + CR	18 (64%)	20 (74%)
Total	28	27

Table 4. Treatment results in patients with viscera as the
dominant site of disease. (Review committee/local
investigator).

	CMF	CMF + TAM
PD	4 (12%)	8 (29%)
NC	6 (18%)	9 (32%)
PR	16 (49%)	10 (36%)
CR	7 (21%)	1 (4%)
PR + CR	23 (70%)	11 (39%)
Total	33	28

Table 5. Treatment results in patients with bone as the
dominant site of disease. (Review committee/local
investigator).

	CMF	CMF + TAM
PD	8 (47%)	5 (29%)
NC	5 (29%)	1 (6%)
PR	3 (18%)	10 (60%)
CR	1 (6%)	1 (6%)
PR + CR	4 (24%)	11 (65%)
Total	17	16

extramurally. As appears from the table the
addition of tamoxifen significantly improved
the treatment results. It is still too early
to analyse the duration of response in the
two treatment groups. Subdivision of these
results into patients with dominant site of
disease in soft tissue, bone and viscera
shows the same trend in all groups; however,
it is still too early to draw any definite
conclusions (Tables 3-5).

Figure 1 shows the time to progression by
treatment group. Using the log-rank test
the difference between these curves is
significant with a p-value of 0.04, thus
indicating that the addition of tamoxifen
significantly increases the duration of time
until progression occurs.

The toxicities to treatment are shown in
Tables 6 and 7.

Haematologic as well as non-haemetologic

side effects occured with equal frequency
in the two treatment groups.

DISCUSSION

Nine centers participated in the study.
It was expected that there might be some
disagreement between assessment by the
review committee and the assessment by local
investigators, however, not to the extent
that actually occured. Because it is too
early to evaluate the response in all the
cases the results must be considered preliminary and more time has to pass and a
more extensive review has to be done before
the trial results can be finalyzed. However,
the conclusion that tamoxifen significantly
improves the treatment results will hardly
be changed. Among 143 cases entered from

122   H. T. Mouridsen *et al.*

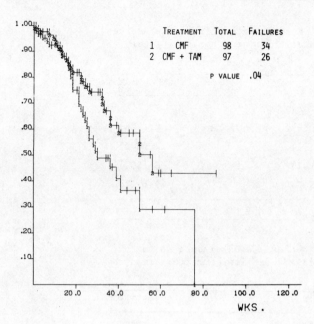

TREATMENT	TOTAL	FAILURES
1 CMF	98	34
2 CMF + TAM	97	26

P VALUE .04

Fig. 1. Time to relapse.

one of the participating centers (Finsen-institute) similar differences between the two treatment groups were observed and among 20 of these cases which were reviewed, the assessment by the local investigator was changed in only 1 case by the review committee (from complete to partial remission). The value of tamoxifen is also supported by the fact that the time until progression was significantly different between the two treatment groups. This analysis is less dependent on the differences in the evaluation of the response by the local investigator and the review committee as it depends only upon the time to progression. It is thus a more reliable indicator that tamoxifen significantly improves the treatment results with CMF.

Table 6. Hematological toxicity. Median nadir values.

	CMF	CMF + TAM
WBC	2.800	2.800
Platelets	182.000	165.000

Table 7. % of patients with toxicity.

	CMF	CMF + TAM
nausea	81	71
anorexia	67	33
vomiting	58	40
mucous membr.	33	27
weakness	33	35
other	60	51

REFERENCES

1. S. K. Carter, Integration of chemotherapy into combined treatment of solid tumors. VII Adeno-Carcinoa of the breast. *Cancer Treatm. Rev.* 3, 141 (1976).
2. M. Rozencweig, J. C. Heuson, D. D. von Hoff, W. H. Mattheiem, H. L. Davis and F. M. Muggia, Breast Cancer. In *Randomized Trials in Cancer. A Critical review by Sites.* (Edited by M. J. Staquet) p. 231. New York, Raven Press (1978).
3. H. T. Mouridsen, T. Palshof, S. Patterson and L. Battersby, Tamoxifen in advanced breast cancer. *Cancer Treatm. Rev.* 5, 131 (1978).
4. J. J. van Dyk and G. Falkson, Estended survival and remission rates in metastatic breast cancer. *Cancer* 27, 300 (1971).
5. D. L. Ahmann, M. S. O'Connell, R. G. Hahn, H. F. Bisel, R. A. Lee and J. H. Edmonson, An evaluation of early or delayed adjuvant chemotherapy in premenopausal patients with advanced breast cancer undergoing oophorectomy. *New Engl. J. Med.* 297, 356 (1977).
6. K. W. Brunner, R. W. Sonntag, P. Alberto, H. J. Senn, G. Martz, P. Obrecht and P. Maurice, Combined chemo- and hormonal therapy in advanced breast cancer. *Cancer* 39, 2923 (1977).
7. R. E. Lloyd, S. E. Jones, S. E. Salmon, Comparative trial of low-dose adriamycin plus cyclophosphamide with or without additive hormonal therapy in advanced breast cancer. *Cancer* 43, 60 (1979).

8. K. W. Brunner, R. W. Sonntag, P. Alberto,
   H. J. Senn, G. Martz, P. Obrecht and
   P. Maurice, Combined chemo- and hormonal
   therapy in advanced breast cancer. *Cancer*
   39, 2923 (1977).

9. J. L. Hayward, P. P. Carbone, J.-C. Heuson,
   S. Kumaoka, A. Segaloff and R. D. Rubens,
   Assessment of response to therapy in
   advanced breast cancer. *Europ. J. Cancer*
   13, 89 (1977).

Hormono-Chemotherapy versus Hormonotherapy Followed by Chemotherapy in the Treatment of Disseminated Breast Cancer

F. Cavalli[1], P. Alberto[2], F. Jungi[3], K. Brunner[4], and G. Martz[5]
for the Swiss Group for Clinical Cancer Research (SAKK)

[1]Division of Oncology, Ospedale San Giovanni, Bellinzona
[2]Division of Oncology, Hôpital Cantonal, Genève
[3]Division of Oncology, Kantonsspital, St. Gallen
[4]Division of Oncology, Inselspital, Bern
[5]Division of Oncology, Kantonsspital, Zürich

Correspondence to F. Cavalli, M.D., Division of Oncology, Ospedale San Giovanni,
6500 Bellinzona, Switzerland

Abstract—372 *previously untreated patients (pts.) with disseminated breast carcinoma were stratified as regards known prognostic factors and randomized to oophorectomy (premenopausal pts.) or to receive tamoxifene (postmenopausal pts.), either with concurrent combination chemotherapy or alone, chemotherapy being delayed for at least 6 weeks. After this observation time, combination chemotherapy was started unless hormonotherapy had already shown tumor regression: if so, chemotherapy was further delayed to the occurrence of a new tumor progression.*

Patients were further randomly allocated to 3 different chemotherapy regimens (1mfp, LMP/FVP, LMFP/ADM), including chlorambucil (L), methotrexate (M), fluorouracile (F), vincristine (V), adriamycin (ADM) and prednisone (P).

311 cases are already evaluable. In the premenopausal group remissions were seen in 24/42 (57%) pts. with a concurrent hormono-chemotherapy and in 17/38 (45%) pts. if chemotherapy is delayed. The corresponding results in the postmenopausal pts. are 52/118 (44%) and 46/113 (40%).

Concerning the combination chemotherapy the response rates are: 27/94 (28%) for 1mfp, 42/88 (48%) for LMP/VFP and 50/86 (58%) for LMFP/ADM (1mfp vs. LMFP/ADM, p < 0.05).

No difference in survival exists between concurrent hormono-chemotherapy and delayed chemotherapy as well as among the different chemotherapy regimens.

INTRODUCTION

Chemotherapy and hormonal therapy act by different mechanisms and have different spectra of toxicity. It would seem promising to combine both modalities of treatment in advanced breast cancer with the hope to improve the results, since combination chemotherapy seems to have reached an apparent plateau (1,2).

In a previous study of the Swiss Group for Clinical Cancer Research (SAKK) the combined modality approach with simultaneous poly-chemotherapy and hormonal treatment did not produce statistically significant better results than chemotherapy alone (3). However there was a clear-cut tendency for better remission, longer remission duration and survival when chemotherapy was combined with oophorectomy in premenopausal patients.

Our present study was therefore directed toward the next question: Should combination chemotherapy be delayed until primary failure under hormonal therapy or should both treatments be started simultaneously?

The second question of our still ongoing trial relates to the correlation between "aggressiveness" of the chemotherapy and

therapeutic results. In fact there have been suggestions (4), that even a low-dose chemotherapy can achieve results similar to those produced by more toxic combinations. Moreover, as already mentioned, in breast cancer chemotherapy seems to have reached a plateau in their effectiveness. We designed therefore our study in order to be able also to answer the following question: How aggressive should be the first combination chemotherapy used in previously untreated patients with metastatic breast cancer?

MATERIAL AND METHODS

The protocol (SAKK 2/75) was activated within the participating institutions (Division of Clinical Oncology of the Cantonal and University Hospital of Geneva, Lausanne, Bern, Basel, Zürich, St. Gallen and Bellinzona) late in 1975.

The study design is outlined in Table 1. Before randomization patients were stratified according to the menopausal status and the "risk-group". They were classified as "low" or "high" risk, based on a retrospective evaluation of the previous SAKK-studies (5).

Table 1. Study design.

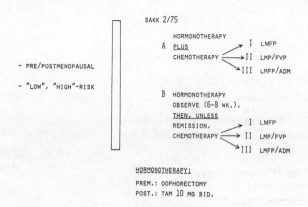

SAKK 2/75

HORMONOTHERAPY
A PLUS
   CHEMOTHERAPY → I   LMFP
                → II LMP/FVP
                → III LMFP/ADM

B HORMONOTHERAPY
   OBSERVE (6-8 WK.),
   THEN, UNLESS
   REMISSION,   → I   LMFP
   CHEMOTHERAPY   → II LMP/FVP
                        → III LMFP/ADM

HORMONOTHERAPY:
PREM.: OOPHORECTOMY
POST.: TAM 10 MG BID.

The following cases were considered to be "low-risk":
- Free interval (FI) mastectomy-diagnosis of the first metastasis of at least 2 years and only contra-lateral, loco-regional nodal metastases.
- FI at least 2 years and only bony metastases.
- Maximally 2 out of the following parameters:
  a) lung or liver metastases (not both!) with a FI of at least 4 years
  b) an isolated bony metastasis with a FI of at least 2 years
  c) scattered skin metastases (not cancer en cuirasse!) and/or an ipsilateral malignant pleural effusion of at least 2 years
  d) ipsilateral loco-regional nodal metastases and FI of at least 2 years

All other patients were considered "high-risk".

Patients were randomized to A (concurrent chemo- and hormonotherapy) or B: Hormonotherapy, observe 6-8 weeks, start than chemotherapy, *unless* hormonotherapy has already shown tumor regression. If so, combination chemotherapy was started in B only upon new progression of the tumor parameters.

At the time of the randomization to A or B, patients were also randomly allocated to 3 different chemotherapy regimens: I, II, III. Dosage and schedule of the 3 regimens are shown in Table 2.

Table 2. Chemotherapy regimens.

I "MINIMAL" (LMFP)
CLB 5 MG/M²/D   D 1-14 P.O.
MTX 10 MG/M²/W D 1+8   P.O. (1 DOSE!)
5-FU 500 MG/M²/W D 1+8   P.O.
PDN 30 MG/M²/D D 1-14 THEN
Q 4 WKS. = INTERMITTENT

II "MEDIUM" (LMP/FVP)
CLB AS IN I
MTX 15 MG/M²/D SUBDIVIDED IN 3 DAILY DOSES D 1-3, D 8-10 P.O.
PDN 30 MG/M²/D D 1-14
5-FU 500 MG/M²/W D 15+22 I.V.
VCR 1.2 MG/M²/W D 15+22 I.V.
PDN 30 MG/M²/D D 25-28 THEN
Q 4 WKS. = CONTINUOUS

III "MAXIMAL" (LMFP/ADM)
CLB AS IN I
MTX 40 MG/M²/W D 1+8   I.V.
5-FU 600 MG/M²/W D 1+8   I.V.
PDN 30 MG/M²/D D 1-14, THEN
ADM 60 MG/M²   D 28
Q 8 WKS. = INTERMITTENT

Regimen I (LMFP, "minimal") is a peroral, intermittent combination designed in a pilot study carried out in St. Gallen (6). In all regimens we used chlorambucil instead of cytoxan, in order to avoid some of the toxicities related to the latter. In a previous study the SAKK has shown that both drugs are equivalent in the treatment of breast cancer (7).

Regimen II (LMP/FVP, "medium") corresponds to the "Swiss version" (3,7) of the "Cooper regimen". Regimen III (LMFP/ADM, "maximal") is an alternating combination with adriamycin and LMFP (= CMFP, but with chlorambucil instead of cytoxan).

At the last evaluation (15.2.1979) 372 patients were entered into the study: All had measurable, previously untreated, advanced breast cancer. At this cut-off 311 cases were already evaluable (> 6 weeks of treatment): 31 were too early for evaluation and 30 were not evaluable (protocol violations, refusal of patients, early death, etc.). Only death within 4 weeks are considered early death: Later they are accounted as failure.

The distribution of the pretreatment patients characteristics is shown in Table 3: Only evaluable cases are accounted for. We analysed age, free interval, menopausal status (80 pre-, 231 postmenopausal), risk group of 7 sites of predominant metastases (loco-regional, skeletall, loco-regional + pleural effusion, loco-regional + skeletall, visceral + loco-regional, visceral + skeletall, visceral only).

As it can be seen from Table 3 there is a very similar distribution of all characteristics between A/B and also among the regimens I/II/III.

Table 3. Pretreatment patient characteristics.

	A	B	I	II	III
MEDIAN AGE (Y.)	57	59	59	58	57
MEDIAN F.I. (MT.)	26,5	26	29	22	23,5
< 12 MT.*	27	36	26	39	31
12-60 MT.*	56	47	60	45	49
> 60 MT.*	17	17	14	16	20
PREMENOPAUSAL* (N= 80)	26	25	28	26	27
POSTMENOPAUSAL* (N= 231)	74	75	72	74	73
HIGH RISK*	23	26	26	25	23
LOW RISK*	77	74	74	75	77
SITE OF METASTASES*					
LOCO-REGIONAL	7	13	11	9	9
SKELETALL	18	18	18	17	22
LOCO-REGIONAL+PLEURAL	4	4	3	5	5
LOCO-REGIONAL+SKELETALL	18	20	12	21	21
VISCERAL+LOCO-REGIONAL	12	7	14	6	10
VISCERAL+SKELETALL	27	25	24	31	20
VISCERAL	14	13	18	11	13

* = PERCENTAGE

Criteria of response were the same as those now used internationally (PR, NC, PD), except that we still use the category minor response (MR), in order to compare the current results with our previous studies. A MR is defined as a clear-cut tumor shrinkage, which does not reach the limit of 50% in the sum of the product of the 2 largest diameters of all measurable lesions.

Performance status (0-4) and toxicity (0-2) were recorded according to ECOG-scale. The same grading was used in order to reduce the dosage in presence of myelo-suppression (toxicity 1 = reduction 50%, toxicity 2 = reduction 100%).

Rather than duration of remission, whose onset can always conceal a subjective error, we analyse responding patients (PR, MR and NC) according to the time from the beginning of the treatment till appearance of new progression (time to progression). Survival and time to progression were calculated based on the method of Kaplan and Meyer (8).

RESULTS

Of the 311 evaluable patients, 160 were randomized in A (concurrent hormono- and chemotherapy) and 151 in B ("delayed" chemotherapy). In this latter group 38 patients underwent an oophorectomy and 113 postmenopausal patients received tamoxifen. The therapeutic responses to oophorectomy were as follows: 7 PR (19%) and 4 MR (11%). Tamoxifen elicited 20 PR (18%) and 8 MR (6%). Both treatments are known to produce in unselected patients a remission in about 1/4 of the cases. This percentage is reached in our study, if we add PR and MR. The rather low rate of PR is probably due to the stringent criteria of our protocol.

The median time to progression for patients responding to hormonotherapy only (PR + MR) was 17,0 months, after oophorectomy and 19,4 months after tamoxifen.

Table 4 presents the remission rate for A and B. For the latter group the results achieved with the "delayed" chemotherapy are added to the tumor regressions produced by the hormonotherapy. But patients who achieved a second chemotherapy-induced remission after a first hormono-therapy-induced regression, are accounted for only once.

Table 4. Therapeutic results.

		NO OF PTS.	PR	MR	NC	PD
PREMENOPAUSAL	A	42	24 (57%)	4 (10%)	6 (14%)	8 (19%)
	B	38	17 (45%)	8 (21%)	9 (24%)	4 (10%)
POSTMENOPAUSAL	A	118	52 (44%)	15 (13%)	26 (22%)	25 (21%)
	B	113	46 (40%)	16 (14%)	20 (18%)	31 (28%)

A = CONCURRENT HORMONO-CHEMOTHERAPY
B = "DELAYED" CHEMOTHERAPY

The results are very similar in the postmenopausal group with 44% PR, 13% MR, 27% NC in A and 40% PR, 14% MR and 18% NC in B. However there is a clear trend toward better remissions for A in premenopausal women (24/42 = 57%) versus 17 PR out of 38 patients (= 45%) in B: This difference lacks statistical significance. On the reverse in B there are more (21%) MR than in A (10%).

The median survival in months is 13,0 for A and 10,5 for B (p = 0,619).

Figs. 1 and 2 show the actuarial survival curves for A/B according to menopausal status. In the premenopausal group there is a statistically not significant difference

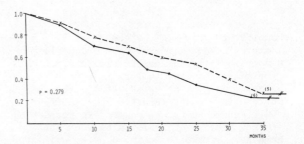

Fig. 1. Survival in postmenopausal patients. A (simultaneous), •——•, median 17,8 months. B (wait) x----x, median 25,6 months.

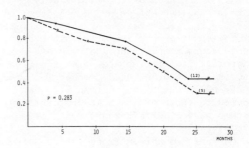

Fig. 2. Survival in postmenopausal patients. A (simultaneous), •——•, median 22,5 months. B (wait) x----x, median 20,4 months.

(p = 0,283) in favor of A (22,5 months median survival vs. 20,4), whereas in the postmenopausal group an essentially similar difference (p = 0,279) is found for B (25,6 months) versus A (17,8 months).

In Table 5 are summarized the remission rates according to the chemotherapy regimens (I = LMFP, II = LMP/FVP, III = LMFP/ADM) for the 268 patients who are already evaluable as regards this treatment modality. These 268 cases encompass essentially all evaluable patients of the concurrent hormono-

Table 5. Therapeutic results:
          chemotherapy.

REGIMEN	NO OF PTS.	PR	MR	NC	PD	
I	94	28	15	25	31	= 100%
II	88	48	16	19	17	= 100%
III	86	58	11	15	16	= 100%
	268					

I vs. II   p = 0,1. BUT < 0,05 BY ONLY R
I vs. III   p = < 0,05
II vs. III   p = 0,4
I vs. (II+III) p = < 0,005

I = LMFP ("MINIMAL")
II = LMP/FVP ("MEDIUM")
III = LMFP/ADM ("MAXIMAL")

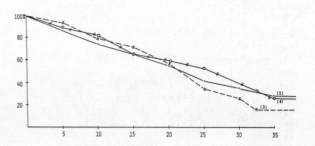

Fig. 3. Survival according to chemotherapy.
        I (LMFP, MINIMAL) ·———·, median
          22 months.
        II (LMP/FVP, MEDIUM) x----x,
          median 21,7 months.
        III (LMFP/ADM, MAXIMAL) o-#-#-o,
          median 25,7 months.

chemotherapy group (A), whereas for B
("delayed" chemotherapy) we recorded all
chemotherapy treated cases, either after
primary or secondary failure to hormonotherapy. It must be noted, that although
the results are not reported here, we found
no difference so far as regards response
rate and time to progression between the
chemotherapy results achieved after primary
and those observed after secondary hormonal
failure in group B.

As it can be seen from Table 5, there are
significant more PR and MR (p < 0,05) in
regimen III than in I. The "maximal"
regimen (III) and "medium" regimen (II)
together are superior (p < 0,005) to the
"minimal" chemotherapy (I), whereas regimen
I and II are different (p < 0,05) only
regarding the percentage of PR. A detailed
report of the side-effects of the 3 different
chemotherapy regimens is not possible here.
We note however, that haematologic and non-
haematologic toxicities are both significantly
(p < 0,05) more pronounced, concerning frequency and intensity in regimen III when
compared to those of the LMFP-chemotherapy.
The combination LMP/FVP shows an intermediate
score of toxicity.

A coherent comparison among the chemotherapy
regimens as regards the time to progression
is chiefly possible in the group A. Considering only PR, we have following median
values in months: 17,2 for AI, 14,5 for AII
and 17,3 for AIII (p = 0,498).

Fig. 3 shows the actuarial survival curves
for the 3 chemotherapy regimens. The median
survival time in months is 22,0 for I, 21,7
for II and 25,7 for III: These results are
essentially similar (p = 525).

Marked differences are found, if the time
to progression and survival are compiled
according to the therapeutic results. The
median time to progression is 16,8 months
for PR, 7,0 months for MR and 5,8 months for
NC. The median survival in months is 32,5
for PR, 19,1 for MR, 15,9 for NC and 6,0
for PD. All differences concerning time to
progression and survival are statically significant but between PR and NC.

Even if a detailed report is not possible
within the limit of this paper, we note, that
other significant differences in median

survival were found in the analysis of
following parameters:

Free interval (FI ≤ 12 months: 17,8,
FI ≥ 60 months: 30,8), site of metastases
(longest median survival with 26,8 months for
bony metastases, shortest for visceral and
skelettal localisation with 16,7 months),
risk-group ("high"-risk: 20,7, "low"-risk
28,0 months).

DISCUSSION

We present here an interim evaluation of a
still ongoing trial. We are continuing the
study mainly, because we hope, that by
accruing more patients, we could be able to
substantiate some differences in different
subsets of patients.

For the time being, we can only partially
confirm two previous reports, in which premenopausal patients fared significantly
better, when combination chemotherapy was
immediately added to oophorectomy (9,10).
In our study in fact the differences as
regards remission rate, time to progression
and survival are in favour of the group with
concurrent oophorectomy-chemotherapy: But
the disadvantage for the premenopausal
patients with "delayed" chemotherapy lacks
statistical significance. However it must
be underlined, that also in at least one of
the two mentioned reports (9), statistically
significant differences were found only
after exclusion of the group with early progression. The other paper was so far presented only as an abstract without elaborate
statistical analysis (10).

We want also to stress a methodological
difference between our trial and the above
mentioned studies. In our study the "delayed"
chemotherapy was begun, *unless* tumor regression was apparent 6-8 weeks after oophorectomy or start of tamoxifen, in postmenopausal
women. The two other studies called for the
beginning of "delayed" chemotherapy *only* in
case of evident tumor progression after

oophorectomy.

We are not aware of a similar study in postmenopausal patients. Contrary to the first evaluation of our trial (11), at present we have essentially the same remission rate for patients treated simultaneously with tamoxifen and chemotherapy and for cases with "delayed" chemotherapy. However as regards survival there is an advantage emerging in favor of the group with "delayed" chemotherapy. The difference lacks so far statistical significance, but is becoming more evident by each subsequent analysis of our trial.

The second question in our study relates to the intriguing problem of dose-response relationship in the treatment of advanced breast cancer (12). The interpretation of our present results is difficult. In fact we have clear differences with more and better tumor regressions in favour of the more aggressive and toxic regimens. In the overall study population we have also a stringent relationship between the grade of the therapeutic response and the median survival. But the survival curves are so far similar for all 3 chemotherapy regimens. A possible answer to this intriguing question could be a different therapeutic response to the subsequent treatments among relapsing patients. It is in fact possible, that the great majority of patients relapsing after a "maximal" chemotherapy (in our study LMFP/ADM) will be resistant to a secondary treatment. On the reverse we have some hints in favour of the hypothesis, that at least a significant subset of the patients receiving a "minimal" chemotherapy (in our study LMFP) is still responsive to a later, more intensive combination chemotherapy. But to answer properly this question, we have to await the final and thorough evaluation of our study.

REFERENCES

1. P. P. Carbone, M. Bauer, P. Band and D. Tormey, Chemotherapy of disseminated breast cancer. Current status and prospects. *Cancer* 39, 2916 (1977).

2. P. P. Carbone and T. E. Davis, Medical treatment for advanced breast cancer. *Seminars in Oncology* 4, 417 (1978).

3. K. W. Brunner, R. W. Sonntag, P. Alberto, H. J. Senn, G. Martz, P. Obrecht and P. Maurice, Combined chemo- and hormonal therapy in advanced breast cancer. *Cancer* 39, 2923 (1977).

4. R. H. Creech, R. B. Catalano, M. J. Mastrangelo and P. F. Engstrom, An effective low-dose intermittent cyclophosphamide, methotrexate and 5-fluorouracil treatment regimen for metastatic breast cancer. *Cancer* 35, 1101 (1975).

5. K. W. Brunner, Stand der Hormon- und Chemotherapie beim Mammakarzinom. *Schweiz. Med. Wschr.* 108, 1338 (1978).

6. H. J. Senn, M. Fopp and R. Amgwerd, Divergent effect of adjuvant chemo-immunotherapy on recurrence rates in node-negative and -positive breast cancer patients. *Proceedings ASCO* 20, 393 (1979).

7. K. W. Brunner, R. W. Sonntag, G. Martz, H. J. Senn, P. Obrecht and P. Alberto, A controlled study in the use of combined drug therapy for metastatic breast cancer. *Cancer* 36, 1208 (1975).

8. E. L. Kaplan and P. Meier, Nonparametric estimation from incomplete observations. *J. Amer. Stat. Ass.* 53, 457 (1958).

9. D. L. Ahmann, M. J. O'Conell, R. G. Hahn, H. F. Bisel, R. A. Lee and J. H. Edmonson, An evaluation of early or delayed adjuvant chemotherapy in premenopausal patients with advanced breast cancer undergoing oophorectomy. *N. Engl. J. Med.* 297, 356 (1977).

10. G. Falkson, H. C. Falkson, L. Leone, O. Glidwell, V. Weinberg and J. F. Holland, Improved remission rates and durations in premenopausal women with metastatic breast cancer. A Cancer and Acute Leukemia Group B study. *Proceedings ASCO* 19, 416 (1978).

11. F. Cavalli, P. Alberto, F. Jungi, G. Martz and K. W. Brunner, Tamoxifene alone or combined with multiple drug chemotherapy in disseminated breast cancer. X. International Congress of chemotherapy, p. 1286. Current Chemotherapy (1978).

12. M. H. Tattersall and J. S. Tobias, Are dose response relationships relevant in clinical cancer chemotherapy? In *Recent advances in cancer treatment* (edited by H. J. Tagnon and M. J. Staquet), p. 227. Raven Press, New York (1977).

Use of an Antiosteolytic Agent in Treatment of Patients with Bone Metastases from Breast Cancer

P. J. Dady[1], R. C. Coombes[2], I. E. Smith[1], C. A. Parsons[3],
H. T. Ford[4], J. C. Gazet[5], J. M. Henk[4], A. G. Nash[6] and
T. J. Powles[7]

[1]Department of Medicine, Royal Marsden Hospital, Sutton, Surrey
[2]Ludwig Institute for Cancer Research (London Branch), Unit of Human Tumour
Biology, Royal Marsden Hospital, Sutton, Surrey
[3]Department of Diagnostic Radiology, Royal Marsden Hospital, Sutton, Surrey
[4]Department of Radiotherapy, Royal Marsden Hospital, Sutton, Surrey
[5]Department of Surgery, Royal Marsden Hospital, Sutton, Surrey
[6]Department of Surgery, St. Helier Hospital, Carshalton, Surrey
[7]Institute of Cancer Research, London, S.W.3

Correspondence to P. J. Dady, Department of Medicine, Royal Marsden Hospital,
Sutton, Surrey, UK

Abstract—18 patients with advancing bone metastases from breast cancer were
treated with a combination of Adriamycin, Vincristine and the antiosteolytic
agent mithramycin in an attempt to control tumour in bone and reverse tumour
induced osteolysis. 16 patients had pain as a major symptom and in 81% this
was relieved, completely or partially. Bone marrow infiltration was reduced
and there was evidence of regression of disease at other sites. Biochemical
evidence suggested that treatment affected osteolysis in some patients, and
radiological evidence of increased net bone repair was seen. The effect of
this treatment on survival was negligible. Mithramycin caused vomiting in
33% of patients, but in no case was this severe enough to necessitate
discontinuing treatment.

INTRODUCTION

Eighty-four percent of a group of patients
with advanced breast cancer have been shown
to have evidence of skeletal metastases (1).
Many of these patients develop bone pain,
which, if localised may be relieved by radiotherapy, and if generalised may respond to
hormone manipulation, although eventual
relapse is inevitable.

A combination of vincristine, adriamycin
and prednisolone has been shown to have useful activity against metastatic breast
cancer in soft tissue and visceral sites (2)
and bone marrow (3). In general, however
little radiological evidence of remission in
bone occurred (15).

In vitro, tumour mediated osteolysis is
inhibited by the antibiotic mithramycin (4),
and in vivo it reduces bone destruction by
myeloma (5). Mithramycin has been used
successfully in the management of hypercalcaemia caused by skeletal metastases from
breast cancer (6). A further report from
this unit (7) suggested that mithramycin
could be used to obtain relief of pain due
to bone metastases, and in a small number of
cases biochemical and radiological evidence
of regression of bone disease was obtained.
Hitherto the application of this drug in
anticancer therapy has been virtually confined to the treatment of testicular teratoma
(8).

We have studied a combination of adriamycin,
vincristine and mithramycin given to patients
with skeletal metastases from breast cancer
in order to determine its antitumour and
bone healing effects.

METHODS

Chemotherapy was given on a 28 day cycle.
In the first treatment cycle patients
received adriamycin 50-70mg and vincristine
1.5-2.0 mg. intravenously, on days 0 and 7.
In subsequent courses the dose of adriamycin
was modified according to blood counts taken
on day 21 of each cycle. Mithramycin 1 mg.
in 200 mls normal saline, was infused over
2 hours, at weekly intervals, starting on
day 0. Treatment was continued until either
the cumulative dose of adriamycin reached
550 mg/m^2 or there was evidence that the
metastatic disease was progressing.

Investigations before and on completion of
treatment included radiological survey of
the axial skeleton, skull, femora, humeri
and chest. Plasma calcium, alkaline phosphatase and in most cases of glutamyl transpeptidase were measured. Fasting early
morning urine specimens were taken, as
described by Powles et al. (9), for measurement of hydroxyproline excretion, which was
expressed as a ratio of urinary hydroxyproline (mg/ml) × 100/urinary creatinine (mg/ml).
Technetium polyphosphate bone scintigraphy
(bone scan) and liver scan and/or ultrasound

were performed. Platelets, white cells and
haemoglobin were measured and bone marrow
was examined for metastatic tumour, the
marrow was aspirated from the iliac crest,
irrespective of the sites of radiological
bone involvement.

All patients were clinically examined and
the extent of the disease was charted, visible
tumour deposits were photographed. A careful
assessment was made of pain and details of
the nature, site and severity were recorded
when the patient was seen, as was the
Karnofsky performance status (10) before,
during and after treatment. Radiographs were
reviewed by an independant radiologist, whose
assessment followed the proposals recommended
by the UICC (10), as did the assessment of
response of other measurable disease. Bone
scan improvement was said to have occurred
of the areas of increased uptake decreased
by $\geq$ 25% increase in number, a similar
increase was taken to represent deterioration.

Eighteen patients, all female, with histologically proven breast cancer were included
in the study, between January 1977 and
December 1978. Ages ranged from 41 to 69
years, with a mean of 53.5 and a median of
51 years.

All patients had had previous treatment
for metastatic disease. In the majority
(89%) this had included some form of hormone
manipulation, although not within 4 weeks of
the start of chemotherapy.

None had known endocrine, renal or metabolic bone disease, or received other specific anticancer treatment during the period
of study.

RESULTS

1. Radiology

All patients had radiological evidence of
tumour deposits in bone. 10 patients had
purely lytic lesions, 1 purely sclerotic
and 7 had a mixture of lytic and sclerotic
deposits. Response was assessed in 16
patients (2 having died before this could
be done). 4 (25%) showed partial response,
5 (31%) were unchanged and in 7 (44%) there
was radiological progression of disease.

2. Pain Relief

16 patients had pain attributable to bony
metastases, which had been recorded on two
or more consecutive occasions immediately
before treatment. Chemotherapy produced
complete remission of pain in 9 cases (56%),
partial remission in 4 (25%) and in a further
3 (19%) pain was unchanged or deteriorated
during treatment. Pain relief generally
occurred before or during the second course
of treatment, although in 2 cases 3 courses
were required.

Two patients died, pain free, 10.5 months
after pain control and the 5 surviving
patients in the study are all pain free.
The shortest pain free interval was 1 month.

3. Karnofsky Status

The changes in performance status, resulting from treatment, are shown in Table 1.
At the start of treatment the grades were
recorded as follows: grade 4, 3 patients;
grade 3, 10 patients; grade 2, 1 patient;
grade 1, 1 patient.

4. Bone Scan

16 out of 17 pretreatment bone scans
showed areas of increased uptake, although
these did not necessarily correspond with
bone lesions on radiographs. The normal
bone scan was from the patients with radiologically sclerotic bone lesions, which were
widely distributed throughout the vertebral
column and pelvis.

Thirteen post treatment scans were
assessed for response. 3 (23%) had improved,
1 (8%) had deteriorated and 9 (69%) were
unchanged. The 3 improved scans were from
patients who had complete relief of pain,
although bone scan changes did not relate
well to radiological response.

5. Bone Marrow

Of the 18 pretreatment bone marrow samples,
tumour was found in 11, the other 7 were
clear. Fourteen were repeated after treatment, 8 had previously been positive, of
these, 6 (75%) showed no evidence of tumour,
in 2 (25%) tumour persisted. Six samples,
which had been negative before treatment
were repeated, 5 (83%) remained free of
tumour, but 1 (17%) had developed definite
evidence of tumour during treatment.

In all cases where clearance of tumour
from the marrow was not achieved, or infiltration developed, there was radiological
deterioration, disease at other sites progressed, and survival was brief.

6. Calcium

The upper limit of normal for plasma calcium is given as 2.60 mmol/1 in our laboratory. Five patients started treatment with
plasma calcium > 2.80 (albumin was within
the normal range). A marked fall in plasma
calcium occurred in all these cases, and
was maintained whilst these patients were on
chemotherapy (Fig. 1).

Whenever radiological improvement occurred
plasma calcium level fell. Calcium rose to
abnormal levels in 2 patients.

7. Hydroxyproline Excretion

At the start of treatment the urinary
hydroxyproline/creatinine ratio was > 200
in 2 patients, (Fig. 2), in both cases this
fell markedly during treatment. Both patients
were hypercalcaemic before chemotherapy and
became normocalcaemic.

Table 1. Performance status was graded according to the
modification of the original Karnofsky system as
proposed by the U.I.C.C. (10) before and after
treatment. Changes in the grade are shown in the
top line and the number of patients showing these
changes is shown below and below that in parenthesis
this number is shown as a percentage of all patients.

Change in Karnofsky status				
Deterioration	No change	Improvement		
+1	0	-1	-2	-3
3	3	3	5	4
(17%)	(17%)	(17%)	(27%)	(22%)

CALCIUM RESPONSE

HYDROXYPROLINE
EXCRETION RESPONSE

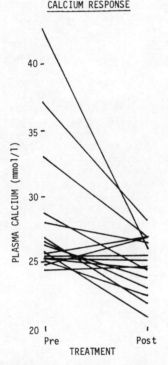

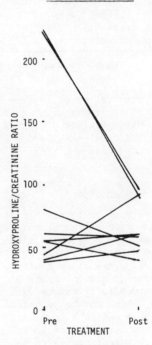

Fig. 1. Plasma calcium was measured before
and on completion of treatment
(pre and post treatment). Each
line indicates the change in value
obtained for 1 patient. The time
interval between pre and post
treatment samples was variable.

Fig. 2. Urinary hydroxyproline excretion,
related to creatinine excretion in
the same sample, was measured
before and on completion of treatment (pre and post treatment) in a
series of patients. The time
interval between the two determinations was variable.

8. Response at Other Sites

Other sites of measurable disease included
lung parenchyma, skin and liver. The results
of treatment could be measured in 9 cases,
there were objective improvements in 5 (55%),
no change in 1 (11%) and deterioration in 3
(33%).

Deterioration in disease at sites other
than bone, correlated with radiological
deterioration in all 3 patients, and in 2,
whose bone marrow response was documented,
there was failure to clear tumour cells from
the marrow or tumour infiltration developed.

9. Survival

The survival of patients included in this

study is shown in Fig. 3, median survival was
42 weeks. 5 patients survive at 23, 26, 28,
30 and 45 weeks after starting treatment.
Of the 4 patients who showed radiological
improvement, 2 are still alive at 30 and 26
weeks and 2 died at 56 and 63 weeks.

10. Side Effects

One third of these patients were troubled
by vomiting after mithramycin, which in
general lasted only one day and was at least
partially controlled by antiemetics. The
vomiting in some cases started one day after
the drug was given. Vomiting was in no case
severe enough to cause treatment to be
discontinued.

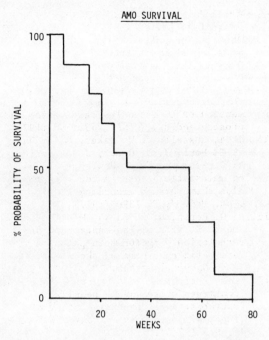

Fig. 3. Survival in weeks from the start
of treatment with Adriamycin,
Mithramycin and Vincristine
(Oncovin) (AMO) was plotted using
actuarial analysis.

DISCUSSION

The pattern of skeletal metastasis in
breast cancer tends to follow the distribution of red marrow in bone (11) and bone
metastases almost certainly originate in the
marrow (12). This study confirms the observation (3) that a combination of vincristine
and adriamycin is effective against tumour
in marrow, although the potential sampling
errors involved in the examination of small
samples from the iliac crest are considerable, where tumour persisted in the marrow
the prognosis was inevitably poor.

It has been suggested (13) that two processes, one due to increased osteoclastic
activity, the other not, are involved in
tumour induced bone destruction. A role
for prostaglandins, as at least one mediator
has been suggested (14). Bone destruction
may lead to hypercalcaemia and increased
hydroxyproline excretion, although hypercalcaemia does not relate to the extent of
bone destruction (1). Hypercalcaemia of
malignant disease is effectively controlled
by mithramycin (6), possibly acting as an
inhibitor of prostaglandin synthesis. Reduction in high circulating levels of calcium
and decreased hydroxyproline excretion may
represent a twofold effect of mithramycin
and reduction in tumour mass due to adriamycin
and vincristine.

Pain was the major cause of morbidity in
this series of patients. In the absence of
obvious causative factors such as fractures,
or evidence of nerve compression, the precise
mechanism by which bone pain arises is uncertain. One explanation has been that an
expanding tumour volume within the bone

causes pressure on the periostium, although
pain relief in several patients in whom all
other available evidence indicated progression of disease, suggests that chemotherapy
was inhibiting some other, possibly biochemical causative factor.

Bone scans were found to be more useful in
the initial detection of bone metastases than
in the assessment of response to treatment.
Scans were unchanged in many cases where
there was distinct radiological evidence of
improvement or deterioration.

A problem encountered in the interpretation of radiological response was that of
the patient who at the start of treatment had
mixed sclerotic and lytic lesions. The overall response of bone to tumour invasion is a
balance between tumour induced osteolysis and
bone production in the normal process of
bone repair and the radiograph shows this
quite accurately (12). Although accurate,
radiology is relatively insensitive means of
detecting osteolysis, since 50-70% of the
invaded bone must be destroyed before the
lesion is seen (1). Where there was a mixed
sclerotic and lytic radiograph before treatment, and after treatment there was progression of lytic disease with an apparent
increase in sclerotic lesions, this was taken
to represent deterioration, whereas this
could possibly represent healing of previously
undetectable lytic deposits.

The radiographs of a similar group of
patients, treated with a combination of
vincristine, adriamycin and prednisolone (15),
were re-reviewed, and the same response
criteria were applied. Only 7% showed radiological partial response, against 25% in
this study. The deletion of prednisolone
and addition of mithramycin appears to have
reduced the amount of bone destruction, at
least in some patients.

The survival data are disappointing, the
mean survival from the start of treatment
was 8 months, and the median survival was
9.5 months. Schurman and Anstutz (11)
reported mean survival in patients who had
developed long bone neoplastic fracture as
10.1 months or 6.5 months, depending on the
site. Other workers have reported 8 months
(16) and 7 months (17) respectively mean
and median survival, following pathological
fractures in long bones.

REFERENCES

1. C. S. B. Galasko, Skeletal metastases
   and mammary cancer ann. *Roy. Coll. Surg.
   Engl.* 50, 3 (1972).
2. J. A. Russell, J. W. Baker, P. J. Dady,
   H. T. Ford, J. C. Gazet, J. A. McKinna,
   A. G. Nash and T. J. Powles, Combination
   chemotherapy of metastatic breast cancer
   with vincristine, adriamycin and prednisolone. *Cancer* 41, 396 (1978).
3. P. J. Dady, J. C. Gazet, H. T. Ford and
   T. J. Powles, Combination chemotherapy
   for thrombocytopenia with bone marrow
   metastases from breast cancer. *Brit.
   Med. J.* 1, 554 (1977).
4. M. Dowsett, PhD Thesis, London University
   (1976).

5. T. C. B. Stamp, J. A. Child and P. G. Walker, Treatment of osteolytic myelomatosis with mithramycin. *Lancet* 1, 719 (1975).

6. I. Smith and T. J. Powles, Mithramycin for hypercalcaemia in cancer. *Brit. Med. J.* 1, 268 (1975).

7. R. C. Coombes, A. M. Neville and T. J. Powles, In *Symposium Proceedings: Bone Disease and Calcitonin*. (Edited by J. A. Kanis) p. 103. Armour Pharmaceutical Co. Ltd. (1976).

8. T. J. Priestman, In *Cancer Chemotherapy*. p. 54. Montedison Pharmaceuticals Ltd. (1977).

9. T. J. Powles, G. Rosset, C. L. Leese and P. K. Bondy, Early morning hydroxyproline excretion in patients with breast cancer. *Cancer* 38, 2564 (1976).

10. International Union against Cancer. Assessment of response to therapy in advanced breast cancer. *Brit. J. Cancer* 35, 292 (1977).

11. D. J. Schurman and H. C. Amstutz, Orthopaedic management of patients with metastatic carcinoma of the breast. *Surg. Gynecol. Obstet.* 137, 831 (1973).

12. R. A. Milch and G. W. Changus, Response of Bone to Tumour invasion. *Cancer* 9, 340 (1956).

13. C. S. B. Galasko, Mechanisms of bone destruction in the development of skeletal metastases. *Nature* 263, 507 (1976).

14. C. S. B. Galasko and A. Bennet, Relationship of bone destruction in skeletal metastases to osteoclast activation and prostaglandins. *Nature* 263, 508 (1976).

15. J. A. Russell, J. W. Baker, P. J. Dady, H. T. Ford, J. C. Gazet, J. A. McKinna, A. G. Nash and T. J. Powles, Response of metastatic breast cancer to combination chemotherapy according to site. *Brit. Med. J.* 2, 1390 (1977).

16. A. G. Coran, H. H. Banks, M. A. Aliapoulis and R. E. Wilson, The management of pathological fractures in patients with metastatic carcinoma of the breast. *Surg. Gynecol. Obstet.* 127, 1225 (1968).

17. F. F. Parish and J. A. Murray, Surgical treatment for secondary neoplastic fractures: a retrospective study of ninety-six patients. *J. Bone Joint Surg.* 52, 665 (1970).

A Phase III Study of Prednimustine (LEO 1031) in Advanced Breast Cancer. A Preliminary Report

M. Rørth*, J. Løber*, P. Dombernowsky**, D. Krusenstjerna-Hofstrom***, W. Mattsson**** and H. T. Mouridsen*

*Finseninstitute, Copenhagen, Denmark
**Med. Dept. C/T, Bispebjerg Hospital, Copenhagen, Denmark
***Odense Sygehus, Odense, Denmark
****Allmänna Sjukhus, Malmö, Sweden

Correspondence to Mikael Rørth, M.D., Radiumstationen, Finseninstitute, Strandboulevarden 49, DK-2100 Copenhagen Ø, Denmark

Abstract—Prednimustine is an experimental drug with a certain activity in human breast cancer. In this study 61 patients with advanced breast cancer, previously treated with chemotherapy and endocrine therapy were treated in a randomized fashion with a) chlorambucil + prednisolone, b) intermittent prednimustine or c) continuous prednimustine. The response rates in the prednimustine groups were 23% and 21%, respectively, while the response rate in the chlorambucil + prednisolone group was 5%.
  The main toxicity problem was myelosuppression. This was most pronounced in the group receiving continuous prednimustine. Future studies should aim at defining the role of prednimustine in combination chemotherapy.

INTRODUCTION

Prednimustine is a prednisolone-ester of chlorambucil. Theoretically, a conjugation of an alkylating agent with a glucocorticoid molecule should lead to an increased intracellular uptake of the cytotoxic compound maybe selectively in cells with steroid-receptors. Intracellular hydrolysis will liberate the cytotoxic agent, in casu chlorambucil, followed by cell killing because of the high intracellular concentration of the agent (1). Prednimustine is absorbed from the gastrointestinal tract to a varying degree, depending mainly on the general condition of the patient (2). The bio-availability is probably around 50-60% when the compound is given by mouth. The extracellular hydrolysis is limited, and indirect evidence indicate that intracellular concentration and hydrolysis take place.

The drug has been found active in several experimental animal tumours and in human neoplastic diseases (3-6). Notably, activity has been demonstrated in cases, which were clinically resistant to other alkylating agents. A recent phase II study in human breast cancer thus indicated a nearly 40% response rate in patients with advanced disease of which all the premenopausal patients had received at least one line of polychemotherapy (7). Earlier studies (2,5) have shown that prednimustine is fairly well tolerated, giving rise to moderate side effects due to the chlorambucil (mainly myelosuppression) as well as prednisolone.

In view of the earlier reported effect in breast cancer, experimentally and clinically, we have undertaken a study of prednimustine in advanced breast cancer with the objectives 1) to compare the effect of prednimustine with that of chlorambucil and prednisolone given as separate drugs, and 2) to compare the efficacy and toxicity ("therapeutic index") of an intermittent dose schedule with the formerly used continuous dose schedule. The study started in 1978 and is still ongoing. The following report is thus preliminary, and the final conclusions have to await the entrance of more patients and longer observation periods.

MATERIAL AND METHODS

The criteria of eligibility are given in Table 1. The different participating institutions used different combination chemotherapy as first and second line treatment, but most of the patients < 68 years had received treatment with CMF, CMFVP or CAF. Endocrine therapy included in all cases tamoxifen, but in some cases also estrogen or gestagen. The patients were randomized to one of 3 treatment arms:

  I: chlorambucil 8 mg/m^2 + prednisolone 8 mg/m^2 daily
  II: prednimustine 160 mg/m^2 d 1-5, cycle repeated every 3 weeks
  III: prednimustine 40 mg/m^2 daily

The relative doses were adjusted according to hematological toxicity as follows: B-leucocytes 3 · 10^9/1 and thrombocytes 100 · 10^9/1: 100% of dose, B-leucocytes 2-3 · 10^9/1 and/or B-thrombocytes 75-100 · 10^9/1: 50% of dose, B-leucocytes 1-2 · 10^9/1

Table 1. Criteria of eligibility.

1) Advanced breast cancer

2) Measurable and/or evaluable disease

3) Patients ≤ 68 hears resistant to a) one or more lines of polychemotherapy (always
   including an alkylating agent) and to b) endocrine therapy.
   Patients < 68 years resistant to at least one line of endocrine therapy

4) Performance status 3

5) B-leucocytes ≥ 3 · $10^9/1$, B-thrombocytes ≥ 100 · $10^9/1$

6) Verbal informed consent

Table 2. Patient characteristics.

Treatment group	No. randomized	No. evaluable	Median age	Median disease-free interval (years)
I = chlorambucil + prednisolone	25	20	50 (31-75)	1 (0-15)
II = intermittent prednimustine	26	22	57 (29-78)	2.5 (0-10)
III = continuous prednimustine	25	19	57 (30-74)	1.5 (0-25)

Table 3. Preliminary treatment results.

	PD	NC	PR	CR	CR+PR	Median duration of responses (months)
I = chlorambucil + prednisolone	45%	50%	5%	0%	5%	3+
II = intermittent prednimustine	18%	59%	18%	5%	23%	4+
III = continuous prednimustine	53%	26%	21%	0%	21%	4+

PD = progressive disease
NC = no change
PR = partial remission
CR = complete remission

and or B-thrombocytes 50-75 · $10^9/1$: 25% of
dose. More pronounced myelosuppression lead
to temporary discontinuation of treatment.
The response to treatment was evaluated
according to the UICC criteria (8).

RESULTS

So far 76 patients have entered the study,
15 were not evaluable either because of too
short treatment period (9 patients) or
because of death from progressive disease
within the first 2-3 weeks after start of
treatment.
The patient characteristics are shown in
Table 2, and Table 3 summarizes the preliminary evaluation of the treatment results.
Chlorambucil + prednisolone had only marginal activity as only one patient obtained
a partial remission, while the response
rates in regimen II and III were 23 and 21%,
respectively. There is no significant
difference between the response rates in the
2 prednimustine arms, whereas the response
rates for prednimustine treatments are significantly different from the chlorambucil +

prednisolone treatment.
In Table 4 the previous treatments and
responses of the prednimustine responders
are given. Table 5 summarizes responses
related to metastatic sites.
The toxicity due to the chlorambucil moiety
of the prednimustine molecule and to chlorambucil is mainly myelosuppression. Table 6
gives an overview of the registrated nadir
values of B-leucocytes and thrombocytes.
Gastrointestinal toxicity (nausea and
vomiting) was noted in 10-15% of the patients
and was of moderate severity. In no case
was glucosuria recorded. Psychic disturbances (confusion, restlessness) were experienced in all 3 treatment groups (10-15%)
but were generally mild and reversible.

DISCUSSION

Prednimustine has antitumour activity in
advanced breast cancer, however in the present study with a response rate which is
somewhat lower than previously found (7).
The activity of the compound does indeed
seem to be related to its conjugated nature,

Table 4. Previous treatments and responses to that treatment in
patients responding to present treatment.

	1. line	2. line	3. line
I = chlorambucil + prednisolone	1. TAM (CR)		
II = intermittent prednimustine	1. CMCc (CR)	TAM (NC)	DES (NC)
	2. VACM (CR)	TAM (NC)	
	3. CVMF (NC)	CAF (NC)	TAM (NC)
	4. MFV (PR)	CAF (PR)	DES + TAM (PD)
	5. CMFVP (Adj.)	TAM (Adj.)	
III = continuous prednimustine	1. CcMeMP (PD)	CAF (CR)	TAM (PD)
	2. T (NC)	TAM (PD)	
	3. VAC (PD)	TAM (PD)	
	4. TAM + DES (NC)		

TAM = Tamoxifen, C = Cyclophosphamid, M = Methotrexate
Cc = CCNU, DES= diethylstilboestrol, V = Vincristine,
A = Adriamycin, F = 5-Fluoro-uracil, P = Prednisone,
T = Testosteron, Me = Melphalan
Adj. = Adjuvant therapy

Table 5. Response related to metastatic sites.

	Soft tissue	Bones	Viscera
I = chlorambucil + prednisolone	1/17	0/8	0/10
II = intermittent prednimustine	4/13	2/9	0/12
III = continuous prednimustine	4/10	0/8	1/10

Table 6. Haematological toxicity.

Study arm	Nadir values of B-leucocytes ($\times 10^9$/1)				Nadir values of B-thrombocytes ($\times 10^9$/1)			
	3.0	2.0-3.0	1.0-2.0	1.0	100	75-100	50-75	50
I = chlorambucil + prednisolone	35%	35%	25%	5%	65%	5%	20%	10%
II = intermittent prednimustine	32%	54%	9%	5%	73%	9%	9%	9%
III = continuous prednimustine	37%	11%	26%	26%	37%	11%	21%	31%

since the two molecular constituents given as separate drugs have very little activity in breast cancer patients, who previously have received systemic treatment. The hematological toxicity of prednimustine given in an intermittent dose schedule is similar to the toxicity seen with treatment with prednisolone + chlorambucil ("equitoxic treatments"), while continuous prednimustine treatment leads to an undesirably high incidence of severe myelosuppression.

Obviously more firm conclusions should not be drawn before the study has ended. Pre-liminarily, we suggest that prednimustine is a tolerable, reasonably active drug in the treatment of breast cancer. The intermittent dose schedule should probably be used. The more exact role of the compound in the armamentarium of antineoplastic drugs, active in breast cancer must be defined through studies with combination regimes including prednimustine as one of the alkylating agents.

REFERENCES

1. R. Wilkinson, P. O. Gunnarsson, G. Pym-
   Forshell, J. Renshaw and K. R. Harrap,
   The hydrolysis of prednimustine by
   enzymes from normal and tumour tissues.
   Exc. Medica Int. Con. Ser. 420, 260 (1978).

2. I. Könyves, B. Nordenskjöld, G. Pym-
   Forshell, A. de Schryver and H. Westerberg-
   Larsen, Preliminary clinical and absorp-
   tion studies with Prednimustine in
   patients with mammary carcinoma. *Eur. J.
   Cancer* 11, 841 (1975).

3. J. Brandt and I. Könyves, Prednimustine
   in adult acute myeloid leukaemia. *Cancer
   Chemother. Pharmacol.* 2, 133 (1979).

4. B. Fredholm, K. Gunnarsson and J. Müntzing,
   Mammary tumour inhibition and subacute
   toxicity in rats of prednimustine and of
   its molecular components chlorambucil and
   prednisolone. *Acta Pharmacol. Toxicol.*
   42, 159 (1978).

5. K. R. Harrap, P. G. Riches, E. D. Gilby,
   S. M. Sellwood, R. Wilkinson and
   I. Könyves, Studies on the toxicity and
   antitumour activity of prednimustine, a
   prednisolone-ester of chlorambucil.
   Eur. J. Cancer 13, 873 (1977).

6. W. Mattsson, F. von Eyben, I. Turesson
   and S. Wählby, Prednimustine (NSC-134087,
   Leo 1031) treatment of lymphocytic and
   lymphocytic-histiocytic lymphomas.
   Cancer 31, 112 (1978).

7. H. T. Mouridsen, D. Kristensen, J. H.
   Nielsen and P. Dombernowsky, Phase II
   trials of prednimustine, L 1031 (NSC-
   134087) in advanced breast cancer. *Cancer*,
   in press (1979).

8. J. L. Hayward, P. P. Carbone, J.-C.
   Heuson, S. Kumaoka, A. Segaloff and R. D.
   Rubens, Assessment of Response to
   Therapy in Advanced Breast Cancer.
   Europ. J. Cancer 13, 89 (1977).

Variations in Responsiveness and Survival of Clinical Subsets of Patients with Metastatic Breast Cancer to Two Chemotherapy Combinations*

R. V. Smalley* and A. A. Bartolucci**
for the Southeastern Cancer Study Group

*The Department of Medicine, Temple University School of Medicine,
Philadelphia, Pennsylvania, U.S.A.
**The Department of Biostatics, University of Alabama School of Medicine,
Birmingham, Alabama, U.S.A.

Correspondence to R. V. Smalley, The Department of Medicine, Temple University
School of Medicine, 3401 North Broad St., Philadelphia, Pennsylvania 19046, U.S.A.

Abstract—*Two-hundred and thirteen evaluable patients were treated with either a 3 drug combination (CAF) containing doxorubicin or a low dose intermittently administered 5 drug non-doxorubicin containing combination (CMFVP). CAF induced more responses, achieved a greater degree of disease control, induced a greater period of unmaintained response and led to improved survival in patients with loco-regional recurrence, lymph node metastases and/or nodular lung metastases. No superiority for either combination was demonstrable in patients with pleural disease, lymphangitic lung involvement or widespread but predominantly liver metastasis. Patients with metastases confined to bones, although not randomized, achieved a greater degree of disease control with CAF than did patients with other patterns of recurrent or metastatic disease.*

INTRODUCTION

Cytotoxic chemotherapy has been demonstrated to be effective in the management of patients with metastatic breast carcinoma. Combinations of agents have usually been noted to be superior to the use of single agent therapy in terms of response induction (1-5) and improved survival of patients with liver metastasis, (4,5) although other studies have failed to confirms this (6,7). More recently a number of studies have indicated that combinations containing doxorubicin are superior to non-doxorubicin combinations in terms of response induction (8-11) and perhaps in terms of survival; (11) however, these gains have been marginal and have been obtained at the expense of significant added morbidity. An analysis was therefore undertaken of the number of responses, the duration of disease control, including periods of unmaintained response, and the survival of clinical subsets of patients entered into a study in which a three drug doxorubicin combination was compared to a five drug low dose non-doxorubicin combination. The two treatment approaches were evaluated and compared as to their effect on these subsets, separated on the basis of their pattern of recurrent or metastatic disease, in an attempt to determine which, if any might warrant being treated with the doxorubicin combination.

PATIENTS AND METHODS

Two hundred and thirteen evaluable patients were prospectively randomized without stratification to either cyclophosphamide + doxorubicin + 5-fluorouracil (CAF) or cyclophosphamide + methotrexate + 5-fluorouracil + vincristine + prednisone (CMFVP) (Table 1).

All patients had measurable metastatic or recurrent breast carcinoma and had not received prior cytotoxic chemotherapy. Other eligibility criteria are as previously reported (8). Patients with metastasis confined to bone (total - 34) were not randomized and were all treated with CAF. They are in addition to the 213 evaluable patients. All patients were continued on treatment until either progression of disease or until they had completed twenty-four to thirty weeks of treatment (seven to ten doses) at which time treatment was discontinued and the patient followed until progression was evident.

Response criteria are those of the Southeastern Cancer Study Group as previously reported and as amended to conform to the recommendations of the treatment subcommittee of the Breast Cancer Task Force (8). Nearly all patients were evaluated prior to treatment with a physical examination, chest x-ray, liver scan and bone scan as well as a complete blood count and a chemistry screen and were then reevaluated eight to twelve weeks later

---

*Supported in part by grant nos. CA-07961-14 and CA-24456-01 from the National Institutes of Health, Bethesda, Maryland, U.S.A.

Table 1. Treatment regimens.

Treatment A

C	Cyclophosphamide	500 mg/M^2 IV	
A	doxorubicin (Adriamycin^R)	50 mg/M^2 IV	q 21 days
F	5-fluorouracil	500 mg/M^2 IV	× 7-9 courses

Treatment B

C	Cyclophosphamide	400 mg/M^2/wk × 2	
M	Methotrexate	30 mg/M^2/wk × 2	
F	5-fluorouracil	400 mg/M^2/wk × 2	q 28 days
V	Vincristine	1 mg/wk × 2	× 6-7 courses
P	Prednisone	20 mg q.i.d. × 7d	

Table 2. Patterns of recurrence.

Pattern 1	Patients with bone-only metastases
Pattern 2	Patients with loco regional recurrence; may have bone metastases
Pattern 3	Patients with pleural involvement (ipsilateral); may have bone metastases; may have large ulcerative chest wall lesion
Pattern 4A	Patients with pulmonary nodular metastasis; may have bone metastasis
Pattern 4B	Patients with lymphangitic pulmonary metastases
Pattern 5A	Patients with widespread metastases; always with liver metastasis; usually with pulmonary and bone involvement; occasionally with contralateral breast and distant skin involvement
Pattern 5B	Patients presenting with Pattern 1 or 2 and then progressing subsequently (mean 18 mos.) with liver metastasis

for response and then every twelve to twenty-four weeks throughout the course of their disease.

The duration of disease control is defined as that period of time between the onset of treatment and the first evidence of progression of disease. The period of survival in this study is as measured from the onset of treatment. A chi square analysis was used to statistically analyze response rates and other variables in Table 3 and 5 while the Gehan adaptation of the Wilcoxon Test was used to compare the duratation of disease control and survival curves which were plotted by the Kaplan-Meier technique. All p values were computed using a two tailed test of hypothesis.

Patients were divided into 5 major and 2 minor subsets based on their clinical pattern of first recurrence (Table 2) following primary therapy for their breast carcinoma. This is a slight variation of that previously reported (12). Patients with pattern 1 are those presenting with metastases to bone only. Patients with pattern 2 (loco-regional disease) are defined as those presenting with either chest wall recurrence and/or axillary or supraclavicular nodal involvement. An occasional patient also had distal nodal involvement and was included in this group. 50% of these patients also had bone metastasis in addition to loco-regional recurrence. Pattern 3 represents those patients who present with ipsilateral pleural masses and/or pleural effusion. These patients

frequently have bulky, ulcerative chest wall disease in addition and may on occasion present in this manner subsequently developing pleural effusion. Their disease free interval (DFI) is nearly always greater than 30 months while the DFI of patients with pattern 2 is usually less than 24 months (12). One-third of these patients also had bone metastatsis. Patients with pattern 4 present with pulmonary metastasis either nodular (4A) or lymphangitic (4B). Patients with pattern 5A are those presenting with liver metastases. They generally demonstrate widespread metastatic disease in addition to their liver metastasis with pulmonary and/or bone and/or distant skin metastasis usually present. Patients with pattern 5B are those who initially presented with either loco-regional and/or bone metastasis and then subsequently progressed with liver metastasis. This progression usually occured 18-20 months (mean) after initial presentation and followed periods of hormonal and/or radiotherapy.

Patients presenting with Stage III or Stage IV disease and receiving cytotoxic chemotherapy as their primary treatment were also eligible for this study and were therefore entered and randomized. These patients were not subclassified into a pattern of recurrence but are considered separately.

RESULTS

Two hundred and thirteen evaluable patients

Table 3. Treatment results.

	Total	CR	PR	S	%R	%R & S
CAF	107	19	46	19	60%	78%
CMFVP	106	8	36	25	42%	65%
				p = < .05		

CR = complete response   %R = %CR + PR
PR = partial response   %R + S = %CR + PR + S
S = Stable

Table 4. Response (PR + CR) according to pattern of recurrence and treatment.

	CAF			CMFVP		
	No.	R	%	No.	R	%
Pattern 2	27	23	85%	26	14	54%
Pattern 4A	24	12	50%	14	4	28%
Pattern 5B	9	5	55%	8	2	25%
Subtotal	60	40	67%	48	20	42%
Pattern 3	13	5	34%	12	5	40%
Pattern 4B	7	3	42%	9	3	33%
Pattern 5A	10	5	50%	17	7	41%
Subtotal	30	13	43%	38	15	39%
Primary therapy	17	12	71%	20	9	45%
Total	107	65	61%	106	44	42%

No. = Total number of patients.
R   = Response (PR + CR).

were randomized. The overall results are noted in Table 3. CAF induced a significantly greater number of responses than did CMFVP (p = < .05). The effect of treatment on the subsets of patients by pattern of metastasis was next evaluated and the results are listed in Table 4. CAF induced responses in 50% or more patients with patterns 2, 4A, 5A and 5B and in patients receiving chemotherapy as their primary treatment. CMFVP induced responses in 50% or more of patients with pattern 2 only. The duration of disease control (DDC) curves were analyzed by pattern for each treatment modality. CAF induced a DDC with a median in excess of 6 months in patients with patterns 2, 4A, and 5B as well as in patients with pattern 1. For patients treated with CAF, the DDC curve for patients with either pattern 1 or 2 was significantly greater (p = < .02) than for either pattern 3 or 4B while the curve for pattern 4A was greater than for pattern 3 (p = < .03) (curves not shown). Although the DDC curve for pattern 5B overlapped those for patterns 1, 2 and 4A, it was not statistically superior to the curve for either patterns 3 and 4B to the small number of patients. The curve for pattern 5A fell in

between these two groups.

CMFVP induced a DDC with a median in excess of 6 months only in patients with pattern 4A. When all DDC curves for the different patterns in patients treated with CMFVP were compared with each other, no individual superiority could be demonstrated.

Because of the relatively long median DDC for patterns 2, 4A, and 5B achieved with CAF, these patterns were considered together as a "good risk" group and the effect of the two treatment modalities compared with each other in patients with either "good risk" (2, 4A, 5B) or "poor risk" patterns (3, 4B, 5A). Thirty-one of 60 patients with "good risk" patterns receiving CAF maintained disease control through 24-30 weeks of treatment and therefore had their treatment discontinued compared to 15 of 48 receiving CMFVP (P < .05). 22% (13 of 60) of CAF treated patients with "good risk" patterns were still in unmaintained response at one year compared to only 2% (1 of 48) of "good risk" pattern patients receiving CMFVP (P < .005) (Table 5).

The effect of the two treatment arms in inducing unmaintained remission in patients with patterns 3, 4B, 5A and in those

Table 5. Patients with good risk patterns of metastases.
Ability of chemotherapy to induce an unmaintained
response.

Patterns 2, 4A, 5B

	Total	R	Stop therapy	In response at 12 mos.
CAF	60	40	31	13
CMFVP	48	20	15	1

R = Response (PR + CR)
Stop therapy = those patients reaching 24 to 30 weeks of treatment without
disease progression.
In response at 12 mos. = those patients still in response 12 months
after initiating therapy and 6 months after
stopping therapy.

Table 6. Patients with poor risk patterns of metastasis.
Ability of chemotherapy to induce an unmaintained
response.

Pattern 3, 4B, 5A

	Total	R	Stop therapy	In response at 12 mos.
CAF	30	13	7	1
CMFVP	38	15	9	2
Primary therapy				
CAF	17	12	5	2
CMFVP	20	9	1	1
Total	105	49	22	6

receiving chemotherapy as primary therapy is
presented in Table 6.

Less than 25% of these patients were in
disease control 24-30 weeks after starting
chemotherapy and less than 6% remained in
unmaintained remission at 12 months regardless of treatment approach.

The effect of the two treatment modalities
on the DDC and survival of patients with
either "good risk" or "poor risk" patterns
were compared (Figs. 1 and 2).

CAF induced both a longer DDC (P = .008)
and survival (P = .06) in patients with
patterns 2, 4A, 5B but no superiority for
either combination was demonstrable in
patients with poor risk patterns (curves not
shown).

DISCUSSION

Various approaches are available for and
useful in the treatment of metastatic breast
cancer. Cytotoxic chemotherapy initially
utilized as sequential single agent therapy
and more recently as combinations of drugs
with or without doxorubicin has been quite
effective in obtaining palliation and in
prolonging life. Initial and preliminary
reports indicated nondoxorubicin containing

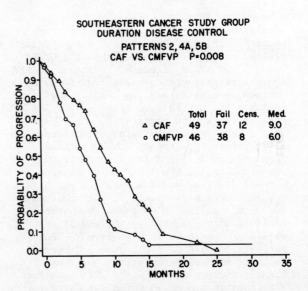

Fig. 1. Duration of disease control curves
for patients with good risk
patterns 2, 4A, 5B receiving
either CAF or CMFVP.

combination therapy induced significantly
more responses than sequentially administered
single agent therapy (1-5) and led to an
improved duration of survival for certain
subsets (4,5). A recent report which
included nearly complete survival data from
two large cooperative group studies confirmed
that only patients with liver metastasis
benefitted with an improved survival from
non-doxorubicin combination chemotherapy
when compared to sequential single agent
therapy (13).

Combinations of three and five drugs containing doxorubicin as one agent have been
utilized more recently and have in general
been found superior to nondoxorubicin containing combinations in their ability to
induce responses (8-11) and to prolong the
duration of disease control (8) and survival
(10). These gains have been, however, at
the expense of increased morbidity and
toxicity. Analyses have been performed in
an attempt to define which prognostic variables may be influential in determining
likelihood of response to chemotherapy
(2,14-16). To date, however, no clear cut
recommendations are available as to the type
of chemotherapy most likely to benefit
subsets of patients with metastatic breast
cancer.

This report subclassifies patients on a
clinical basis and indicates those subsets
which are benefitted by an aggressive doxo-
rubicin-containing combination in terms of
the number of responses, the duration of
disease control, time spent in treatment-
free, disease-free life and in overall
survival from onset of chemotherapy. Those
patients presenting with chest wall recurrence and/or draining lymph node involvement
with or without bone metastasis and those
patients with nodular lung metastasis also
with or without bone metastasis had a 50 to

90% chance or responding, a 50% chance of
maintaining this response through twenty-
four weeks of treatment and a 20% chance of
continuing this response through at least
an additional six months of treatment free
time when treated with CAF. In each of
these parameters, the doxorubicin combination, CAF, was superior to a low dose relatively non-toxic non-doxorubicin containing
combination. Furthermore CAF, although not
directly compared with the CMFVP regimen in
patients with bone only metastasis, induced
clinical response (i.e., loss of pain,
improvement in performance status) in 94% of
patients and induced a symptom-free treatment-
free period in excess of 6 months in over
half.

It is recognized that these subsets of
patients have disease which is biologically
less aggressive, but nevertheless they do
significantly better, both clinically and
statistically, when treated with an aggressive cytotoxic chemotherapeutic approach.
Although the morbidity in terms of nausea
and vomiting, granulocytopenia and alopecia
is greater with CAF than with the intermittent CMFVP approach, the increased survival,
in many instances including a substantial
disease-free treatment-free period of time,
would appear to counter-balance this
increase in morbidity and warrants the recom-
mendation for aggressive chemotherapy in
these patients. It is of interest to note
that patients presenting initially with one
of these good risk patterns but subsequently
progressing with liver metastasis, also
appear to be relatively responsive to and
have a reasonable chance of longterm control
with CAF therapy. This raises the possibility
that there may be a histologic or biochemical means of defining and separating these
groups.

Patients with a "poor risk" subset, i.e.,
either those with lymphangitic pulmonary
spread, those with pleural disease, or those
with widespread metastatic disease, do
equally as well with either intermittent
CMFVP or with CAF and would not therefore
appear to warrant aggressive chemotherapy.
This report represents an interim report
and is an update on the initial report
previously published. Although this study
is now closed, additional patients are undergoing analysis and a final summary is to be
published as the data matures.

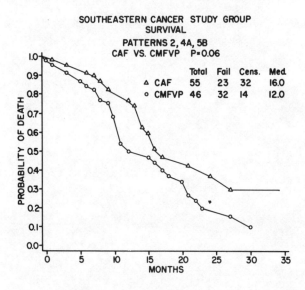

Fig. 2. Survival curves for patients with
        good risk patterns 2, 4A, 5B
        receiving either CAF or CMFVP.

REFERENCES

1. R. V. Smalley, S. Murphy, C. M. Huguley,
   Jr., A. A. Bartolucci, Combination
   versus sequential five-drug chemotherapy
   in metastatic carcinoma of the breast.
   Cancer Research 36, 3911 (1976).
2. G. P. Canellos, S. J. Pocock, S. G.
   Taylor, III, M. E. Sears, D. J. Klaasen
   and P. R. Band, Combination chemotherapy
   for metastatic breast carcinoma. *Cancer*
   38, 1882 (1976).
3. B. Hoogstraten, S. L. George, B. Samal,
   S. E. Rivkin, J. J. Costanzi,

J. D. Bonnet, T. Thigpen and H. Braine, Combination chemotherapy and adriamycin in patients with advanced breast cancer. *Cancer* 38, 13 (1976).

4. R. Chlebowski, L. Irwin, R. Pugh, L. Sadoff, R. Hestorff, J. Weiner and J. Bateman, Survival of patients with metastatic breast cancer treated with either combination or sequential chemotherapy. *Cancer Research* (1978) (Submitted).

5. H. T. Mouridsen, T. Palshof, M. Brahm and I. Rabek. Evaluation of single drug versus multiple drug chemotherapy in the treatment of advanced breast cancer. *Cancer Treatment Rep.* 61, 47 (1977).

6. L. H. Baker, C. B. Vaughn, M. Al-Sarraf, M. L. Reed and V. K. Vaitkivicius, Evaluation of combination versus sequential cytotoxic chemotherapy in the treatment of advanced breast cancer. *Cancer* 33, 513 (1974).

7. R. D. Rubens, R. K. Knight and J. L. Hayward, Chemotherapy of advanced breast cancer: controlled randomized trial of cytoxan versus four-drug combination. *Br. J. Cancer* 32, 730 (1975).

8. R. V. Smalley, J. Carpenter, A. A. Bartolucci, C. Vogel and S. Krauss, A comparison of cyclophosphamide, adriamycin, 5-fluourouracil (CAF) and cyclophosphamide, methotrexate, 5-fluorouracil, vincristine and prednisone (CMFVP) in patients with metastatic breast cancer. *Cancer* 40, 625 (1977).

9. J. M. Bull, D. C. Tormey, S. Li, P. P. Carbone, G. F. Falkson, J. Blom, E. Perlin and R. Simon, Randomized comparative trial of adriamycin versus methotrexate in combination drug therapy. *Cancer* 41, 1649 (1978).

10. D. Tormey, L. Leone, M. Perloff and C. Bloomfield, Evaluation of intermittent versus continuous and of adriamycin versus methotrexate five drug chemotherapy regimens for breast cancer. *Proceedings AACR* 19, 320 (1978).

11. H. B. Muss, D. R. White, F. Richards, M. R. Cooper, J. J. Stuart, D. V. Jackson, L. Rhyne and C. L. Spurr, Adriamycin versus methotrexate in five-drug combination chemotherapy for advanced breast cancer. *Cancer* 42, 2141 (1978).

12. R. V. Smalley, Five clinical patterns of recurrence of Ca of the breast. *Proceedings AACR* 17, 173 (1976).

13. R. Chlebowski, R. Smalley, J. Weiner, L. Irwin, A. Bartolucci and J. Bateman, Combination vs. sequential single agent chemotherapy in advanced breast cancer: relationship between survival and metastatic site. *Proceedings AACR and ASCO* 20, 436 (1979).

14. S. L. George and B. Hoogstraten, Prognostic factors in the initial response to therapy by patients with advanced breast cancer. *J N C I* 60, 731 (1978).

15. P. Valagussa, C. Brambilla and G. Bonadonna, Advanced breast cancer: Are the traditional stratification parameters still of value when patients are treated with combination chemotherapy? *Proceedings AACR* 19, 363 (1978).

16. R. V. Smalley, Prognostic factors indicating likelihood of response to combination chemotherapy in patients with metastatic breast cancer. *Proceedings AACR* 17, 285 (1976).

Adjuvant Systemic Treatment

Trials of Adjuvant Chemotherapy in Breast Cancer. The Experience of the Istituto Nazionale Tumori of Milan*

**A. Rossi, G. Bonadonna, G. Tancini, E. Bajetta, S. Marchini,
P. Valagussa and U. Veronesi**

Istituto Nazionale Tumori, Milan, Italy

Correspondence to G. Bonadonna, Istituto Nazionale Tumori, 20133 Milan, Italy

Abstract—*The paper reviews the strategic approach and the updated results of ongoing adjuvant studies designed for operable breast cancer during the past six years. In the first CMF program (control vs 12 CMF cycles), the 4-year results confirmed that postoperative chemotherapy significantly increased both relapse-free (RFS) and total survival rates. In both pre and post-menopausal women the therapeutic results were influenced by the amount of drug administered. In premenopausal women there was no significant correlation between CMF-induced amenorrhea and RFS. Thus, the schematic concept that the effect of adjuvant chemotherapy is limited to premenopausal patients and that favorable results are primarily due to chemical castration finds no support by our updated results. In the second CMF program the 3-year analysis showed that there was no statistical difference in the RFS and survival rates between patients treated with 12 or 6 cycles, regardless of number of axillary nodes, drug-induced amenorrhea and estrogen receptor status. CMF produced no severe acute or delayed morbidity. In particular, there was no evidence of organ damage nor of increased incidence of second neoplasms. More recent trials were designed in premenopausal women to better define the prognostic importance of bone scan, estrogen receptors and hormone profile as well as to evaluate in postmenopausal patients the efficacy of more intensive drug regimen (CMFP → AV) and of combined chemotherapy-hormone therapy (CMF plus tamoxifen).*

INTRODUCTION

Preliminary results on the value of multi-modal therapy for high-risk patients with operable breast cancer became available during the last few years. Controlled studies testing new combined strategies have consistently reported a significant improvement in the relapse-free (RFS) and total survival, at least for some subsets of patients (1). The importance for regular updating clinical results derives primarily from the need to understand the impact of initital favorable findings on long-term analysis as well as to derive new directions for future trials. Adjuvant studies are long-term experiments but, to a certain extent, intermediate-term results can predict for long-term results.

The scope of this paper is to provide updated results on the adjuvant trials for operable breast cancer being performed at the Istituto Nazionale Tumori during the last six years. The protocol design of more recent adjuvant studies will also be described in order to provide the new lines of therapeutic research selected by our group.

FIRST CMF PROGRAM: CONTROL VS 12 CYCLES

The first CMF adjuvant program was started in Milan on June 1973. Details on study protocol have been described in previous publications (2,3). In short, patients with operable breast cancer (T_1, T_2, T_{3a}, N_0, N_1 according to the International UICC Classification) and histologically positive axillary nodes were randomized to receive either no further treatment (control group) or 12 monthly cycles of CMF after radical (RM) or extended radical mastectomy (ERM). When, in September 1975, patient accrual was discontinued 386 patients were evaluable (179 controls, 207 treated with CMF). Known prognostic variables other than those included in the stratification parameters (age, type of surgery, and number of positive nodes) in particular T extent, histology, and meno-pausal status were comparable between the two treatment groups. Results have been updated as of February 1, 1979, median time on study being 49 months. All patients have been followed for a minimum of 36 months.

*Presented in part at the Second Breast Cancer Working Conference, Copenhagen, May 31 to June 2, 1979.
Supported in part by Contract No. NO1-CM-33714 with DCT, NCI, NIH.

A. Rossi *et al.*

1. Therapeutic Results at Four Years

Table 1 reports the essential data on relapse free and total survival rates in the two treatment groups after four years from surgery.

Adjuvant CMF significantly improved both RFS and total survival irrespective of the extent of axillary node involvement. Adjuvant chemotherapy reduced the incidence of local-regional recurrence (control 11.3%, CMF 8.1%). This was particularly true in premenopausal women (control 10.5%, CMF 6.4%). CMF chemotherapy significantly improved the RFS in women subjected to Halsted RM ($P = 0.004$) and ERM ($P = 0.01$), as well as in patients with negative ($P = 0.09$) and positive ($P = 0.02$) internal mammary lymph nodes. The same applies to RFS in patients with T_{2a} and T_{3a} primary tumor. However, in this particular series the percent difference in RFS of women with T_{1a} lesions was not significant and this was probably due to the limited number of patients with this tumor size (Table 2).

The breakdown of results related to age showed a significant advantage in terms of RFS for all age groups treated with CMF but those of 56-65 and > 65 years (Table 3).

2. Influence of Drug Dosage

The influence of the percent of optimal dose administered in various subsets on RFS was recently evaluated. First of all, it should be recalled that in all patients doses of all three drugs were temporarily reduced 50% in the presence of moderate (Grade 1) marrow suppression detected on day 1 and 8 of each course (1,2,3). Drug dosage was also reduced in the presence of stomatitis (methotrexate, fluorouracil), chemical cystitis (cyclophosphamide) or prolonged gastrointestinal disturbanced (all drugs). Furthermore, 31 of 49 women older than 60-65 years were started on a low dose CMF (cyclophosphamide 100 mg/m^2, methotrexate 30 mg/m^2, fluorouracil 400 mg/m^2). Thus, the total percent of patients receiving more than 75%

Table 1. First CMF program: Comparative percent 4-year relapse-free and total survival (Actuarial analysis as of February 1, 1979).

	Control			CMF			P^o	
	No.	RFS	Surv.	No.	RFS	Surv.	RFS	Surv.
Total	179	47.3	74.0	207	63.1	83.7	0.0001	0.04
1-3 nodes	126	52.7	73.6	140	71.4	88.5	0.0007	0.07
> 3 nodes	53	35.2	57.1	67	44.8	70.4	0.03	0.10

^{o}On time distribution.

Table 2. Comparative percent 4-year relapse-free and overall survival related to tumor extent.

	Control			CMF			P	
	No.	RFS	Surv.	No.	RFS	Surv.	RFS	Surv.
T_{1A}	22	72.4	86.4	18	68.4	94.5	0.46	0.37
T_{2A}	136	45.9	75.7	153	65.4	85.9	< 0.0001	0.04
T_{3A}	21	33.4	55.6	36	50.0	72.0	0.04	0.20

Table 3. Comparative percent 4-year relapse-free and overall survival related to age.

Age (yrs)	Control			CMF			P	
	No.	RFS	Surv.	No.	RFS	Surv.	RFS	Surv.
≤ 35	7	9.5	53.6	15	60.1	80.0	0.05	0.28
36-45	45	50.2	81.7	50	67.5	88.1	0.05	0.29
46-55	63	44.5	69.5	70	67.7	89.2	0.0005	0.006
56-65	34	51.4	78.8	50	60.1	79.7	0.28	0.45
> 65	30	55.6	75.6	22	41.9	65.9	0.25	0.25

of the planned dose for all three drugs was higher in the premenopausal group (67 of 103 or 65%) compared to the postmenopausal group (33 of 104 or 32%).

Figure 1 illustrates that all women receiving ≥ 75% of the optimal dose for each drug showed a higher 4 year RFS (69.6%) compared to women who received a lower dose level (56.0%). Both groups showed a RFS which was superior compared to that of control patients. The same was true for the subgroup of premenopausal women (≥ 75%: 75.2%, < 75%: 58.8%, control: 43.4%) (Fig. 2).

Table 4 presents the results of a similar type of analysis for postmenopausal patients.

Compared to our previous report (4), present findings represent a more detailed analysis on the actual amount of drugs administered. Also in this subgroup the RFS was influenced by the percent of dose administered, although none of the comparative findings was statistically significant. However, it is important to emphasize that in this subset women started on a regular CMF regimen and receiving < 75% of the planned dose as well as those started on a low dose CMF showed a RFS which was similar to that of control women. It should also be noted that within each subset RFS was always related to the extent of nodal involvement. In patients with > 3 nodes and started on low dose CMF the 4-year RFS was low (22.2%)

but not significantly different from the corresponding (women > 3 nodes, age > 60–65 years) control group (41.0%). The reasons for reducing the CMF dose during the courses of treatment were as follows: low dose regimen 44%, drug toxicity 25%, downward adjustment of drugs plus mild toxicity 17%, refusal to complete CMF 14%.

3. Influence of Drug-induced Amenorrhea

As breast cancer is a hormone responsive tumor, hormonal modifications related to drug administration may have therapeutic relevance. Chemotherapy, especially with alkylating agents, is known to produce a high incidence of ovarian failure. The incidence of amenorrhea in premenopausal women given CMF and its relationship with RFS are reported in Table 5.

In the course of CMF therapy 71.6% of menstruating women developed amenorrhea defined as absence of menstrual periods for a minimum of three months. This finding was more frequent in the age group older than 40 years (91.6%). Furthermore, in this group CMF-induced amenorrhea was rarely reversible (4.5%). On the contrary, in 42.9% of women 40 years old or younger normal menstrual function was resumed after temporary amenorrhea. In both age groups, however,

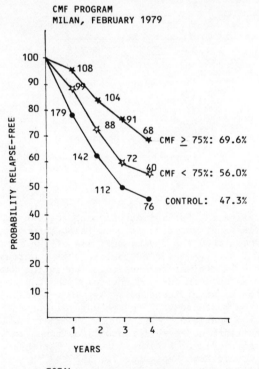

CMF ≥ 75% VS CONTROL P=0.00007
CMF < 75% VS CONTROL P=0.07
CMF ≥ 75% VS CMF < 75% P=0.01

Fig. 1. Four year relapse free survival related to the level of drug dosage (all CMF patients vs controls).

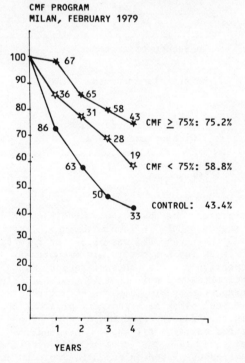

CMF ≥ 75% VS CONTROL P < 0.00001
CMF < 75% VS CONTROL P=0.04
CMF ≥ 75% VS CMF < 75% P=0.05

Fig. 2. Four year relapse free survival related to the level of drug dosage in premenopausal women vs controls.

Table 4. Relapse-free survival in postmenopause related to drug
dosage administered.

Optimal dose	Total		1-3 nodes		> 3 nodes	
	No.	RFS (%)	No.	RFS (%)	No.	RFS (%)
≥ 75%	33/104 (32%)	62.8	22/72 (31%)	67.3	11/32 (34%)	54.4
< 75%	71/104 (68%)	52.2	50/72 (69%)	59.0	21/32 (66%)	41.8
Started on low dose	31/49° (63%)	46.1	22	57.3	9	22.2
Control	93	51.7	66	55.0	27	43.6
		P		P		P
≥ 75% vs control		0.09		0.25		0.20
≥ 75% vs < 75%		0.18		0.29		0.24
≥ 75% vs low dose		0.08		0.31		0.06
< 75% vs control		0.39		0.37		0.46
< 75% vs low dose		0.34		0.44		0.28
Lose dose vs control		0.45		0.47		0.30

°Patients > 60-65 years.

Table 5. CMF-induced amenorrhea in premenopausal patients.
Incidence and relation to relapse-free survival.

	Total	≤ 40 years	> 40 years
Incidence of amenorrhea	58/81 (71.6%)	14/33 (42.4%)	44/48 (91.6%)
Reversible amenorrhea	8/58 (13.8%)	6/14 (42.9%)	2/44 (4.5%)
4-year RFS			
With CMF amenorrhea	73.3%	54.7%°	80.9%°°
Without amenorrhea	56.2%	50.7%°	75.0%°°

° P = 0.26
°°P = 0.43

the presence or absence of amenorrhea failed
to significantly influence the RFS. Furthermore, the 4-year RFS was 58.3% for reversible
and 76.9% for non reversible amenorrhea,
respectively. Also this difference was not
statistically significant (P = 0.28). Finally,
therapeutic ovariectomy was effective also in
women relapsing after surgery plus CMF and
this occurred irrespective of CMF-induced
amenorrhea (4). All above-mentioned results
seem to exclude that drug-induced ovarian
suppression played an essential role in the
therapeutic effectiveness of adjuvant CMF.

Since overall survival is also influenced
by treatments administered after first treatment failure, Table 6 shows that secondary
therapies after first relapse were comparable
between the two treatment groups.

SECOND CMF PROGRAM: 12 VS 6 CYCLES

The study was designed with the intent to

define the optimal duration of adjuvant CMF.
The study was discontinued in postmenopausal
women when the 3-year analysis of the first
CMF program revealed that in this subgroup
the initial difference observed in the failure
rate between CMF and control group was no
longer significant (3). Within 2-4 weeks
from mastectomy 325 premenopausal patients
with operable breast cancer and positive
axillary nodes were randomly assigned to
receive 12 or 6 cycles of CMF. Patients were
accrued from September 11, 1975 to May 31,
1978. Nearly 70% of women had a T_{2a} lesion
and nearly 60% of patients had 1-3 positive
nodes. Data were analyzed as of March 15,
1979. Median follow up was 22 months (12
CMF) and 21 months (6 CMF). The essential
findings of the 3-year analysis are reported
in Table 7.

There was no statistical difference in
RFS and overall survival between patients
treated with 12 and 6 cycles, regardless of
size of primary tumor and number of involved

Table 6. First CMF program. Therapies applied at first relapse.

Secondary therapy	Primary therapy			
	RM		RM + CMF	
	No.	%	No.	%
Total with metastases[o]	88		72	
Polychemotherapy	61	69	42	58
Monochemotherapy	1	1	1	1
Endocrine therapy	19	22	22	31
Local radiotherapy	3	3	3	4
Supportive therapy only	4	5	4	6
Second breast tumors[o]	4		2	
Mastectomy ± chemotherapy	3		2	
Radiotherapy → hormone therapy	1[oo]		–	

[o] Within 4 years from mastectomy.
[oo]Locally advanced breast cancer.

Table 7. Second CMF program: 12 vs 6 cycles in premenopausal
women. Comparative 3-year relapse free and total
survival (Actuarial analysis as of March 15, 1979).

	Mastectomy + 12 CMF (%)	Mastectomy + 6 CMF (%)	p[o]
Total RFS	85.4	82.6	0.29
1-3 nodes	92.3	88.3	0.22
> 3 nodes	69.7	71.0	0.45
Total survival	86.2	85.1	0.49

[o]On time distribution.

axillary nodes (5). The analysis also showed
that CMF-induced amenorrhea occurred more
often in patients treated with 12 cycles
(90%) compared to patients given 6 cycles
(70%). However, the percent of women with
reversible amenorrhea was comparable between
the two treatment groups (10% vs 11%). In
both groups the 3-year RFS was not statistically influenced by CMF-induced amenorrhea.
The RFS was also not significantly influenced
by the estrogen receptor status. This was
true for both nodal subgroup as well as for
women with and without CMF-induced amenorrhea
(5). The findings confirm the limited therapeutic importance of "chemical castration".

ACUTE AND DELAYED TOXICITY OF CMF

Acute toxic manifestations of CMF have
been described in details in previous publications (1,2,3). Myelosuppression was the
most common side effect. However, severe
myelosuppression associated to infective
and hemorragic complications has never
occurred. Gastrointestinal disturbances
and stomatitis were mild to moderate
in degree. Various degrees of hair loss

were fairly common, but complete alopecia
was less than 10%. As discussed before,
amenorrhea was frequently reported in menstruating women. Endocrine studies demonstrated that menstrual changes were of ovarian
origin (6,7).

As far as late toxic signs are concerned,
neither chronic organ damage nor increased
incidence of second cancers has so far been
observed. In particular, chronic liver
damage secondary to methotrexate administration was not evident. Investigations to
detect possible minor liver abnormalities
are in progress. Whereas no second neoplasm
was observed in patients treated with the
second CMF program, in the first CMF study
3 women in the control group and 4 women in
the CMF group, respectively, developed a
second solid tumor other than breast carcinoma. No acute leukemia was so far
observed.

Table 8 schematically reports the observed
incidence of second (contralateral) breast
carcinoma and second non breast carcinoma,
respectively. Second neoplasms other than
breast cancer included cervical carcinoma
(in situ), melanoma and leiomyoblastoma of
uterus in the group treated with radical

Table 8. Second breast and non breast tumors.

Primary Therapy	Breast ca.	Non breast ca.
RM	4 (2.2%)	3 (1.7%)
RM + CMF	2 (1.0%)	4 (1.9%)

mastectomy and gastric carcinoma (2 cases), cystosarcoma phyllodes and pancreatic carcinoma in the group given adjuvant CMF, respectively. Three of four neoplasms observed so far in the chemotherapy group developed in women who, because of refusal, received a minimal amount (3-4 cycles) of CMF. This fact minimizes the possibility that tumors were drug-induced (4).

OTHER ONGOING ADJUVANT STUDIES

Preliminary and intermediate results of the first and second CMF program provided the basis for current adjuvant studies at the Istituto Nazionale Tumori. For premenopausal women a prospective trial was actived on June 1, 1978 with the intent to better define the prognostic significance of estrogen receptor status, bone scan and endocrine profile in women treated with 12 cycles of CMF. So far, 72 patients were accrued.

For postmenopausal women the attempt is to overcome the limits of current adjuvant programs by testing the efficacy of a more intensive chemotherapy regimen. Only postmenopausal women less than 65 years old were considered eligible for this trial. The rationale of the study is mainly based on the concept that selection and overgrowth of drug resistant tumor cells is the major cause of chemotherapy failure (H. Skipper, unpublished data). With the intent to overcome selective drug resistance, the chemotherapy program includes two non cross-resistant combinations administered sequentially for a total of ten cycles (CMFP 6 cycles → AV 4 cycles). Furthermore, the effect of progressive dose intensification is randomly compared to conventional dose schedule in order to test in the clinic the mathematical hypothesis of tumor cell kinetics proposed by Norton and Simon (8). Nearly 100 patients entered the study so far. In postmenopausal women older than 65 years the current therapy program includes 12 cycles of CMF plus tamoxifen (20 mg/day for one year). More than 60 patients have entered into the study. Due to the short period of observation for all above mentioned studies, no meaningful data can be provided. Finally, a fourth protocol is devoted to pre and postmenopausal women with T_1 primary lesion. Since March 1976 T_1 patients entering the randomized study of Halsted RM versus quadrantectomy plus axillary dissection and radiotherapy to the breast were given 12 cycles of adjuvant CMF when found to have histologically positive axillary nodes (9). The theraputic results of CMF in this particular subgroup of patients are under evaluation. Should conservative surgery plus radiotherapy followed by adjuvant CMF be confirmed effective in T_1N+ lesions at the 5-year analysis, the results will provide the baseline for a similar strategic approach to be applied in selected T_2N+ tumors.

CONCLUSIONS

The updated results of the two CMF programs confirm that postoperative chemotherapy when applied to patients with high-risk of minimal residual disease can improve both relapse free and total survival rates over optimal curative surgery. Thus the strategy of combined therapy proved to be correct and needs now to be further expanded and improved. The results of other studies (10,11,12,13,14) are in line with this conclusion. Progress analysis allows to revisit specific aspects of given series, detect new findings and raise new questions. The most important aspect of present analysis is that CMF is indeed active also in postmenopausal women provided the amount of dose administered is reasonably high. For a number of reasons, but especially because of the extreme caution with which combination chemotherapy was administered during our first adjuvant experience, only 32% of postmenopausal women did receive ≥ 75% of the optimal dose. In fact, after the first year of study, to minimize possible side effects in elderly patients the initial dose of methotrexate and fluorouracil were reduced in women older than 60-65 years. However, in reality severe leukopenia and thrombocytopenia were never a problem. It was primarily the planned conservative attitude of protocol modification and of research physicians the major factors yielding to a higher number of postmenopausal patients who received < 75% of the optimal dose compared to premenopausal patients. Although there is no statistically significant difference between RFS of women receiving ≥ 75% and either those given < 75% of the optimal dose or those started on the low-dose CMF, in our opinion the trend is enough to alert physicians that a dose-response relationship also must exist in an adjuvant setting. The analysis of other trials will further elucidate this important aspect. Most probably other, yet undefined, biological reasons could be involved in the fact that postmenopausal women (even those given > 75% of the optimal dose) responded less to adjuvant CMF compared to premenopausal women (e.g. high incidence of tumors with low growth fraction, selective drug resistance, endocrine factors).

About concomitant endocrine factors, present analysis definitely rules out the hypothesis that chemical castration played an important role in the therapeutic effect of CMF in premenopausal women. Not only was amenorrhea not correlated with RFS in both CMF studies, but in the second CMF program the free interval was not significantly influenced by the estrogen receptor status and this occurred regardless of nodal sub-group with or without drug-induced amenorrhea. These clinical findings cannot exclude that in some women the therapuetic benefit of adjuvant CMF was also exerted through ovarian suppression. However, chemical castration probably represented only a minor therapeutic effect of adjuvant combination chemotherapy. The results of other studies utilizing a variety of therapeutic regimens (10,12,13, 14) also support our conclusions from this point of view since no difference is being observed in the RFS of pre versus postmeno-pausal women.

The lack of significant differences in the 3-year RFS and overall survival between the groups of patients treated with 6 and 12 CMF cycles raises once more the unsolved problem of optimal duration of adjuvant treatment. Present results with 6 cycles appear encouraging but they should not yet be considered mature to recommend the routine use of 6 cycles instead of 12 cycles. How-ever, there could be the possibility that there is not much to gain by prolonging treat-ment with the same chemotherapy (provided the dose levels were sufficiently high) beyond the sixth month. Theoretically, after this length of time it would be more impor-tant to apply a non-cross resistant regimen to affect neoplastic cells resistant to the first treatment. Should the 4-year analysis confirm that there is no signifi-cant difference between 6 and 12 cycles, sequential combination chemotherapy (e.g. CMF → AV) will be tested in the attempt to further improve present results. This strategy is currently being applied in our Institute for postmenopausal patients. Adriamycin remains today the most effective single agent in the treatment of advanced breast cancer. An adriamycin-containing regimen could also be applied in an adjuvant setting provided the study is carried out, under strictly controlled basis, by research institutions or research groups and the total dose for this agent does not expose poten-tially curable patients to the risk of cardio-myopathy. In our current regimen for post-menopausal women (6 cycles of CMFP followed by 4 cycles of AV) the total dose of adriamy-cin does not exceed 250 mg/m^2. Similar cautious attitudes are followed in trials conducted elsewhere (12,13). Adjuvant treat-ment with non-cross resistant combinations would also limit the prolonged administration of alkylating agents and, therefore, minimize the potential risk for treatment-induced second neoplasms, especially acute leukemia (15,16).

Present experience with adjuvant chemo-therapy has immensely contributed to develop a strategic attitude for primary breast cancer. Although present results indicate that both RFS and total survival were significantly improved by most of the current drug regimens, much remains to be done to further improve current results and to trans-late present findings into wide clinical application. These goals can be achieved only through prospective controlled clinical trials. We fully support the appeal of Edelstyn et al. (17): "Whatever our own personal prejudices and doubts, it is only in supporting trials that facts can be sub-stituted for opinion. Non-participation in clinical trials is a decision not to contri-bute to medical progress and this, surely, is morally, if not professionally, indefen-sible."

ACKNOWLEDGEMENT

The authors wish to thank T. Busacca, T. Pulejo and R. Terulla for their effective cooperation during the follow up of study patients as well as Drs. J. L. Hayward and R. D. Rubens from Guy's Hospital, London, for critically reviewing the 165 patients alleged to have recurred as of November 1978 (first CMF program).

REFERENCES

1. G. Bonadonna, P. Valagussa, A. Rossi, R. Zucali, G. Tancini, E. Bajetta, C. Brambilla, M. De Lena, G. Di Fronzo, A. Banfi, F. Rilke and U. Veronesi, Are surgical adjuvant trials altering the course of breast cancer? *Seminars Oncol.* 5, 450 (1978).
2. G. Bonadonna, E. Brusamolino, P. Vala-gussa, A. Rossi, L. Brugnatelli, C. Bram-billa, M. De Lena, G. Tancini, E. Bajetta, R. Musumeci and U. Veronesi, Combination chemotherapy as an adjuvant treatment in operable breast cancer. *N. Engl. J. Med.* 294, 405 (1976).
3. G. Bonadonna, A. Rossi, P. Valagussa, A. Banfi and U. Veronesi, The CMF program for operable breast cancer with positive axillary nodes. Updated analysis on the disease-free interval site of relapse and drug tolerance. *Cancer (Philad.)* 39, 2904 (1977).
4. G. Bonadonna, P. Valagussa, A. Rossi, G. Tancini, E. Bajetta, S. Marchini and U. Veronesi, CMF adjuvant chemotherapy in operable breast cancer. In *Adjuvant Therapy of Cancer II* (Edited by S. E. Salmon and S. E. Jones) Grune & Stratton, New York (1979, in press).
5. G. Tancini, E. Bajetta, S. Marchini, P. Valagussa, G. Bonadonna and U. Vero-nesi, Operable breast cancer with positive axillary nodes (N+): results of 6 vs 12 cycles of adjuvant CMF in pre-menopausal women. *Prod. Am. Assoc. Cancer Res.* 20, 172 (1979).
6. D. P. Rose and T. E. Davis, Ovarian function in patients receiving adjuvant chemotherapy for breast cancer. *Lancet* 1, 1174 (1977).
7. C. Recchione and A. Rossi, Hormonal study in patients developing amenorrhea

during chemotherapy for breast cancer.
Tumori 65, 93 (1979).

8. L. Norton and R. Simon, Tumor size,
sensitivity to therapy, and design of
treatment schedules. *Cancer Treat. Rep.*
61, 1307 (1977).

9. U. Veronesi, Value of limited surgery for
breast cancer. *Seminars Oncol.* 5, 395
(1978).

10. B. Fisher, Breast Cancer: studies of the
National Surgical Adjuvant Primary Breast
Cancer Project (NSABP), In *Adjuvant
Therapy of Cancer II* (Edited by S. E.
Salmon and S. E. Jones) Grune & Stratton,
New York (1979, in press).

11. D. L. Ahmann, W. S. Payne, P. W. Scanlon,
J. R. O'Fallon, H. F. Bisel, R. G. Hahn,
J. H. Edmonson, J. N. Ingle, S. Frytak,
M. J. O'Connell and J. Rubin, Repeated
adjuvant chemotherapy with phenylalanine
mustard or 5-fluorouracil, cyclophosphamide, and prednisone with or without
radiation, after mastectomy for breast
cancer. *Lancet* 1, 983 (1978).

12. A. U. Budzar, G. R. Blumenschein, J. U.
Gutterman, C. K. Tashima, G. N.
Hortobagyi, T. L. Smith, L. T. Campos,
W. L. Wheeler, E. M. Hersh, E. J.
Freireich and E. A. Gehan, Postoperative
adjuvant chemotherapy with 5-fluorouracil,
adriamycin, cyclophosphamide and BCG.
A follow-up report. *JAMA* (1979, in press).

13. A. G. Wendt, S. E. Jones, S. E. Salmon,
G. F. Giordano, R. A. Jackson, R. S.
Miller, R. S. Heusinkveld, T. E. Moon,
Adjuvant treatment of breast cancer with
adriamycin-cyclophosphamide with or
without radiation therapy. In *Adjuvant
Therapy of Cancer II* (Edited by S. E.
Salmon and S. E. Jones) Grune & Stratton,
New York (1979, in press).

14. H. Glucksberg, S. E. Rivkin and
S. Rasmussen, Adjuvant chemotherapy for
Stage II Breast Cancer: a comparison of
CMFVP versus L-PAM. In *Adjuvant Therapy
of Cancer II* (Edited by S. E. Salmon and
S. E. Jones) Grune & Stratton, New York
(1979, in press).

15. H. J. Lerner, Acute myelogenous leukemia
in patients receiving chlorambucil as
long-term adjuvant chemotherapy for
Stage II breast cancer. *Cancer Treat.
Rep.* 62, 1135 (1978).

16. P. Valagussa, R. Kenda, F. Fossati-
Bellani, F. Franchi, A. Banfi, F. Rilke
and G. Bonadonna, Incidence of second
malignancies in Hodgkin's disease after
various forms of treatment. *Proc. Am.
Soc. Clinical Oncol.* 20, 360 (1979).

17. G. A. Edelstyn and K. D. Macrae, Trials
of adjuvant chemotherapy in breast cancer.
Lancet 1, 324 (1979).

Adjuvant Chemotherapy with Chlorambucil and 5-fluorouracil in Primary Breast Cancer (Cooperative Study Heidelberg)

M. Kaufmann[1], D. V. Fournier[1], H. Sievers[2], I. Staib[3],
P. Wöllgens[4], R. Nedden[5], H. Lochbühler[6], W. Queisser[7],
D. Christmann[8], R. Bühner[9], P. J. Pfuhl[10], B. Henningsen[11],
H. Kuttig[12], S. Wysocki[13], D. Thüre[14], C. Köhler[15] and
P. Drings[9]

[1]Univ.-Frauenklinik Heidelberg (Director: Prof. Dr. F. Kubli)
[2]Med. Kliniken I. II Darmstadt (Prof. Dr. Anschütz, Prof. Dr. T. Pfleiderer)
[3]Städt. Kliniken Darmstadt, Chir. Klinik (Prof. Dr. I. Staib)
[4]Radiologie II im Strahleninstitut der Städt. Krankenanstalten Darmstadt (Dr. P. Wöllgens)
[5]Elisabethen-Krankenhaus Chirurg. Klinik Darmstadt (Dr. A. Hüffell) and Med.
Klinik (Prof. Dr. T. Fuchs)
[6]Chir. Univ.-Klinik Heidelberg - Mannheim (Director: Prof. Dr. M. Trede)
[7]Onkologisches Zentrum der Städt. Krankenanstalten Mannheim (Prof. Dr. W. Queißer)
[8]Geburtsch.-Gynökolog. Abt. des Diakonie-Krankenhauses, Schwäbisch Hall (Prof. Dr. R. Blobel)
[9]Med.-Univ.-Klinik Heidelberg (Director: Prof. Dr. Drs. h.c. G. Schettler)
[10]Marienkrankenhaus, Chir. Abteilung Darmstadt (Dr. Dr. H. Strack) and
Gynäkolog. Geburtsch. Abt. (Dr. P. J. Pfuhl)
[11]Chir. Univ.-Klinik Heidelberg (Director: Prof. Dr. Drs. h.c. F. Linder)
[12]Univ.-Strahlenklinik Heidelberg (Director: Prof. Dr. K. zum Winkel)
[13]Chirurg. Abt. des Krankenhauses Salem, Heidelberg (Prof. Dr. St. Wysocki)
[14]Alice-Hospital Chirurg. Abt. Darmstadt (Dr. Paulus) Innere Abt. (Dr. D. Thüre)
[15]Institut für Dokumentation, Information und Statistik am DKFZ Heidelberg
(Director: Prof. Dr. G. Wagner)

Correspondence to Prof. Dr. P. Drings, Krankenhaus Rohrbach, Klinik für
Thoraxerkrankungen, D 6900 Heidelberg, Federal Republic of Germany

Abstract—One hundred patients (pts.) (age $\leq$ 65) with primary breast cancer
and histologically positive axillary lymph nodes ($T_{0-3}N_{1-2}M_0$) were evaluated
by a prospective, randomized, clinical cooperative study. Primary treatment
was modified radical mastectomy and radiotherapy followed by either observation only (47 pts.) or prolonged adjuvant chemotherapy (chlorambucil =
CLB/fluorouracil = 5 FU) orally for two years in six-week intervals (53 pts.).
After 24 months (Nov. 1976 - Nov. 1978) treatment failures occured in
20.8 per cent (11/53) of the control patients, and in 12.8 per cent (6/47)
of the patients with adjuvant chemotherapy. In women age $\leq$ 50 years treatment failure is 16.7% (5/30) of the treated vs. 31.3% (10/32) of the
control group. The mean time of appearance of recurrance is 13.8 vs. 9.7
months in the control population.

Toxicity was minimal.

The observed preliminary trends with benefit to women age $\leq$ 50 are in
agreement with other earlier and more extensive studies. Long term effects
and prolonged survival rates for this drug regimen, however, remain to be
determined.

INTRODUCTION

Adjuvant breast cancer treatment is a
challenging problem in cancer treatment
today. In the past few years many randomized adjuvant chemotherapy studies with
different treatment regimens were started
and are going on (1-7). Only a few, however,
have controlled follow-up more than four
years (8-11).

On the basis of the known data in 1976
we started a prospective controlled adjuvant
trial with various Departments of the University Hospital of Heidelberg and regional
hospitals. In this study we have compared
the results of mastectomy and radiotherapy
with or without interval adjuvant chemotherapy. A drug regimen was chosen, which
seemed to be appropriate for easy application
with minimal toxicity.

MATERIAL AND METHODS

1. Patients Selection

Of 113 randomized patients entered in the
study since November 1976, 100 were evaluable
and were willing to take part in this clinical
trial. All patients who had potentially
curable breast carcinoma had modified radical mastectomies followed by radiotherapy
(^{60}Co 4.500 rads to supraclavicular, parasternal (when localized medially) and axillary areas without chest wall; begin of
radiation 2 weeks post mastectomy). Extent
of primary tumor and axillary -lymph node
metastases as entry criteria were $T_{0-3}N_{1-2}$
(histologically positive M_0 (TNM staging
system, UICC). Criteria for ineligibility
were as follows: age > 65, pregnant or lactating, previous or concurrant second cancer,
serum creatinine > 1,5 mg/dl, WBC < 2.500,
platelets < 150.000, bilirubin > 4 mg/per
100 ml, chemotherapy begin > 6 weeks of
mastectomy, bilateral breast cancer.

2. Drug Treatment Administration

The 2-drug combination chemotherapy
consisted of a orally given cyclic administration of chlorambucil (CLB: day 1-14) and
5-fluorouracil (5 FU: day 1,8,15). The first
cycle started between 4-6 weeks post mastectomy. The next cycle was started after a
four-week rest period, and the regimen is
continued in the same sequence for two
years.

> 150.000; 50%: WBC 4-2.500, platelets
150-100.000; therapy stop: WBC < 2.500,
platelets < 100.000).

4. Study Parameters

The patients were assessed by physical
examination every six weeks. X-ray (chest:
PA and lateral) and scan examination (bone,
liver) were performed every six months.
Suspicious osseous lesions were controlled
by X-rax studies and liver lesions by sono-
graphy. Blood chemical studies (bilirubin,
SGPT, alkaline phosphatase, serum calcium,
BUN or serum creatinine) were carried out
every six weeks; HGB, WBC and platelets
every two weeks.

5. End Point

Treatment failure is the major point of
this trial, which is defined as presence of
tumor in loco-regional or distant sites.
Loco-regional recurrence has to be confirmed
by biopsy and pathological examination, distant recurrance by X-ray or radioisotopic
evidence.

6. Statistical Analysis

To determine the significance of treatment
failures the chi-square-test was calculated
in each subgroup of patients. The comparison
of the failure-time distribution in both

Table 1. Preliminary results (Nov. 76-Nov. 78) of the
Heidelberg Cooperative Breast Cancer Adjuvant Study:
Characteristics of 53 control patients and 47 patients
treated with chlorambucil (CLB) and 5-fluorouracil (5 FU)

	Control (No. of relapses/No. treated) (%)	CLB/5 FU (No. of relapses/No. treated) (%)
Total	11/53 (20.8)	6/47 (12.8)
Mean follow-up period (months)	12.4	10.8
Mean time of relapse (months)	9.7	13.8
Age		
≤ 50	10/32 (31.3)	5/30 (16.7)
> 50	1/21 (4.8)	1/17 (5.9)
Stage		
T_1	3/14 (21.4)	2/20 (10.0)
T_2	7/34 (20.6)	4/20 (20.0)
T_3	1/5 (20.0)	0/7 (0)

3. Dose Modifications

Dose modifications were done according to
body weight (≤ 70 kg: CLB: 5 mg, 5 FU:
500 mg; > 70 kg: CLB: 7,5 mg, 5 FU: 750 mg
and according to haematologic toxicity
(calculated dose 100%: WBC > 4.000, platelets

groups was carried out by the log rank test
(12). Further on a failure time regression
model (13) with prognostic factors was
applied.

RESULTS

L. Effect of Treatment

Out of 100 patients evaluable 53 (age: $\leq$ 50 yr = 32, > 50 yr = 21) were observed after radiotherapy without further treatment 47 women (age: $\leq$ 50 yr = 30, > 50 yr = 17) were given CLB/5 FU. Table 1 shows the results summarized for all patients. Of 53 control patients 11 (= 20,8%) have relapsed, whereas 6 (= 12,8%) of the 47 patients treated with CLB/5 FU relapsed. The difference in patients $\leq$ 50 in the total rate of treatment failure (31,3% vs. 16,7%) is striking, but not significant ($p = 0,2$), whereas relapses in patients age > 50 (4,8% vs. 5,9%) are without different trends.

The mean time until relapse was also different (9,7 control group vs. 13,8 months treated group). Treatment-failure time distribution for all patients is presented in Fig. 1.

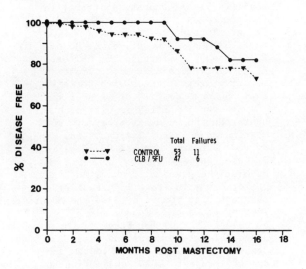

Fig. 1. Treatment-failure time distribution in all evaluable patients (statistical analysis: log rank test).

2. Site of Recurrence

In spite of radiotherapy, the most frequent initial relapses seen, were loco-regional recurrences (control group: 8 ipsilateral chest wall, 2 lymph nodes recurrences vs. treated group: 2 ipsilateral chest wall recurrences). 4 distant recurrences (3 bone, 1 lung metastases) were documented in the CLB/5 FU group, and only 1 liver metastasis in the control group.

3. Toxicity

Chemotherapy was well tolerated in all patients without any severe toxicities. Nausea was documented once, and vomiting in 3 cases. Not a single case of loss of hair or infection was seen. WBC < 3.000 was limited to 5 patients without thrombocytopenia < 100.000. No toxicity was stated in 94 patients.

DISCUSSION

In this trial lymph node positive breast cancer patients with CLB/5 FU adjuvant chemotherapy following mastectomy and radiotherapy show longer disease free intervals. Benefit of this therapy regimen is obvious in women $\leq$ 50 years, but statistical significance is not stated, neither for all the women, nor for subgroups.

Our findings are according to those of other authors (10,11,14-17), who found a significant benefit in premenopausal and young women. The results, however, are contradictionary to other reports (8,9,18-23), who described equivalent benefit in pre- and postmenopausal patients. Till now the cytotoxic suppressive effect of adjuvant chemotherapy on ovarian hormonal function remains unsolved.

The orally administered adjuvant chemotherapy regimen is appropriate for easy application and shows no severe toxicities.

The only long term results with relatively mild adjuvant chemotherapy are those of Nissen-Meyer et al. (8,9), who found a significant difference of recurrences in patients also 12 years after adjuvant chemotherapy treatment. However, the basic difference between the Scandinavian and this trial is beginning of the adjuvant chemotherapy. This regimen was started immediately intra- and postoperatively for a short time; our regimen starts immediately post radiotherapy, respectively during the rest period of postoperative administered radiotherapy for a longer period.

Till now long term effects of postoperative adjuvant chemotherapy are unknown problems, because observation time of the ongoing studies is too short. Optimal cytotoxic drug combinations with tolerable side effects, as well as duration and time of application of adjuvant chemotherapy are unsolved questions in breast cancer patients (24).

To make further progress, stratification should be done according to clinical and histological stage and prognostic factors, e.g. age, obesity, menopausal status, lymph node status, cytotoxic chemoresistance (25) and steroid hormone receptor content (26).

REFERENCES

1. V. T. DeVita, Jr., Carcinoma of the breast: Status of adjuvant medical treatment. In *Breast Cancer. Frontiers in Radiation Therapy of Oncology*. (Edited by J. M. Vaeth), Vol. 11, p. 42. Karger, Basel (1976).
2. C. G. Schmidt, Adjuvante chemotherapie beim mammakarzinom. *Med. Welt (Stuttg.)* 27, 1033 (1976).
3. Multicentre Breast Cancer Chemotherapy Group, Multimodal therapy for histological stage - II breast cancer. *Lancet* II, 396 (1977).

4. S. E. Salmon and S. E. Jones, *Adjuvant Therapy of Cancer*. Elsevier/North Holland, Biomed. Press, Amsterdam (1977).

5. M. Kaufmann, F. Kubli, P. Drings and G. Lammers, Zur adjuvanten (prophylaktischen) postoperativen Chemotherapie beim Mammakarzinom. *Dtsch. med. Wschr.* 103, 1881 (1978).

6. Eastern Cooperative Oncology Group (ECOG), Protocol EST 5177: "An adjuvant clinical trial to compare CMF to CMF P with or without tamoxifen in premenopausal women with stage II breast cancer." Jan. 1978.

7. Ludwig Breast Cancer Studies I, II, III, IV: Search for optimal adjuvant therapies, combining hormone and chemotherapy, in operable breast cancers. Study protocol. July 1978.

8. R. Nissen-Meyer, K. Kjelligren, K. Malmio, B. Mansson and T. Norin, Surgical adjuvant chemotherapy. *Cancer* (Philad.) 41, 2088 (1978).

9. R. Nissen-Meyer, One short chemotherapy course in primary breast cancer: 12-year follow-up in series 1 of the Scandinavian Adjuvant Chemotherapy Study Group. Abstract, Int. Conference on the Adjuvant Therapy of Cancer, Tucson (1979).

10. Breast Cancer: Studies of the National Surgical Adjuvant Primary Breast Cancer Project (NSABP). Abstract, Int. Conference on the Adjuvant Therapy of Cancer, Tucson (1979).

11. G. Bonadonna, A. Rossi, G. Tancini, E. Bajetta and P. Valagussa, CMF adjuvant chemotherapy in operable breast cancer. Abstract, Int. Conference on the Adjuvant Therapy of Cancer, Tucson (1979).

12. R. Peto, M. C. Pike, P. Armitage, N. E. Breslow, D. R. Cox, S. V. Howard, N. Mantel, K. McPherson, J. Peto and P. G. Smith, Design and analysis of randomized clinical trials requiring prolonged observation of each patient. II. Analysis and examples. *Brit. J. Cancer* 35, 1 (1977).

13. D. R. Cox, Regression models and life tables (with discussion). *J. Roy. Statist. Soc.* B 34, 187 (1972).

14. B. Fisher, P. Carbone, S. G. Economou, R. Frelick, A. Glass, H. Lerner, C. Redmond, M. Zelen, P. Band, D. L. Katrych, N. Wolmark and E. R. Fisher (and other cooperating investigators), L-Phenylalanine mustard (L-PAM) in the management of primary breast cancer. *New Engl. J. Med.* 292, 117 (1975).

15. G. Bonadonna, E. Brusamolino, P. Valagussa, A. Rossi, L. Brugnatelli, C. Brambilla, M. De Lena, G. Tancini, E. Bajetta, R. Musumeci and U. Veronesi, Combination chemotherapy as an adjuvant treatment in operable breast cancer. *New Engl. J. Med.* 294, 405 (1976).

16. D. L. Ahmann, W. S. Payne, P. W. Scanlon, J. R. O'Fallon, H. F. Bisel, R. G. Hahn, J. H. Edmonson, J. N. Ingle, S. Frytak, M. J. O'Connell and J. Rubin, Repeated adjuvant chemotherapy with phenylalanine mustard or 5-fluorouracil, cyclophosphamide and prednisone with or without radiation, after mastectomy for breast cancer. *Lancet*, I 893 (1978).

17. D. Tormey, G. Falkson, R. Weiss, M. Perloff, O. Glidewell and J. F. Holland, Postoperative chemotherapy with/without immunotherapy for mammary carcinoma. Abstract, Int. Conference on the adjuvant therapy of cancer, Tucson (1979).

18. A. U. Buzdar, J. V. Gutterman, G. R. Blumenschein, G. N. Hortobagyi, C. K. Tashima, L. T. Campos, T. L. Smith, E. M. Hersh, E. J. Freireich, E. A. Gehan, Intensive postoperative chemoimmunotherapy for patients with Stage II and Stage III breast cancer. *Cancer (Philad.)* 41, 1064 (1978).

19. H. J. Senn, Behandlungsfortschritte durch multimodale Therapie beim Mammakarzinom? *Schweiz. med. Wschr.* 108, 1938 (1978).

20. H. J. Senn, W. F. Jungi and R.A Amgwerd, Divergent effect on chemo-immunotherapy with LMF/BCG in node-negative and node-positive breast cancer. Abstract, Int. Conference on the Adjuvant Therapy of Cancer, Tucson (1979).

21. S. E. Salmon, A. Wendt, S. E. Jones, R. Jackson, G. Giordano, R. Miller, R. Heusinkveld and T. Moon, Treatment of early breast cancer with adriamycin-cyclophosphamide with or without radiation therapy: initial results of a brief and effective adjuvant program. EORTC Meeting on Adjuvant Therapies and Markers of Post-Surgical Minimal Residual Disease, Paris (1978).

22. H. Glucksberg and S. Rivkin, Adjuvant chemotherapy in Stage II breast cancer. Abstract, Int. Conference on the Adjuvant Therapy of Cancer, Tucson (1979).

23. A. Hubay, Therapy for Stage II and Stage III carcinoma of the breast. Breast Cancer Task Force Program and Related Projects DHEW Publication No. (NIH) 79-1869, p. 95 (Jan. 1979).

24. S. K. Carter, Adjuvant chemotherapy in breast cancer: critique and perspectives. *Cancer Chemoth. Pharmacol.* 1, 178 (1978).

25. M. Kaufmann, K. Klinga, B. Runnebaum and F. Kubli, Hormone receptor assay and prediction test of tumor response to chemotherapy in primary breast cancer. *New Engl. J. Med.* 300, 1052 (1979).

26. W. L. McQuire, Steroid receptors in human breast cancer. *Cancer Research* 38, 4289 (1978).

ACKNOWLEDGEMENT

The authors thank all colleagues and heads of the participating hospitals for their excellent interdisciplinary cooperation.

Adjuvant Chemotherapy with Four Drugs for Stage 2 Breast Cancer

T. K. Wheeler on behalf of Multicentre Breast Cancer Chemotherapy Group
G. A. Edelstyn (Chairman), T. S. Bates, D. Brinkley, R. G. B. Evans, G. Kitchen, K. D. MacRae, N. T. Nicol, M. Spittle and T. K. Wheeler

Addenbrookes Hospital, Cambridge, U.K.

Correspondence to T. K. Wheeler, 1 Spens Avenue, Cambridge, U.K.

Abstract—*A report of multimodal therapy for clinical stage 2 breast cancer is given with particular reference to toxicity. One hundred and twenty five of two hundred and fifty two patients had adjuvant chemotherapy, with Vincristine, Cyclophosphamide, Methotrexate and 5-Fluorouracil monthly for six months after surgery.*

The preliminary data on the rate of recurrence suggest an advantage for those patients reeiving chemotherapy which is significant at twelve, twenty four and thirty six months.

INTRODUCTION

Fisher et al. (1), Bonadonna et al. (2), and Ahman et al. (3) have published results indicating that adjuvant therapy is notably effective in pre-menopausal patients, in whom only 1-3 axillary nodes are involved by disease. Ahman et al. (3) have suggested that radio-therapy still has a place after surgery for breast cancer and reduces the risk of local recurrence even when chemotherapy is planned.

The interesting and valuable study by Nissen-Meyer et al. (4) has shown that the timing of chemotherapy is probably all important.

The Mayo Clinic and the South West Oncology Group (SWOG) have used schedules where Prednisone in short intermittent doses is combined with cytotoxic drugs. The benefit of cortico-steroid therapy in advanced disease is well known and Meakin et al. (5) have shown that small regular doses of Prednisone enhance the benefit of castration in increasing the disease free interval in pre-menopausal patients.

The aim of the present study was to assess the efficacy and the acceptability of adjuvant chemotherapy with a combination of CMF plus Vincristine.

MATERIALS AND METHODS

The trial was started in 1975. Participants in the Multicentre Breast Cancer Chemotherapy Group (MBCCG) entered their patients from eighteen hospitals. Two hundred and ninety one patients presented with stage 2, T1 or T2, N1a, N1B Mo adenocarcinoma of the breast. Of these, thirty nine patients were excluded because chemotherapy could not be given within ten weeks of surgery. All patients were less than seventy years old.

Staging was by clinical examination, radiography, bone scanning and liver function tests. Primary treatment was deemed to be curative in conventional terms but was the standard for each participating clinician.

The Secretariat in Belfast under the direction of the Chairman (G.E.) stored and analysed the data, but allocation to the treatment or control groups was made in a random manner at each referring hospital using sealed envelopes from the Secretariat. This method ensured distribution of various primary managements in the adjuvant and control groups, and therefore comparability.

The object of this study was to assess acceptability of a combination of cytotoxic drugs in the primary management of operable breast cancer. Given that this aim has been achieved it should be stated at this point that future studies should define criteria of entry more strictly to avoid incomparable subsets of patients emerging from the design.

The chemotherapy used in this study had been designed from earlier trials in advanced disease (6): the final schedule of Vincristine, Cyclophosphamide, Methotrexate and 5-Fluorouracil had achieved 70% remission rates in stage 4 breast cancer.

Norton and Simon (7) have described the theoretical solution to the problems of adjuvant chemotherapy in which rising doses of drugs should be given. A number of trials have published preliminary results of adjuvant combinations of cytotoxic drugs and the authors note that the schedules cannot always be given in full dose.

In order to spare the patients in this trial some of the known toxicity reported in the studies in advanced disease the doses prescribed are given in Table 1.

The dose of Cyclophosphamide was reduced to 200mg and of Methotrexate to 25mg if the patient weighed less than 54kg.

Treatment was started within ten weeks of

Table 1. Treatment regimes.

Cyclophosphamide	300mg
Vincristine	0.65mg
5-fluorouracil	500mg
4-6 days later	
Cyclophosphamide	300mg
Vincristine	0.65mg
Methotrexate	37.5mg

operation, given by rapid intravenous injection and the aim was to give paired injections each month for six months.

RESULTS

Maguire et al. (8) have drawn specific attention to the problems of side effects faced by a patient who has treatment for breast cancer.

In this MBCCG study only four of one hundred and twenty five patients could not co-operate with their clinicians. One refused after the first injection and another after the second.

In all, thirteen of the one hundred and twenty-five patients did not complete six months chemotherapy; the causes are listed in Table 2.

Table 2. Reasons for incomplete treatment in 13 of 125 patients.

Non-cooperation	4
General malaise	1
Nausea and vomiting	1
Neurotoxicity	2
Marrow toxicity	2
Intercurrent illness	3

For nine patients the clinicians withdrew further treatment to reduce side effects. No patient needed a wig. Two patients suffered leucopenia below 2.5 cells/dl but there were no serious complications of this problem.

The details of toxicity are summarised in Table 3, and were reported in 1978 (9).

The preliminary results have been published (10).

Selected data is reproduced to form the basis of the discussion, summarised in Table 4.

The advantage for the patients given chemotherapy show an actual difference, 16.7% at twelve months which is significant, (p = <0.001, by the Log Rank test). The actuarial result at thirty six months is also significant, those patients given chemotherapy gained an advantage compared with controls. Overall thirty-seven patients have recurred in the

Table 3. Toxicity, percentage of 125 patients.

Hgb. less than 12	11
WBC less than 2.5	6
Platelets less than 150	4
Nausea and vomiting	45
Diarrhoea	7
Stomatitis	4
Epilation	10
Neuropathy	6

chemotherapy group and fifty six in the control, (p = <0.01).

In one hundred and seven patients who were menopausal adjuvant chemotherapy significantly reduced the rate of recurrence at twelve months. 91.8% were disease free at that time compared with 76.4% of controls, (p = <0.005).

When patients with positive node histology only are examined the advantage for those given chemotherapy is still found. There were ninety-seven node positive patients given cytotoxic drugs and ninety eight controls, the respective disease free rates were 88.4% and 69.8% (p = <0.001) at one year.

DISCUSSION

In common with other early studies the preliminary results indicate that chemotherapy can significantly reduce the rate of recurrence following surgery for stage 2 breast cancer.

Further study must be undertaken to solve the following questions:

1. Does the surgical technique used to treat Stage 2 breast cancer influence the prognosis when chemotherapy is to be given?

2. Does a short course of cytotoxic chemotherapy in the immediate post-operative period confer equal benefit when compared with prolonged therapy? A positive finding would reduce the risks associated with the cytotoxic schedules used currently in practice.

3. Should intermittent courses of Prednisone be added to cytotoxic drug combinations irrespective of menopausal status? Holland (11) indicated that the original study by Cooper was effective in young and older patients, this finding is confirmed by SWOG.

4. Finally, the theoretical model devised by Norton and Simon (2) will have to be tested in practice. The question here is: Does more therapy, or the addition of different drugs into the schedule achieve better results than a simpler, shorter course of treatment? Is the theoretical advantage in cell killing lost through toxicity or unacceptability rendering it impossible to give treatment as planned? Surely one of the criteria for adjuvant therapy in the future must be that it can be administered

Table 4. Survival, free from recurrence at January 1, 1979.

Months of observation	Chemotherapy			Control		
	No.	%	SE	No.	%	SE
12	125	88.6	2.9	127	71.9	4.0
24	107	66.7	4.8	87	53.7	4.8
36	60.5	62.2	5.5	48	49.2	8.4

universally.

5. Strict protocols will be necessary to eliminate incomparable characteristics of management and this may prove to be the hardest problem to solve although for patients, doctors and researchers, one of the most important.

REFERENCES

1. B. Fisher, A. Glass, C. Redmond, E. R. Fisher, B. Barton, E. Such, P. Carbone, S. Economou, R. Foster, R. Frelick, H. Lerner, M. Levitt, R. Margoleses, J. MacFarlane, D. Plotkin, H. Shibata and H. Volk, L-Phenylalamine mustard (L-PAM) in the management of primary breast cancer. *Cancer* 39, 2883 (1977).

2. G. Bonadonna, A. Rossi, P. Valagussa, A. Banfi and U. Veronesi, The CMF program for operable breast cancer with positive axillary nodes. *Cancer* 39, 2904 (1977).

3. D. L. Ahmann, P. W. Scanlon, H. F. Bisel, J. H. Edmonson, S. Frytak, W. S. Payne, J. R. O'Fallon, R. J. Hahn, J. N. Ingle, M. J. O'Connel and J. Rubin. Repeated adjuvant chemotherapy with Phenylalamine mustard, or 5 Fluorouracil, Cyclophosphamide and Prednisone with or without radiation after mastectomy for breast cancer. *Lancet* 1, 893 (1978).

4. R. Nissen-Meyer, K. Kjellgren, K. Malmio, B. Mansson and T. Norin, Surgical adjuvant chemotherapy: results with one short course with Cyclophosphamide after mastectomy for breast cancer. *Cancer* 41, 2088 (1978).

5. J. W. Meakin, W. E. C. Allt, F. A. Beale, T. C. Brown, R. S. Bush, R. M. Clark, P. J. Fitzpatrick, N. V. Hawkins, R. D. T. Jenkin, J. F. Pringle, W. D. Rider, J. L. Hayward and R. D. Bulbrock, Ovarian irradiation and Prednisone following surgery for carcinoma of the breast. In *Adjuvant Therapy of Cancer* (edited by S. E. Salmon and S. E. Jones (p. 95. Amsterdam, North-Holland Publ. (1977).

6. G. A. Edelstyn, T. Bates, D. Brinkley, K. D. Macrae, M. Spittle and T. Wheeler, Short-course cyclical chemotherapy in advanced breast cancer. *Lancet* 1, 592 (1977).

7. L. Norton and R. Simon, Tumour size and sensitivity to therapy and design of treatment schedules. *Cancer Treatment Reports* 61, 1307 (1977).

8. G. P. Maguire, E. G. Lee, D. J. Bevington, C. S. Kuchemann, R. J. Crabtree and C. E. Cornell, Psychiatric problems in the first year after mastectomy. *Br. Med. J.* 7, 963 (1978).

9. G. A. Edelstyn, T. Bates, D. Brinkley, G. Kitchen, K. D. MacRae, N. T. Nicol, M. Spittle and T. Wheeler, Multimodal therapy for Stage 2 breast cancer. *Lancet* 2, 1092 (1978).

10. T. K. Wheeler, G. A. Edelstyn, T. S. Bates, D. Brinkley, R. G. B. Evans, G. Kitchen, K. D. MacRae, N. T. Nicol and M. Spittle, Four drug combination following surgery for breast cancer. In *Adjuvant Therapy of Cancer* II (edited by S. E. Salmon and S. E. Jones) in press.

11. J. F. Holland, Treatment of early breast cancer. *Lancet* 2, 1148 (1978).

Adjuvant Intermittent Chemo-Immunotherapy of Breast Cancer. A Prospective Study*

W. Schreml*, M. Betzler**, M. Lang*, H.-P. Lohrman*, P. Kubitza*, P. Schlag**, H.-D. Flad*** , Ch. Herfarth** and H. Heimpel*

*Department of Internal Medicine, Haematology and Oncology, University of Ulm, Federal Republic of Germany
**Department of Surgery, University of Ulm, Federal Republic of Germany
***Laboratory of Immunology, University of Ulm, Federal Republic of Germany

Correspondence to W. Schreml, Department of Internal Medicine, Haematology and Oncology, University of Ulm, D7900 Ulm, Federal Republic of Germany

Abstract—*Fifty patients operated for breast cancer were treated with 6 monthly courses of adjuvant aggressive chemotherapy (Adriamycin-Cyclophosphamide) and were randomized to receive either immunotherapy with Levamisole or no additional therapy. Probability of disease-free survival for the whole group is 66% at 33 months. The addition of Levamisole did not influence the course of disease nor the changes of the immune status or granulopoiesis during chemotherapy.*

INTRODUCTION

Based on the data on adjuvant chemotherapy of breast cancer published by Bonadonna et al. (1) and Fischer et al. (2), an interdisciplinary study was started in June 1976 with the following aims:

a) to test, in a phase II study, the feasibility of a short-term (6 months) highly aggressive chemotherapy regimen of adriamycin (ADR) and cyclophosphamide (CPA) in breast cancer patients;

b) to study, in a phase III setting, the influence of additional immunotherapy with levamisole on the clinical and pathophysiological effects of adjuvant chemotherapy;

c) to perform thorough laboratory investigations on the influence of the chosen chemotherapeutic regimen on the immune status and on the hemopoietic system of patients.

MATERIAL AND METHODS

1. Patients

50 patients < 65 yrs (32 premenopausal and 18 postmenopausal) were entered into the study, after modified radical mastectomy for primary breast cancer. Patients were free of recognizable metastases as judged from thorough clinical check up, laboratory data, liver- and bone scan, but were considered on high risk for recurrence (positive axillary lymph nodes or large primary tumor, i.e. T_3 in lateral location or T_2 in medial or central location). 9 patients were treated for large primary only, 27 had 1 to 3 involved lymph nodes, 14 had 4 or more positive nodes.

2. Chemotherapy

All patients were to receive 6 courses of ADR, 50 mg/m², i.v., and CPA, 500 mg/m², i.v., in 500-1000 ml glucose, as single doses in monthly intervals.

3. Immunotherapy

The patients were randomly assigned by the department of clinical documentation to receive either no additional therapy or additional immunotherapy (levamisole, 150 mg p.o. on days 14, 15, 21 and 22 of each course and on 2 consecutive days every week for 1 1/2 year after completion of chemotherapy).

4. Clinical Studies

Clinical and laboratory studies were done every month during the chemotherapy period, and every 3 months thereafter according to the guidelines established in our group (3). Side effects were noted on a questionnaire.

5. Immunological and Hematological Studies

The special laboratory techniques have been published which were used to determine the immune status (4,5) and the hemopoietic function (6,7,8).

6. Statistical Analysis

The probability of disease-free survival was estimated in three month intervals, by

*Supported by the Deutsche Forschungsgemeinschaft, SFB 112.

the actuarial method (9). The present data
are evaluated in March 79, 33 months after
initiation of the study.

RESULTS

1. Patient Compliance

Two patients were taken off the study
during the first course of chemotherapy, one
for severe bone marrow depression with
leucopenia, thrombopenia and consequent
sepsis and bleeding complications; the
patient recovered and is free of disease up
to now. The second patient refused further
chemotherapy because of side effects and
did not return for follow-up. Of the
remaining 48 patients, 42 have completed
chemotherapy with a total of 252 courses.

In one patient a delay and dose reduction
was necessary in 2 courses because of severe
stomatitis. Levamisole had to be discontinued in 6/24 patients before the scheduled
completion of 2 years for side effects.

2. Disease-free Survival

Probability of disease-free survival for
the whole group is shown in Fig. 1A. At
33 months, this probability is estimated to
be 66%. Pre- and postmenopausal women
(Fig. 1B) did not show any noticeable difference in disease-free survival. The curve
for patients treated with additional immunotherapy did not differ from that of patients
without Levamisole (Fig. 1C).

3. Type of Recurrence

The time course of treatment failures is
indicated in Fig. 1. 8/11 recurrences
occurred during the first 12 months. In
7/11 recurrences, loco-regional metastases
preceded or accompanied the development of
distant metastases. Four patients have
died; in all these 4 cases, central nervous
system metastases were leading to the ter-
minal complications.

4. Side Effects

In order to evaluate clinical side effects,
a questionnaire comprising 10 items was
completed at the end of each course and the
severity of side effects was rated on an
arbitrary scale by the attending physician.
For these items where more than occasional
entries were made, the evaluation is given
in Table 1.

The questions for infection, bleeding,
neurological symptoms, respiratory distress
did not reveal noteworthy side effects of
this therapy. One important complaint which
became apparent during the study was psychological stress and depression in nearly 80%
of the patients, with severe depression
necessitating the consultation of a

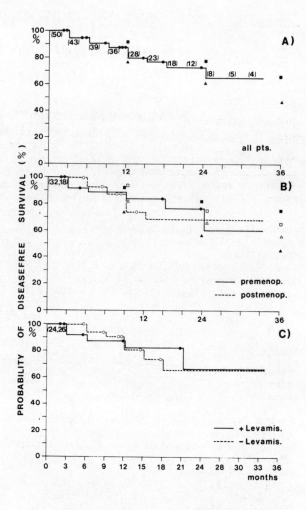

Fig. 1. Probability of disease-free survival for all patients (A), and pre-
and postmenopausal subgroups (B),
and for patients with and without
Levamisole (C). Patients at risk
for each 3 month period in A),
and initially in B) and C) are
given in parenthesis. ●, o:
recurrences.
Corresponding 1, 2 and 3 data
from Bonadonna (12) are indicating
in A) and B): ▲ = Control; ■ = CMF;
black symbols = premenopausal,
open symbols = postmenopausal.

psychiatrist in 3 patients.

The changes in immune function during and
after adjuvant therapy have been described
(4,5).

The hematologic studies of the short-term
effects has allowed to deliniate the pattern
of depletion and repletion of a normal human
granulopoietic system in response to exposure
to the cytotoxic drug combination employed.
With respect to long-term consequences of
such treatment, a persisting defect of
granulopoiesis could be demonstrated (8,10).
Side effects occurring under levamisole after
discontinuation of chemotherapy were rheuma-
toid joint and muscle pain, edematous swelling of hands and feet, malsensations of the

Table 1. Evaluation of clinical side effects by questionnaire.

Side effect	Results of questionnaire
Nausea/vomiting	All patients; moderate to severe (rating: 2.2 ± 0.6*)
Alopecia	All patients; complete or nearly complete
General fatigue	8 patients, mild to moderate (rating: 1.6 ± 0.7*)
Mucous membranes	Mild to moderate, 27 episodes in 11 patients
Diarrhoea	Mild to moderate, 15 episodes in 5 patients
Hemorrhagic cystitis	Mild to moderate, 6 episodes in 4 patients

Arbitrary scale: 0 = no complaints: 1 = mild; 2 = moderate; 3 = severe, 4 = life threatening.
*Mean ± 1 S.D. of 252 (or 48) courses.

taste and general malaise, which necessitated the discontinuation of Levamisole in 6 patients.

Levamisole did not influence the effects of chemotherapy on the immune status (5) or on granulopoiesis (11).

DISCUSSION

The disease-free survival for the whole group and for pre- and postmenopausal patient lies between the control and CMF-group of Bonadonna et al. (12).

Pre- and postmenopausal patients do not show a different behavior in our study. This may be due to the fact that our age limit was 65 years, which made it possible to adhere to the planned dose schedule in most cases. Our phase II study indicates that a 6 month, aggressive adjuvant chemotherapy regimen can be performed with high patient compliance when patient care is given high attention. There were only 2/52 patients lost from the study, both during its early phase.

At the present time, only 8/50 patients are followed for more than two years. Therefore, the confidence limits for the probability of disease-free survival are large and do not yet allow a conclusion, whether this type of adjuvant chemotherapy should be compared in a phase III trial.

Levamisole was added in a randomised trial to the chemotherapeutic regimen in 24/50 patients in order to evaluate a potential additional effect on disease-free survival as described by Rojas et al. for stage III breast cancer after local irradiation (13). No such effect could be observed for the observation period. In addition, our immunologic and hematologic laboratory investigations did not document an effect of levamisole on the immunestatus or granulopoiesis in this setting of combined chemo-immunotherapy.

The documentation of long-lasting side effects, in particular in granulopoiesis, which were detectable not by routine peripheral blood counts but only by studies of the early compartments of granulopoiesis renders such basic studies mandatory for all adjuvant chemotherapy regimens, in order to select the least toxic combination when several cytotoxic combinations with similar clinical effectiveness are available.

REFERENCES

1. G. Bonadonna, E. Brusamolino. P. Valagussa, A. Rossi, L. Brugnatelli, C. Brambilla, M. De Lena, G. Tancini, E. Bajetta, R. Musumeci and U. Veronesi, Combination chemotherapy as an adjuvant treatment in operable breast cancer. *New Engl. J. Med.* 294, 405 (1976).

2. B. Fisher, P. Carbone, S. G. Economon, R. Frelic, A. Glass, H. Lerner, C. Redmond, M. Zelen, P. Band, D. L. Katrych, M. Wolmark and E. R. Fisher, 1-Phenylalanine mustard (L-PAM) in the management of primary breast cancer: a report of early findings. *New Engl. J. Med.* 292, 117 (1975).

3. M. Betzler, P. Schlag, W. Schreml and Ch. Herfarth, Mammakarzinom: Stadieneinteilung, Therapie und Nachsorge. *Med. Klin.* 73, 633 (1978).

4. H.-D. Flad, M. Betzler, W. Schreml, H. Müller, H.-P. Lohrmann, Ch. Herfarth and H. Heimpel; Verhalten lymphatischer Subpopulationen unter zytostatischer Therapie. In *Adjuvante zytostatische Chemotherapie. Zytostatische Therapie als Rezidivprophylaxe?* (Edited by H. Huber, H. J. Senn, M. Falkensammer) Springer-Verlag Berlin, Heidelberg, New York (1978).

5. M. Betzler, H.-D. Flad, W. Schreml, H. Müller, R. Huget, H. Heimpel and Ch. Herfarth, Quantitative and functional studies of lymphocyte subpopulations during adjuvant chemo(immuno)therapy in patients with breast cancer. In *Immunodiagnosis and Immuntherapy of Malignant Tumors.* (Edited by H.-D. Flad, Ch. Herfarth, M. Betzler) Springer-Verlag Berlin, Heidelberg, New York (1979).

6. H.-P. Lohrmann, W. Hansi and H. Heimpel, Human placenta-conditioned medium for stimulation of human granulopoietic precursor cell (CFU-c) colony growth in vitro. *Blut* 36, 81 (1978).

7. H.-P. Lohrmann, Thymidine-suicide of human granulocytic progenitor cells (CFU-C). *Biomedicine* 28, 319 (1978).

8. H.-P. Lohrmann, W. Schreml, M. Lang,
   M. Betzler, T. M. Fliedner and H. Heimpel,
   Changes of granulopoiesis during and
   after adjuvant chemotherapy of breast
   cancer. *Brit. J. Haematol.* 40, 369
   (1978).
9. H. Immich, *Medizinische Statistik.*
   Schattauer Verlag, Stuttgart (1977).
10. W. Schreml and H. P. Lohrmann, Hemato-
    toxicity of adjuvant chemotherapy. In
    Adjuvant Therapy of Cancer II. (Edited
    by S. S. Salmon and S. E. Jones) Grune
    and Stratton, New York (in press).
11. W. Schreml and H.-P. Lohrmann, No effects
    of Levamisole on cytotoxic drug-induced
    changes of human granulopoiesis. *Blut*
    38, 331 (1979).
12. G. Bonadonna, P. Valagussa, A. Rossi,
    R. Zucali, G. Tancini, E. Bajetta,
    C. Brambilla, M. De Lena, G. D. Fronzo,
    A. Banfi, F. Rilke and V. Veronesi,
    Are surgical adjuvant trials altering
    the course of breast cancer? *Sem.
    Oncology* 5, 450 (1978).
13. A. F. Rojas, E. Mickiewicz, J. N.
    Feierstein, H. Glait and A. J. Olivari,
    Levamisole in advanced human breast
    cancer. *Lancet* I, 211 (1976).

Divergent Effect of Adjuvant Chemo-Immunotherapy on Recurrence Rates in Node-Negative and Node-Positive Breast Cancer Patients

W. F. Jungi*, H. J. Senn*, R. Amgwerd**, E. Hochuli***
and East Switzerland Cooperative Oncology Group (OSAKO)

*Medizinische Klinik C, Kantonsspital, St. Gallen
**Klinik für Chirurgie, Kantonsspital, St. Gallen
***Frauenklinik, Thurg. Kantonsspital, Münsterlingen

Correspondence to W. F. Jungi, Medizinische Klinik C, Kantonsspital, CH-9007
St. Gallen, Switzerland

Abstract—In contrast to the innumerable adjuvant studies in node-positive
(N+) patients, virtually none have been performed in node-negative (N-)
breast cancer patients, despite the well known recurrence time curve in this
patient group. Theoretically the 1/3 of N- patients likely to relapse are
the most suitable candidates for adjuvant chemotherapy. We have tested the
protective effect of a simple oral chemotherapy, followed by immunotherapy
in N+ and N- patients with breast cancer stage T 1-3a N 0-1 M 0. After
modified radical mastectomy 254 patients were randomized to observation only
or intermittent oral chemotherapy with Chlorambucil, Methotrexate and
Fluorouracil (LMF) for 6 and BCG skin scarifications for 18 months. After a
median postoperative observation period of 34 months 242 patients (126 N-
and 116 N+) are evaluable. LMF reduces the recurrence rate overall as well
as in all subgroups. However statistically significant difference is reached
only in N- patients. Almost no effect is seen in the high risk group of N-
premenopausal patients. In N+ patients there is only a borderline, in N-
on the contrary a highly significant prolongation of relapse-free survival.
Our experience with a short, extremely well tolerated chemotherapy + BCG in
N+ patients is in contrast to other comparable adjuvant chemotherapy programs.
The protective effect in N- patients is quite remarkable and warrants
further studies in this patient group.

INTRODUCTION

Traditional surgical and radiological
methods of loco-regional treatment of breast
cancer have stagnated for decades and have
not been able to change the eventual outcome
of the disease. The prognosis is before all
dismal for the so-called node-positive (N+)
patients with malignant infiltration of the
regional, mostly axillary nodes. Whereas
early attempts of adjuvant endocrine
manoeuvres have failed, several recent trials
of adjuvant chemotherapy trials have yielded
encouraging results (1-4).

The concept of adjuvant chemotherapy is
theoretically to eradicate residual subclinical tumor after surgical removal of all
visible tumor. Almost all current adjuvant
studies in breast cancer include only patients
with positive axillary nodes with their dis-
tressingly constant high risk of tumor
recurrence (1-3). However, it is well known
that also node-negative (N-) patients
relapse to a significant degree, about 25% at
5 years and 35-40% at 10 years postoperatively.
This recurrence rate seems to be even higher
in Eastern Switzerland (5). If the concept
of adjuvant chemotherapy is correct, node-
negative patients with presumable micrometastases in one third of the cases theoretically are the most suitable candidates for

adjuvant chemotherapy, provided that such a
treatment has no undesirable short or long
term side effects. As long as we have no
prognostic indicators to detect node-negative
patients likely to relapse, we have to conduct adjuvant trials in these patients in a
randomized fashion and have to accept that
we overtreat 2/3 of them. We have tested
the effectiveness of an adjuvant regime consisting of 6 months chemotherapy followed by
18 months BCG-immunotherapy. Evaluated were:
1. Recurrence rate and site, 2. disease-free
interval, 3. survival, 4. early and long-term
toxicity, 5. changes in some immunological
parameters (not reported).

The 3-drug-chemotherapy regimen used in
the present study was found considerably less
toxic, but not significantly inferior in
its antitumor effect compared to more complicated combinations (6,7).

MATERIALS AND METHODS

Two hundred and fifty four patients with
breast cancer stages T1-3a N0-1 M0 entered
the trial between March 1974 and December
1977. After standardized modified radical
mastectomy and routine postoperative staging
patients were stratified according to nodal
status. They were then allocated randomly

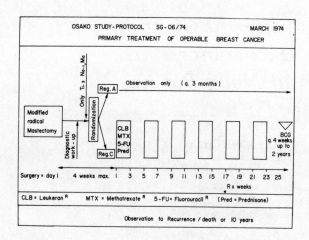

Fig. 1. Patient selection and study design
of OSAKO - study 06/74.

to either the observation group (A) or the
treatment group (C), (Fig. 1). Postoperative
radiation was not given in any case.

Table 1 summarizes the characteristics of
242 evaluable out of the initially randomized 254 women. Fifteen patients were
eliminated due to staging errors, concommit-
ant second tumors and loss to follow-up.

- chlorambucil (Leukeran^R) 6-8 mg po.d. 1-14
- amethopterin (methotrexate^R) 5-7.5 mg
  po.d.1-3, 8-10
- 5-fluorouracil 500-750 mg po.d.1 and 8

The lower doses were given to patients
69 kg, the higher to those 70 kg of body
weight, with usual dose modification.

During the first phase of the study (102
patients) prednisone was added to the above
LMF-regimen: 50 mg daily po. × 14 days
during the first and 10 mg daily po. x 14
days in subsequent cycles. Prednisone was
dropped then due to endocrine and vascular
toxicity. Immunotherapy was given by monthly
BCG-skin-scarifications up to 2 years post-
operatively.

Follow-up examinations (except for the bi-
weekly clinic visits during the initial LMF-
chemotherapy in regimen C) were performed
every 3 months. They included physical
examination, routine laboratory tests. Chest
X-ray was repeated every 6 months and a bone
scan, bone marrow biospy and mammography of
the contralateral breast every 12 months, or
earlier if indicated. In addition, the
study population was subjected to a series of
immunologic tests not referred to here.
Tumor recurrence had to be unequibocally documented.

Statistical comparisons of recurrence
rates and disease-free intervals were
performed by the biostatistical centre of the

Table 1. Adjuvant chemo-immunotherapy in operable breast cancer.
Patient characteristics as of January 1st, 1979.

Patient subgroup	Regimen A (Surg. only)	Regimen C (Surg. + LMF/BCG)	All patients evaluable
All N_- + N_+	124	118	242
N_-	67	58	125
N_+	57	60	117
N_+ (1-3)	37	42	79
N_+ (4)	20	18	38
T_{1-2a}	112	107	219
T_{3a}	13	10	23
Pre + perimenop.	60	58	118
Postmenopausal	64	60	124
Median age (y.)	56.6	53.0	55.3

Lost to follow up 2, refusal 3, staging error 5, randomisation error 4,
2nd malignancy 1.

Recognized risk factors such as nodal
status, tumor size, menopausal and median
age were well balanced in the 2 study regimens. Median follow-up after mastectomy in
both treatment groups (Jan. 1, 1979) is 34
(14-58) months.

The adjuvant chemotherapy regimen given
for 6 monthly cycles after mastectomy consisted of an entirely oral, well tolerated
combination (LMF):

Swiss Group for Clinical Cancer Research
(SAKK, Dr. R. Berchtold). Intermediate
reports are prepared every 6 months.

RESULTS

Overall recurrence rates are presented in
Table 2. Median postoperative observation
time is now 3 years. There is a statistically

Table 2. Adjuvant chemo-immunotherapy in operable breast cancer, overall recurrence rates after median observation of 34 (14-60) mos.

Patient subgroup	Regimen A (Surg. only)	Regimen C (Surg. + LMF/BCG)	P
All N_- + N_+	45/124 = 36.3%	27/118 = 22.9%	0.032
All premenop.	23/60 = 38.3%	15/58 = 25.9%	0.211
All postmenop.	22/64 = 34.3%	12/60 = 20.0%	0.112
N_-	18/67 = 26.8%	4/58 = 6.9%	0.007
N_- premenop.	7/29 = 24.1%	2/29 = 6.9%	0.147
N_- postmenop.	11/38 = 28.9%	2/29 = 6.9%	0.051
N_+	27/57 = 47.4%	23/60 = 38.3%	0.425
N_+ premenop.	16/31 = 51.6%	13/29 = 44.8%	0.789
N_+ postmenop.	11/26 = 42.3%	10/31 = 32.3%	0.611
N_+ (1-3+LN)	17/37 = 45.9%	13/42 = 30.9%	0.256
N_+ (4+LN)	10/20 = 50.0%	10/18 = 55.5%	0.986

borderline decrease of recurrences in the LMF/BCG treated patients (p = 0.03) in the whole population of N-- + N+ cases.

It is evident that node-negative and node-positive women behave differently: There is a clearcut and highly significant lower recurrence rate among node-negative patients receiving LMF/BCG (6.9% vs. 26.8%, p = 0.007) but at best only a marginal trend to fewer recurrences with the same adjuvant regimen in node-positive women (38.3% vs. 47.4%, p = 0.42). We are specially disturbed by the fact, that there is virtually no decrease in recurrence rates by the addition of LMF/BCG in the high risk node-positive premenopausal cases (44.8% vs. 51.6%, p = 0.79) and in women with major axillary inolvement or 4 and more nodes (50.0% vs. 55.5%, p = 0.99).

Pre- and postmenopausal N- women both show definitely lower recurrence rates by LMF/BCG, whereas both menopausal subgroups show at best a similar, very marginal trend to fewer tumor recurrences among N+ patients.

Seventy two women have relapsed so far. The percentage of loco-regional recurrences (45.8%) is somewhat higher than in several comparable studies, but distant or combined metastases prevail (54%). Many cases with initial "locoregional" recurrence will present distant metastases shortly thereafter (60%).

Figure 2 shows the calculated treatment-failure time-distribution curves for node-negative and node-positive patients. There is a highly significant difference in N- women in favour of LMF/BCG treated patients, while this difference is absent in N+ cases. While median disease-free intervals have not yet been reached in N- patients, the respective figures in N+ patients are 27 months for surgical controls and 38 months for the adjuvant LMF/BCG subgroup (p = 0.31).

Survival data show no difference between

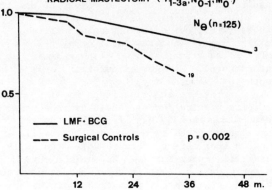

PROBABILITY OF DISEASE-FREE INTERVAL AFTER MODIFIED RADICAL MASTECTOMY (T_{1-3a}, N_{0-1}, M_0)

$N_\ominus$ (n = 125)

—— LMF·BCG
- - - Surgical Controls   p = 0.002

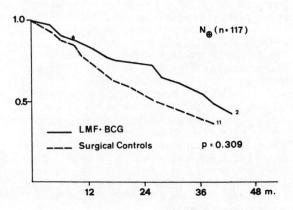

$N_\oplus$ (n = 117)

—— LMF·BCG
- - - Surgical Controls   p = 0.309

Fig. 2. Probability of disease-free interval for N- and N+ patients 3-4 years postop.

the 2 regimens up to 3 years post mastectomy.
The respective survival for surgical controls
and LMF/BCG patients at present are: 92.5%
vs. 96.5% for N- and 80.7% vs. 83.3% for
N+ patients. A trend towards higher survival
rate of LMF/BCG cases seems to slowly emerge
for N- women.

Toxicity was extremely low for the LMF (P)
chemotherapy in general. Only 1 of 118
patients in the adjuvant regimen refused to
complete 6 months of LMF. Temporary dose
reduction of LMF due to moderate hemato-
toxicity was necessary in 40% of women and
a dosage increase was possible in 14%.
Minor transient gastro-intestinal toxicity
was noted in only 25% of study patients,
but virtually no loss of hair.

DISCUSSION

Several other adjuvant trials demonstrate
a significant decrease of early relapse
rates for premenopausal node-positive
patients, but our study using rather short-
term oral LMF-chemotherapy with BCG shows
virtually no beneficial effect in these high
risk patients. Since there exists no major
difference regarding patient selection and
type of initial surgery, the disagreement in
results has to be attributed to variations in
the adjuvant regimens tested. Compared to
others (2,3), our adjuvant regimen differs
in 3 points: 1. entirely oral combination of
LMF. 2. substitution of cyclophosphamide by
chlorambucil. 3. shorter duration, only 6
months of chemotherapy.

In contrast to the experience in N+
patients we have demonstrated that the same
chemo-immunotherapy significantly reduces
tumor recurrences in N- women. Time will
show whether this difference will eventually
result in longer survival and higher cure.
To our knowledge this is the first randomized
adjuvant trial with combination chemotherapy
in N- breast cancer patients. Our experience
confirms earlier, non-randomized data by
Donovoan et al. (8), showing a lower recurrence rate and higher survival after 5 years
in N-, but not in N+ cases, using adjuvant
cyclophosphamide. It can also be compared to
the favorable results with short-term cyclophosphamide in N- and N+ patients by Nissen-
Meyer et al. (10) and Rieche et al. (9).

Thus relatively non-toxic LMF - followed
by BCG, the contribution of which is not
assessable - might turn out to be an effective
way of preventing tumor recurrence in truly
node-negative patients with minimal residual
tumor but a definite risk of relapse and
tumor mortality. As regards the N+ patients
a Swiss National adjuvant study (SAKK 27/76)
is now analyzing whether 6 or 24 months of
the same LMF therapy will be more effective
in N+ patients.

REFERENCES

1. B. Fisher, P. Carbone, S. G. Economou,
   R. Frelick, A. Glass, H. Lerner, P. Band,
   D. L. Katrych, W. Wolmark, E. R. Fisher,
   L-phenylalanine-mustard in the manage-
   ment of primary breast cancer. *New Engl.
   J. Med.* 929, 117 (1975).
2. G. Bonadonna, E. Brusamolino, P. Vala-
   gussa, A. Rossi, L. Brugnatelli,
   C. Brambilla, M. Delena, G. Tacini,
   E. Bajetta, R. Musumeci, U. Veronesi,
   Combination chemotherapy as an adjuvant
   treatment in operable breast cancer.
   New Engl. J. Med. 294, 415 (1976).
3. Multicenter Breast Cancer Chemotherapy
   Group, Multimodal therapy for histo-
   logical stage II breast cancer. *Lancet*
   II, 306 (1977).
4. H. J. Senn, W. F. Jungi, R. Amgwerd,
   Adjuvant chemoimmunotherapy with LMF +
   BCG in node-negative and node-positive
   breast cancer patients. *Antibiot.
   Chemoth.* 24, 213 (1978).
5. F. Mutzner, R. Amgwerd, U. Gessner,
   Prognose des lokalen primären Mamma-
   karzinoms unter der bisherigen Therapie.
   Schweiz. med. Wschr. 107, 992 (1977).
6. F. Cavalli, P. Alberto, W. F. Jungi,
   K. Brunner, G. Martz, Hormonochemotherapy
   vs. hormonotherapy followed by chemotherapy in disseminated breast cancer.
   Europ. J. Cancer (in press).
7. A. C. Mayr, W. F. Jungi, H. J. Senn,
   Oral combination chemotherapy with LMFP
   in advanced breast cancer. Wellcome
   Symposium in Cancer Chemotherapy, London,
   1979 (in press).
8. S. Donovan, J. Powell, J. A. H. Water-
   house, D. M. Morissey, A prolonged course
   of cyclophosphamide as an adjunct to
   mastectomy in the primary treatment of
   breast cancer. *Br. J. Surg.* 63, 871
   (1976).
9. K. Rieche, H. Berndt, B. Prahl, Continuous
   postoperative treatment with cyclophosphamide in breast carcinoma - a randomized
   clinical study. *Arch. Geschwulstforsch.*
   40, 349 (1972).
10. R. Nissen-Meyer, K. Kjellgren, K. Malmio,
    B. Mansson, T. Norin, Surgical adjuvant
    chemotherapy. Results with one short
    course of cyclphosphamice after mastectomy
    for breast cancer. *Cancer* 41, 2083 (1978).

Surgical Adjuvant Trials in the United States

M. Rozencweig*, D. D. Von Hoff**, J. C. Allegra** and F. M. Muggia**

*Service de Médecine et Laboratoire d'Investigation Clinique, Département de Chimiothérapie, Institut Jules Bordet, Brussels, Belgium
**Division of Cancer Treatment, National Cancer Institute, Bethesda, Maryland

Correspondence to M. Rozencweig, Investigational Drug Section, Department of Chemotherapy, Internal Medicine, Institut Jules Bordet, 1, rue Héger-Bordet, B-1000 Brussels, Belgium

Abstract—It has been almost 7 years since the NSABP initiated the L-PAM study and encouraging results persist in premenopausal women with 1-3 positive nodes. Several surgical adjuvant trials with L-PAM and with drug combinations have been undertaken subsequently by the NSABP and other cooperative groups in the United States. Most adjuvant regimens are currently investigated without untreated controls. Preliminary data are suggestive of a superiority of combination chemotherapy over L-PAM in terms of disease-free interval.

The large number of trials carried out by the cooperative groups in the United States illustrates some of the treatments and concepts currently available for adjuvant studies. Patient entry is terminated in several of these but final conclusions must await longer follow-up periods.

INTRODUCTION

A large number of adjuvant studies have been undertaken in early breast cancer following the encouraging results initially reported by Fisher et al. (1) and Bonadonna et al. (2). Few of the trials subsequently activated in the United States have been completed and, generally, available results are still very preliminary. This review is limited to trials carried out in stage II disease by the cooperative groups including Cancer and Leukemia Group B (CALGB), Central Oncology Group (COG), Eastern Cooperative Oncology Group (ECOG), National Surgical Adjuvant Project for Breast and Bowel Cancers (NSABP), Southeastern Cancer Study Group (SEG) and Southwest Oncology Group (SWOG).

The design of these adjuvant studies is relatively uniform. Patients are included after radical or modified radical mastectomy has been performed. Axillary invasion must be histologically demonstrated. Stratification is classifically by age (< 50 versus ≥ 50) or menopausal status and by extent of axillary involvement (1 to 3 versus 4 or more positive nodes). Hormonal receptors are being used for stratification purposes in the most recently activated studies. Adjuvant treatments are commonly started 2 to 10 weeks after mastectomy and are given for 1 to 2 years.

Only a few trials involve untreated controls whereas the vast majority of these trials is aimed at defining optimal systemic regimens. Most studies are comparing various chemotherapy programs with either L-PAM or cyclophosphamide, methotrexate and 5-fluorouracil in the control arm. The remaining trials attempt to clarify the role of hormonetherapy or immunotherapy when given concomitantly with chemotherapy.

TRIALS INVOLVING A PLACEBO GROUP

The L-PAM study of the NSABP has been widely publicized. After stratification according to age and nodal status, patients were randomized within each participating institution to receive L-PAM therapy or a placebo. The drug was given at a dose of 0.15 mg/kg per day for five consecutive days every six weeks for 2 years. A total of 370 patients were entered into this trial between September 1972 and February 1975. Only 5.9% of these were excluded from the analysis.

With a mean time on study of 23 months (3), the disease-free survival rates at 24 months were 68.4% in the placebo group and 76.2% in the L-PAM group (p = 0.009). An analysis by stratification criteria revealed a significant effect of L-PAM in patients under 50 with one to three positive nodes. The difference was no longer significant with more extensive nodal invasion and in older patients. Of interest, the proportion of locoregional relapses as first site of reported failures was similar in both treatment groups.

These data have been reanalyzed with an average time on study of 52 months ranging from 42 to 92 months (4). Trends noted earlier in the study are still apparent. Partial results have been recently published and indicate a survival rate at 4 years without disease of 47 versus 65% for patients under 50 receiving the placebo or the L-PAM respectively.

In addition to the NSABP trial, 2 other trials use a placebo group (Table 1). These two studies have been activated very recently by ECOG in postmenopausal women. Patients younger than 65 years of age are randomly allocated to receive a placebo or a combination chemotherapy regimen consisting of cyclophosphamide, methotrexate, 5-fluorouracil and prednisone (CMFP) with or without tamoxifen. ECOG had previously demonstrated the superiority of CMFP over CMF in patients with advanced breast cancer in response rate and duration of response (5). Patients assigned to the CMFP combination chemotherapy group receive 12 courses of cyclophosphamide 100 mg/m^2 p.o. days 1 through 14 of each cycle, methotrexate 40 mg/m^2 i.v. days 1 and 8 of each cycle, 5-fluorouracil 600 mg/m^2 i.v. days 1 and 8 of each cycle, and prednisone 40 mg/m^2 p.o. as a single daily dose days 1 through 14 of each cycle. Cycles are repeated at 28-day intervals. Patients assigned to the chemohormonal therapy group receive in addition tamoxifen 10 mg p.o. twice daily continuously for one year. Stratification criteria include the status of estrogen receptors.

Women older than 65 years of age are included in another protocol of ECOG comparing tamoxifen alone and placebo. Tamoxifen is given at a dose of 10 mg twice daily. Treatments are administered continuously for 2 years. Patients with negative estrogen receptor status are excluded from entry on this trial.

COMPARISON OF CHEMOTHERAPY REGIMES

Following the early success of the L-PAM study, the NSABP embarked on a series of successive trials testing first the value of L-PAM relative to that of L-PAM plus 5-fluorouracil. Subsequently, the latter combination was investigated versus a regimen consisting of L-PAM, 5-fluorouracil and methotrexate (Table 2).

The design of these studies was similar to that of the initial L-PAM study. As of January 1979, the average time on study was 38 and 26 months for each of those protocols which accrued 672 and 701 patients respectively. Little data have been published on either of these studies (4).

L-PAM has also been compared with combination chemotherapy regimens by two other cooperative groups. COG randomized 265 evaluable patients to either L-PAM (0.15 mg/kg daily × 5 repeated every 6 weeks), or a combination of cyclophosphamide (2 mg/kg p.o. daily for 6 weeks), methotrexate (0.5 mg/kg i.v. weekly x 6), 5-fluorouracil (10 mg/kg i.v. weekly x 6), and vincristine (0.025 mg/kg i.v. weekly x 4) (CMFV). Each 6-week cycle of therapy was followed by a 4-week rest period and both programs were administered for one year. Interim results were reported with a median follow-up of 36 months (6). The relapse rate at 48 months was 40% versus 27% in the L-PAM and the CMFV group respectively. An analysis of the disease-free interval curves showed a significant advantage for the CMFV arm. Data by age indicated that this superiority could be shown only in patients older than 49 years

Table 1. Cooperative trials involving a placebo group.

Cooperative group	Treatment duration (yr)	Treatment options		
		1	2	3
NSABP	2	Placebo	L-PAM	–
ECOG[a]	1	Placebo	CMFP	CMFP + tam
ECOG[b]	2	Placebo	Tam	–

[a]Postmenopausal ≤ 65 yr.
[b]Postmenopausal > 65 yr.

Table 2. Cooperative trials comparing chemotherapy regimens.

Cooperative group	Treatment duration (yr)	Treatment options		
		1	2	3
NSABP	2	L-PAM	L-PAM + 5FU	–
COG	1	L-PAM	CMFV	–
SWOG	2	L-PAM	CMFVP[a]	
NASBP	2	L-PAM + 5FU	L-PAM + 5FU + MTX	–
ECOG[b]	1	CMF	CMF	CMF + tam
CALGB	2	CMF	CMFVP	CMF + MER

[a]CMFVP is given for 1 year.
[b]Premenopausal patients.

of age. Among these, results approach
statistical significance in women with 1 to
3 invaded nodes whereas the p value was 0.05
in women with more extensive nodal invasion.
No difference in therapeutic effectiveness
could be detected in younger patients.

L-PAM was also randomly compared by SWOG
to a combination chemotherapy regimen consisting of cyclophosphamide (60 mg/m^2 p.o. daily),
methotrexate (15 mg/m^2 i.v. weekly, 5-fluor-
ouracil (300 mg/m^2 i.v. weekly), vincristine
(0.625 mg/m^2 i.v. weekly × 10), and prednisone (30-10 mg/m^2 p.o. daily × 42) (CMFVP).
L-PAM (5 mg/m^2 daily for 5 consecutive days)
was given intermittently every 6 weeks for
2 years whereas the combination was given
continuously for 1 year. This CMFVP regimen
emerged from an earlier study performed by
SWOG in advanced disease (7). Patients with
postoperative radiotherapy were eligible but
were randomized separately. Results were
reported for 353 evaluable women on study
with a mean follow-up of 2 years (8).
Relapse rate was 10% for the combination and
28% for the single agent. The disease-free
interval was prolonged in the CMFVP group at
the 0.001 level. Similar figures were
obtained in pre- and postmenopausal women
with either treatment. The largest therapeutic difference was found in premenopausal
patients with 4 or more invaded nodes (13
versus 38%). Toxicity findings were reportedly
mild and transient with both treatments.

A combination of cyclophosphamide, methotrexate and 5-fluorouracil (CMF) serves as
control treatment in a ECOG and a CALGB
trial. The ECOG study is restricted to premenopausal patients and compares CMF to CMFP
and to CMFP plus tamoxifen. Patients are
stratified according to the number of positive axillary nodes and results of estrogen
receptor assay. Drug doses are identical
to those used in postmenopausal patients
(see above) and treatments are given for one
year. This ECOG study has been recently
activated and no results are available yet.

In the CALGB trial, the therapeutic options
are CMF versus CMFVP versus CMF plus MER (9).
During the first 6 weeks, the following dose
schedules are utilized = cyclophosphamide
80 mg/m^2 p.o. daily, methotrexate 40 mg/m^2
i.v. weekly, 5-fluorouracil 500 mg/m^2 i.v.
weekly, vincristine 1.5 mg i.v. weekly,
prednisone 40 mg/m^2 daily for 3 weeks. MER
is administered every other week. Starting
on week 9, ten 4-week cycles are given.
Vincristine, prednisone and MER are discontinued thereafter, patients receiving 6 cycles
of CMF at 8-week intervals in all treatment
groups. Chemotherapy is administered for a
total period of two years. An interim analysis indicated that treatment groups were
similar with respect to age, menopausal
status, primary tumor diameter, proportion
of positive nodes and prior administration
of radiotherapy. Four hundred and forty-nine
patients were entered into the trial, approximately 150 per treatment arm. The MER-
containing regimen was stopped when it
appeared that MER failed to improve disease-
free survival or drug tolerance. Results
obtained with the other regimens are still

coded (P and Q). With a mean follow-up of
17 months and life table plots to three
years, recurrence rates were 10.8%, 17.9%
and 16.0% for P, Q and CMF-MER respectively.
No difference was detectable by menopausal
or nodal categories either.

CHEMOTHERAPY VERSUS CHEMOTHERAPY + HORMONE THERAPY

The ECOG protocols in pre- and postmenopausal patients have been described earlier.
Chemohormonetherapy is also evaluated in a
NSABP trial testing L-PAM, methotrexate,
5-fluorouracil alone or with tamoxifen.
No data are presently available on either of
these trials.

CHEMOTHERAPY VERSUS CHEMOTHERAPY + IMMUNO- THERAPY

In addition to the CALGB study investigating
the value of MER in combination with chemotherapy (see above), two trials are exploring
the role of immunotherapy. NSABP compares
L-PAM, methotrexate, 5-fluorouracil to the
same program given with C. Parvum whereas
SEG compares cyclophosphamide, methotrexate,
5-fluorouracil given for 6 months with the
same regimen plus BCG. Follow-up is still
too short in these latter trials for meaningful assessment.

DISCUSSION

Data presently available indicate that
surgical adjuvant therapy can prolong the
free interval relative to surgical resection
alone. This observation validates the concept of a combined modality approach to
primary tumors at a time when dissemination
is most likely to be present but cannot be
detected by current diagnostic methods.
Whether this control of clinically undetected
metastases truly improves cure rates still
remains a matter of conjecture.

In premenopausal patients with breast
cancer, the problem is no longer whether
adjuvant therapy has a role but new challenging questions have arisen. However, untreated
control arms must still be recommended in
trials involving postmenopausal patients.
Reasons for the apparently different effect
of adjuvant chemotherapy according to menopausal status remain to be clarified (10).

Some of the treatments and concepts currently available for adjuvant approaches have
been illustrated by this review of studies
carried out by the cooperative groups in
the United States. These studies are essentially designed to define optimal adjuvant
regimens. Little attention has been directed
to modifying the extent of local therapy, and
its morbidity, as systemic therapy is added.

Objective antitumor activity achieved in
advanced disease provides the most rational
basis for selecting a regimen in an adjuvant
setting. This is further supported by the
demonstrated superiority of combination

chemotherapy over single agent treatments
in advanced and, it would appear, in early
breast cancer (6,7,11). Of note, although
adriamycin is considered as the most active
single agent in this disease (12), it has not
been used in any trial under the scope of
this review. Adriamycin has however been
incorporated in adjuvant combination chemotherapy regimens by several investigators
(13-I5).

Dose-schedule and duration of treatment
are likely to be critical in adjuvant surgical chemotherapy programs. Intensive regimens and prolonged administrations are widely
advocated. New approaches based on experimental data have been proposed. A major
cause of relapse in cancers that are initially
responsive to chemotherapy seems related to
a selection and overgrowth of specifically
and permanently drug-resistant tumors cells
(16). Sequential administration of effective
drug combinations has been shown to circumvent this phenomenon in murine leukemia (16).
Alternate combinations have also been used
clinically in advanced solid tumors and
should be further explored in adjuvant
programs.

Norton and Simon (17) have recently proposed that the sensitivity to chemotherapy is
a function of the growth rate of the tumors
and not of their growth fraction as commonly
believed. In a Gompertzian growth, it may
be calculated that the growth rate is maximum
when the tumor is about 37% of its maximum
size and it is at this point that chemotherapy would be most effective. In contrast,
the growth rate is smallest, and resistance
to chemotherapy would be the greatest, for
very large and very small tumors. According
to this hypothesis, optimal treatments should
include the administration of a late intensification program at a time when the tumor
is most resistant. This concept is attrac-
give and deserves further testing.

Long-term risks of adjuvant therapy warrant
considerable attention and should be evaluated
in the light of the cure rate that may be
anticipated with surgery alone in a specific
population. Selection of adjuvant chemotherapy regimens should take these risks into
consideration. The possible development of
second malignancies induced by chemotherapy
also requires efforts directed to prevent
carcinogenic effects of anticancer agents.

Chemohormonetherapy trials of the cooperative groups have yielded little data so far.
Encouraging interim results have been reported
by Husbay et al. with the suggestion that the
addition of tamoxifen may increase the efficacy of combination chemotherapy (18). Conflicting data obscure the prognostic significance of hormone receptors for the recurrence
of breast cancer and for the response of the
disease to systemic treatment (20-22).
Current trials with very large patient accrual
should greatly help define the role of these
receptors when designing therapeutic strategies in early breast cancer.

The role of immunotherapy in the treatment
of cancer is being increasingly investigated
(19). Immunotherapy is essentially used with
other modalities since experimental models
have shown its effectiveness to be dependent
upon reduction of tumor cell burden. The
potential of immunotherapy would thus appear
to be most apparent in a surgical adjuvant
situation. Surprisingly, despite a increasing knowledge of the mechanism of action of
immunotherapeutic agents and the greater
scientific basis for their use, most of the
current trials remain largely empirical.
More thorough information on immuntherapeutic
agents is needed to logically build clinical
experience that, in turn, should provide
some clues to important interactions between
a particular immunotherapy, the status of
the host immune system, tumor burden, and
other therapeutic modalities.

In conclusion, results of completed trials,
as well as the variety of therapeutic options
that are being investigated or remain to be
tested, make the entire area of adjuvant
treatments increasingly attractive. Clinical
trial methodology and reporting are fraught
with pitfalls, and theories must eventually
give way to facts. Current trends in adjuvant trials are promising but are essentially
based on early findings. Full assessment
of the actual value of adjuvant treatment
must await additional results. The data
should be expanded and more experience should
be gained in carefully designed and evaluated
therapeutic trials investigating the most
pertinent hypotheses (23).

ACKNOWLEDGEMENTS

This work was supported by Grant no.
3.4535.79 from the "Fonds de la Recherche
Scientifique Médicale" (FRSM, Belgium) and
Contract N.I.H. N 01/CM 53840 from the
National Cancer Institute, Bethesda, MD,
U.S.A.
The authors acknowledge the technical
assistance of Miss G. Decoster in the
preparation of this manuscript.

REFERENCES

1. B. Fisher, P. Carbone, S. G. Economou,
   R. Frelick, A. Glass, H. Lerner,
   C. Redmond, M. Zelen, P. Band, D. L.
   Katryck, N. Wolmark, E. R. Fisher and
   other Co-operating Investigators,
   L-Phenylalanine mustard (L-PAM) in the
   management of primary breast cancer. A
   report of early findings. *N. Engl. J.
   Med.* 292, 117 (1975).
2. G. Bonadonna, E. Brusamolino, P. Vala-
   gussa, A. Rossi, L. Brugnatelli,
   C. Brambilla, M. DeLena, G. Tancini,
   E. Bajetta, R. Musumeci and U. Veronesi,
   Combination chemotherapy as an adjuvant
   treatment in operable breast cancer.
   N. Engl. J. Med. 294, 405 (1976).
3. B. Fisher, A. Glass, C. Redmond, E. R.
   Fisher, B. Barton, E. Such, P. Carbone,
   S. Economou, R. Foster, R. Frelick,
   H. Lerner, M. Levitt, R. Margolese,
   J. MacFarlane, D. Plotkin, H. Shibata,

H. Volk (and other cooperating investigators), L-phenylalanine mustard (L-PAM) in the management of primary breast cancer: An update of earlier findings and a comparison with those utilizing L-PAM plus 5-fluorouracil (5-FU). *Cancer* 39, 2883 (1977).

4. B. Fisher, Breast cancer: Studies of the National Surgical Adjuvant Primary Breast Cancer Project (NSABP). Abstract of the 2nd International Conference on the Adjuvant Therapy of Cancer, Tucson, Arizona, U.S.A. Abstract 48 (1979).

5. P. R. Band, D. C. Tormey and M. Bauer, Induction chemotherapy and maintenance chemohormonetherapy in metastatic breast cancer. *Proc. Am. Assoc. Cancer Res. and ASCO* 18, 228 (1977).

6. H. L. Davis, G. E. Metter, G. Ramirez, T. B. Grage, G. Cornell, W. Fletcher, S. Moss and P. Multhauf, An adjuvant trial of L-phenylalanine mustard (L-PAM) vs cyclophosphamide (C), methotrexate (M), 5-fluorouracil (F) and vincristine (V) -CMF-V following mastectomy for operable breast cancer. *Proc. Am. Assoc. Cancer Res. and ASCO* 20, 358 (1979).

7. B. Hoogstraten, S. L. George, B. Samal, S. E. Rivkin, J. J. Costanzi, J. D. Bonnet, T. Thiggen and H. Braine, Combination chemotherapy and adriamycin in patients with advanced breast cancer. A Southwest Oncology Group study. *Cancer* 38, 13 (1976).

8. S. Rivkin, H. Glusberg and S. Rasmussen, Adjuvant chemotherapy in stage II breast cancer. *Proc. Am. Assoc. Cancer Res. and ASCO* 20, 353 (1979).

9. R. Weiss, D. Tormey, O. Glidewell, G. Falkson, M. Perloff, L. Leone and J. F. Holland, Evaluation of postoperative chemoimmunotherapy in mammary carcinoma. *Proc. Am. Assoc. Cancer Res. and ASCO* 20, 244 (1979).

10. M. Rozencweig, M. Zelen, D. D. Von Hoff and F. M. Muggia, Waiting for a Bus: Does it explain age-dependent differences in response to chemotherapy of early breast cancer? *N. Engl. J. Med.* 299, 1363 (1978).

11. M. Rozencweig, J. C. Heuson, D. D. Von Hoff, H. W. Mattheiem, H. L. Davis and F. M. Muggia, Breast cancer. In *Randomized Trials in Cancer: A Critical Review by Sites* (Edited by M. J. Staquet) p. 231, Raven Press, New York (1978).

12. S. K. Carter, Integration of chemotherapy into combined modality treatment of solid tumors. VII. Adenocarcinoma of the breast. *Cancer Treat. Rev.* 3, 141 (1976).

13. A. U. Buzdar, G. R. Blumenschein, J. U. Gutterman, C. K. Tashima, G. N. Hortobagyi, T. L. Smith, E. M. Hersh, E. J. Freireich and E. A. Gehan, Prolongation of disease-free and overall survival with the adjuvant FAC-BCG in stage II, III breast cancer. *Proc. Am. Assoc. Cancer Res. and ASCO* 20, 352 (1979).

14. A. G. Wendt, R. C. Miller, R. S. Heuksinkveld, G. F. Giordano,

R. A. Jackson, S. E. Salmon and S. E. Jones, Adjuvant treatment of breast cancer with adriamycin - cyclophosphamide ± radiotherapy. Abstracts of the 2nd International Conference on the Adjuvant Therapy of Cancer, Tuscon, Arizona, U.S.A. Abstract 56 (1979).

15. S. Williams and L. Einhorn, Adriamycin (ADR) chemoprophylaxis in high risk breast cancer. Abstracts of the 2nd International Conference on the Adjuvant Therapy of Cancer, Tucson, Arizona, U.S.A. Abstract 57 (1979).

16. H. E. Skipper, Adjuvant chemotherapy. *Cancer* 41, 936 (1978).

17. L. Norton and R. Simon, Tumor size, sensitivity to therapy, and design of treatment schedules. *Cancer Treat Rep.* 61, 1307 (1977).

18. C. A. Hubay, O. H. Pearson, J. S. Marshall, R. Rhodes, E. Mansour, R. Hermann, J. C. Jones, W. Flynn, C. Eckert, W. L. McGuire and S. M. Debanne, Adjuvant chemotherapy, antiestrogen therapy and immunotherapy for stage II, III breast cancer. Abstracts of the 2nd Breast Cancer Working Conference, Copenhagen, Denmark, p. 59 (1979).

19. F. M. Muggia, Immunotherapy of cancer. A short review and commentary on current trials. *Cancer Immunol. Immunother.* 3, 5 (1977).

20. W. A. Knight III, R. B. Livingston, E. J. Gregory and M. L. McGuire, Estrogen receptor as an independent prognostic factor for early recurrence in breast cancer. *Cancer Res.* 37, 4669 (1977).

21. D. T. Kiang, D. H. Frenning, A. I. Goldman, V. F. Ascensao and B. J. Kennedy, Estrogen receptors in responses to chemotherapy and hormonal therapy in advanced breast cancer. *N. Engl. J. Med.* 299, 1330 (1978).

22. M. E. Lippman, J. C. Allegra, E. B. Thompson, R. Simon, A. Barlock, L. Green, K. K. Huff, H. M. T. Do, S. C. Aitken and R. Warren, The relation between estrogen receptors and response rate to cytotoxic chemotherapy in metastatic breast cancer. *N. Engl. J. Med.* 298, 1223 (1978).

23. M. Rozencweig and F. M. Muggia, The delta and epsilon errors in the assessment of cancer clinical trials. *Proc. Am. Assoc. Cancer Res. and ASCO* 20, 321 (1979).

Ovarian Irradiation and Prednisone Following Surgery and Radiotherapy for Carcinoma of the Breast

J. W. Meakin*, W. E. C. Allt*, F. A. Beale*, R. S. Bush*, R. M. Clark*, P. J. Fitzpatrick*, N. V. Hawkins*, R. D. T. Jenkin*, J. F. Pringle*, J. G. Reid*, W. D. Rider*, J. L. Hayward** and R. D. Bulbrook**

*The Princess Margaret Hospital, Toronto, Canada
**The Imperial Cancer Research Fund, London, U.K.

Correspondence to J. W. Meakin, The Ontario Cancer Treatment and Research Foundation, 7 Overlea Boulevard, Toronto, Ontario M4H 1A8, Canada

Abstract—*Following surgery and regional radiotherapy for operable carcinoma of the breast in premenopausal women, ovarian irradiation (2000 rads in 5 daily fractions) plus prednisone (7.5 mg per day) results in delayed recurrence and prolonged survival.*

INTRODUCTION

Because some recurrent breast cancers regress following therapeutic castration, several clinical trials have been carried out to test the value of prophylactic ovarian ablation as part of primary treatment.

In the Manchester Trial (1) ovarian irradiation (450r in 1 fraction), in premenopausal patients with histologically negative and positive axillary nodes, delayed the appearance of distant metastases (P = 0.04) but did not significantly prolong survival (P = 0.07) at 10 years.

In the Oslo Trial (2) ovarian irradiation (1000r in 6 daily fractions) in premenopausal (histologically positive axillary nodes) and postmenopausal (histologically negative and positive axillary nodes) patients delayed recurrence and also prolonged survival at 7 years but the differences were small.

In the Trial of the National Surgical Adjuvant Breast Group (3) oophorectomy did not result in a significant delay in recurrence nor prolongation in survival during 3 to 5 years of follow up in premenopausal patients who had either histologically negative or positive axillary nodes.

Because of the ambiguity resulting from these trials the following study was begun in 1965 to test the hypothesis that prophylactic ovarian irradiation, with or without prednisone, could not only delay recurrence but also prolong survival.

MATERIALS AND METHODS

From 1965 to 1972, following mastectomy, premenopausal and postmenopausal patients, aged 35-70 years, with or without histologically positive axillary nodes, received irradiation to the chest wall and regional nodal areas. They were then randomized to receive no further treatment (NT), or ovarian irradiation to a dose of 2000 rads in 5 days (R), or (if 45 years or more) ovarian irradiation in the same dosage plus prednisone, 7.5 mg daily (R + P) for up to 5 years. Patients, entered on study, have been followed for up to 10 years. Patients were considered premenopausal if their last menses had occurred within 6 months of the date of surgery. Patients who had had a hysterectomy, but not an oophorectomy, were considered premenopausal up to the age of 50 years. Steroid receptor assays were not done.

The generalized Wilcoxen Test (4) has been used to determine the significance of differences in the results.

RESULTS

Of 779 randomized patients 23 were ineligible by protocol and are omitted from all analyses. An additional 51 patients were eligible by protocol but did not receive the randomly-assigned treatment; analyses of the data with or without these patients included has not affected the results. Therefore the following data relate to 705 randomized patients who were eligible by protocol and did receive the assigned treatment as of March 1979. The results of this study as of May 1977 have been previously published in detail (5).

For reporting the patients are divided into 3 groups: (a) premenopausal less than 45 years of age, (b) premenopausal 45 years or more in age, and (c) postmenopausal.

1. Premenopausal Patients Less than 45 Years of Age

(a): In this group (35-44 years) clinical stages (TNM) I, II and III were entered, and were randomized only between NT and R. The two groups were comparable for age and stage. Histologically positive axillary

lymph nodes were identified in 83% of the
NT group and in 91% of the R group.

The recurrence-free and survival curves
(actuarial) are presented in figs. 1 and 2.
Numbers of patients followed to specific
times are recorded on the graphs. While
there is a persistent delay in recurrence
and prolongation of survival the differences
are not statistically significant (P = 0.17
for Fig. 1 and P = 0.24 for Fig. 2).

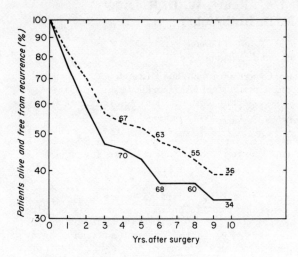

Fig. 1. Premenopausal patients less than
45 years. NT (70 patients) ———,
R (67 patients) -----, (NT vs R,
P = 0.17). No. of patients
followed to specific times are
recorded on the graphs.

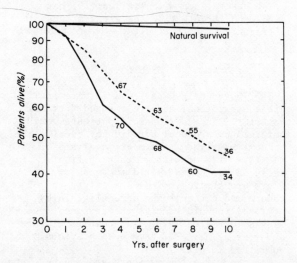

Fig. 2. Premenopausal patients less than
45 years. NT (70 patients) ———,
R (67 patients) -----, (NT vs R,
P = 0.24). Natural survival for
age range shown in heavy line at
top. No. of patients followed to
specific times are recorded on
the graphs.

Separate analyses of the histologically
node-positive patients only from Figs. 1 and
2 reveals a similar degree of delay in

recurrence and improvement in survival
between the NT and R groups as follows:
(a) Fig. 1, P = 0.14; (b) Fig. 2, P = 0.17.

2. Premenopausal Patients 45 Years or more

(b): In this group clinical stages (TNM)
I, II, and III were randomized between NT,
R, or R + P. The three groups were comparable for age and stage. Histologically
positive axillary nodes were identified as
follows: NT - 69%; R - 66%; R + P - 71%.

The actuarial recurrence-free and survival
curves are shown in Figs. 3 and 4. Numbers
of patients, followed to specific times,
are recorded on the graphs.

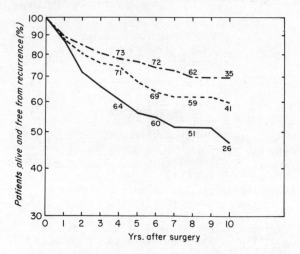

Fig. 3. Premenopausal patients 45 years or
more. NT (64 patients) ———,
R (71 patients) -----, R + P (73
patients) -.-.-., (NT vs R,
P = 0.21; NT vs R + P, P = 0.02;
R vs R + P, P = 0.27). No. of
patients followed to specific
times are recorded on the graphs.

In Fig. 3 while R and R + P are delaying
recurrence, only R + P is doing so to a
statistically significant degree (NT vs
R + P, P = 0.02).

In Fig. 4 R and R + P are prolonging
survival, but only R + P is doing so significantly over the NT group (P = 0.03).

If only the patients with histologically
positive axillary nodes from Figs. 3 and 4
are analyzed the significance of the differences between the NT and R + P groups
decreases to: (a) Fig. 3, P = 0.05;
(b) Fig. 4, P = 0.1.

3. Postmenopausal Patients

(c): No differences in time to recurrence
nor in survival could be demonstrated between
the NT, R and R + P groups.

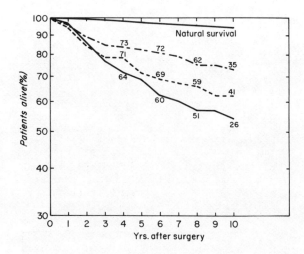

Fig. 4. Premenopausal patients 45 years or
more. NT (64 patients) ———,
R (71 patients) —————, R + P (73
patients) -.-.-., (NT vs R,
P = 0.51; NT vs R + P, P = 0.03;
R vs R + P, P = 0.16). Natural
survival for age range shown in
heavy line at top. No. of patients
followed to specific times are
recorded on the graphs.

DISCUSSION

These data are in agreement with the
Manchester (1) and Oslo (2) Trials in demonstrating an apparent delay in recurrence and
prolongation of survival after adjuvant
ovarian irradiation alone, but were not
statistically significant in this study.

The lack of agreement with the results of
the NSABP Trial (3) of prophylactic oophorectomy is possibly the effect of chance, or
that an irradiated ovary may result in a
different physiologic state from that after
a surgical oophorectomy. Alternatively,
further follow-up data from the NSABP Trial
(3) may demonstrate some value for surgical
oophorectomy, for it may be noted that the
effect of ovarian ablation in our study did
not become firm until after 3 to 5 years
of follow-up.

However the data of this study indicate
that the addition of small doses of prednisone
to ovarian irradiation produces significant
delay in recurrence and prolongation in
survival in premenopausal patients. Whether
the prednisone produced its effect by suppressing estrogen of adrenal origin, or by
some other mechanism is not known. Other
possible mechanisms include a reduction in
prolactin secretion (perhaps mediated by
reduced estrogen production), immunological
factors, or direct anti-tumour effects.
Again it is emphasized that the effect of
ovarian irradiation plus prednisone did not
become definite until after 3 years of
follow-up.

One of the important features of these data
is that ovarian ablation and prednisone were

effective in delaying recurrence in premenopausal patients with histologically positive
axillary nodes. Thus it would seem rational
in future studies to examine the role of
adjuvant hormonal therapy, both as a comple-
ment to, and as an alternative to adjuvant
chemotherapy, particularly in patients with
steroid receptor-positive tumours.

ACKNOWLEDGEMENTS

We are indebted to The Ontario Cancer
Treatment and Research Foundation and the
Imperial Cancer Research Fund for their
financial support, to the many surgeons who
agreed to the entry of their patients into
this study, to Drs. A. Phillips, A. Sellers,
and G.DeBoer for their biostatistical help,
to Drs. A. Alaton and the late Dr. E. Kruyff
for their assistance in the clinical assessment of patients, and to the clinical trials
secretaries who helped monitor the study.

REFERENCES

1. M. P. Cole, Suppression of ovarian function in primary breast cancer. In *Prognostic Factors in Breast Cancer*. (Edited
   by A. P. M. Forrest and P. B. Kunkler),
   p. 146, E. and S. Livingston, Edinburgh
   (1968).
2. R. Nissen-Meyer, Suppression of ovarian
   function in primary breast cancer. In
   Prognostic Factors in Breast Cancer.
   (Edited by A. P. M. Forrest and P. B.
   Kunkler), p. 139, E. and S. Livingston,
   Edinburgh (1968).
3. R. G. Ravdin, E. F. Lewison, N. H. Slack,
   T. L. Dao, B. Gardner, D. State, and
   B. Fisher, Results of a clinical trial
   concerning the worth of prophylactic
   oophorectomy for breast carcinoma. *Surg.
   Gynec. Obstet.* 131, 1055 (1970).
4. E. A. Gehan, A generalized Wilcoxen test
   for comparing arbitrarily singly-sensored
   samples. *Biometrika* 52, 203 (1965).
5. J. W. Meakin, W. E. C. Allt, F. A. Beale,
   T. C. Brown, R. S. Bush, R. M. Clark,
   P. J. Fitzpatrick, N. V. Hawkins, R. D. T.
   Jenkin, J. F. Pringle, J. G. Reid, W. D.
   Rider, J. L. Hayward, and R. D. Bulbrook,
   Ovarian irradiation and prednisone following surgery and radiotherapy for carcinoma
   of the breast. *Can. Med. Assoc. J.* 120
   (1979).

Adjuvant Endocrine Therapy of Primary Operable Breast Cancer. Report on the Copenhagen Breast Cancer Trials*

T. Palshof*,**, H. T. Mouridsen*** and J. L. Daehnfeldt**

University Hospital Gentofte, Dept. R, Copenhagen
University Hospital Glostrup, Dept. D, Copenhagen
University Hospital Bispebjerg, Dept. L, Copenhagen
***The Fibiger Laboratory, Copenhagen*
****Finseninstitute, Copenhagen*

Correspondence to T. Palshof, Dept. R, University Hospital Gentofte, Niels Andersensvej 65, 2900 Hellerup, Copenhagen, Denmark

Participating departments:
Dept. of thoracic surgery R, Amtssygehuset i Gentofte.
Dept. of thoracic surgery L, Bispebjerg Hospital.
Dept. of surgery D, Amtssygehuset i Glostrup.
Dept. of pathology, Amtssygehuset i Gentofte.
Dept. of pathology, Amtssygehuset i Glostrup.
Dept. of radiology, Bispebjerg Hospital.
Dept. of radiology, Amtssygehuset i Glostrup.
Dept. of radiology, Amtssygehuset i Gentofte.
Dept. of clinical chemistry, Amtssygehuset i Glostrup.
Dept. of clinical chemistry, Amtssygehuset i Gentofte.
Dept. of clinical chemistry, Bispebjerg Hospital.
Dept. of gynaecology, Amtssygehuset i Gentofte.
Radiumstationen, Copenhagen.
Dept. of oncology and radiotherapy, Amtssygehuset i Herlev.
Dept. of nuclear medicine, Finseninstitute.
Dept. of surgery, Finseninstitute.
Dept. of medical oncology R II & R V, Finseninstitute.
Dept. of dermatology, Finseninstitute.
Dept. of nuclear medicine, Bispebjerg Hospital.
Dept. of fysiurgi, Amtssygehuset i Gentofte.

Abstract—*The Copenhagen Breast Cancer Trials include propsective randomized trials evaluating the effect of additive endocrine adjuvant therapy to pre- and postmenopausal women with stage I-III breast cancer. The therapeutic effect of 2 years treatment with tamoxifen or placebo to premenopausal, diethylstilboestrol, tamoxifen or placebo to postmenopausal is evaluated by the rate of recurrence and the length of disease free interval. The clinical results are retrospectively correlated to estrogen receptor content of the primary tumor in 332 patients.*

Treatment with tamoxifen and placebo was well tolerated whereas side effects prompted a high rate of discontinuation in the diethylstilboestrol-treated group.

After a median observation time of 3 years a reduced rate of recurrence is observed in both pre- and postmenopausal patients treated with tamoxifen and diethylstilboestrol, especially in those with ER pos. tumors.

INTRODUCTION

The basis for adjuvant additive endocrine therapy in breast cancer was until a few years ago based on a theoretical background. At the beginning of this decade the well known effect of endocrine manipulation in advanced disease was documented to be correlated to hormone dependency of the tumor, defined by the presence of steroid hormone receptors [1,2]. Simultaneously a new potent anti-estrogen, tamoxifen, was introduced, less toxic than estrogens and androgens and with an equal or higher therapeutic efficacy

---

*This investigation has been supported by grants from the Danish Cancer Society (including Scholarship for T. Palshof), the Danish Medical Research Counsil and Mrs. Agathe Neye. Imperial Chemical Industries (ICI), Pharmaceuticals Division has generously supplied the tablet material for this trial.

in advanced disease (3,4). As with other
endocrine treatments the efficacy of this
anti-estrogen is correlated to the hormone
dependency of the tumor.

The aim of the Copenhagen Breast Cancer
Trials is to evaluate the effect of adjuvant
additive endocrine therapy with estrogen and
anti-estrogen and to correlate retrospectively
any change in disease free interval and
survival to the estrogen receptor content of
the primary tumor.

MATERIAL AND METHODS

From 1975-1978 consecutive patients admitted
to three breast cancer clinics in Copenhagen
entered the study.

1. Inclusion Criteria

Women, less than 70 years of age, with
tumors of category T_{1-4}, N_{0-3}, M_0. The M_0-
status was assessed by X-ray of chest, skeleton survey and bone scintigraphy. There
must be no history of previous or concomitant
malignancy, thromboembolic or chronic hepatic
disorders. Hypertension or congestive heart
failure must be corrected before entry to
the study.

2. Definitions

Postmenopausal are patients with at least
five years normal menostasia. Patients
previously hysterectomized, ovariectomized
or with continued menstrual bleedings on
hormonal administration are defined postmenopausal after the age of 55 years. All
other patients are regarded premenopausal
(i.e. this group includes perimenopausal
patients).

3. All Patients had Simple Mastectomy

All patients had simple mastectomy (without
routinely axillary dissection) and post-
operative irradiation either by conventional
or high voltage technique.

Two weeks after surgery patients were
randomized according to menopausal status to
double blind endocrine therapy for two years
(Table 1).

Treatment is discontinued in case of
severe or life-threatening side effects or
in case of recurrence. Patients are considered non-evaluable if treatment was discontinued within three months.

At entry to the study the patients were
informed that they received profylactic
endocrine treatment, but only till later all
patients have been informed about the double
blind technique used in the trial.

4. Clinical Follow-up

Physical examination and clinical chemical
studies were done every three months for
two years and then every 6 months for the
next 3 years. Hereafter patients are seen
once a year for 5 years. Bone scintigraphy
is performed yearly and X-ray of chest and
mammography is performed every 18 months.

5. Estrogen Receptor Determination

Biopsies from the primary tumor were
initially frozen on CO_2-ice and stored at
-80^oC before determination. All ER analysis
were performed at the Fibiger Laboratory
using the dextran-coated charcoal technique
(5,6).

Estrogen receptor positive (ER pos) were
defined by $\geq$ 20 femto moles/mg cytosol
protein (fmol/mg) (Table 2).

Tumors in the interval between 10-20
fmol/mg were considered ER neg including a
few biopsies without histological examination.
Tumors defined ER neg with less than 10
fmol/mg have all been proved to contain
tumor cells in the biopsy for ER determination. Tumors with less than 10 fmol/mg and
without histological examination of the
biopsy are defined ER neg?.

RESULTS

A total of 387 eligible patients entered
the study. Eight patients refused randomization to therapy, 5 have been lost to follow-
up and in 33 treatment was discontinued
within three months due to side effects.

332 patients were evaluable with respect
to treatment and among these 254 were also
evaluable according to ER content of the
primary tumor. As appears from Table 3 the

Table 1. Randomization of pre- and postmenopausal patients
to treatment.

Premenopausal   Tamoxifen 10 mg × 3 daily
Placebo 1 tablet × 3 daily

Postmenopausal   Tamoxifen 10 mg × 3 daily
Diethylstilboestrol 1 mg × 3 daily
Placebo 1 tablet × 3 daily

Table 2. Definitions of ER status in The Copenhagen Breast
Cancer Trials.

Estrogen receptor positive (ER pos):
More than 20 fmol/mg cyt. protein
Estrogen receptor negative (ER neg):
Less than 20 fmol/mg cyt. protein
If less than 10 fmol/mg cyt. protein
malignant histology of the biopsy is required
Estrogen receptor negative? (ER neg?):
Less than 10 fmol/mg cyt. protein
but not proven malignant histology of the biopsy for receptor determination
Estrogen receptor unknown (ER unknown):
No biopsy for receptor determination

Table 3. Distribution of ER pos. and neg. in the patient material
and according to menstrual status.

Pre	ER pos	39%
	ER neg	61%
Post	ER pos	47%
	ER neg	53%
All	ER pos	42%
	ER neg	58%

distribution of ER pos and neg in premenopausal patients is 39% versus 61% and in the postmenopausal 47% versus 53%. In the total material there is a few more ER neg tumors (58%).

After a median duration of observation of nearly three years 91 recurrences have been observed.

It must be emphasized that in all but the ER neg and ER neg? there is an equal distribution of patients according to stage of disease. In the ER neg group there is a higher number of stage III patients which may explain the higher rate of recurrence in this group.

In the premenopausal patients evaluable according to therapy the rate of recurrence in the tamoxifen and placebo groups are 21% and 35% respectively.

As seen in Fig. 1 the present results indicate that ER neg premenopausal patients seems to have a better prognosis than ER pos.

This tendency is specially pronounced in the placebo treated group, but regardless of treatment the rate of recurrence in ER pos premenopausal patients 31% versus 25% in ER neg patients.

In postmenopausal patients evaluable according to therapy a rate of recurrence in the DES tamoxifen and placebo groups is 18%, 24% and 36% respectively. In this group the ER

pos seems to have a better prognosis than ER neg having a recurrence regardless of therapy of 14% in ER pos and 39% in ER neg. It would be reemphasized of this that the ER neg group contain a higher number of stage III patients.

As appears from Fig. 2 there is a dramatic effect of DES in all ER pos categories, but the number of patients in this treatment group is small. Tamoxifen reduced the rate of recurrence if ER pos tumor contain more than 50 fmol/mg.

Generally the treatments have been well tolerated. At present 36% of the premenopausal patients treated with tamoxifen have not reported any side effects compared to 45% in the placebo group. In the postmenopausal patients only 15% treated with DES were without side effects compared to 48% and 53% in the tamoxifen and placebo groups. Treatment had to be discontinued in 17% of all patients. In pre- and postmenopausal patients treatment with tamoxifen and placebo was discontinued in 13% and 10% respectively. Nearly half (42%) of patients treated with DES had discontinuation of treatment and in 17% (8/49) due to thromboembolic events. No deaths have been ascribed to any of the treatments.

Other side effects were in general mild or moderate and the most common reported were hot flushes. Menstrual disturbances

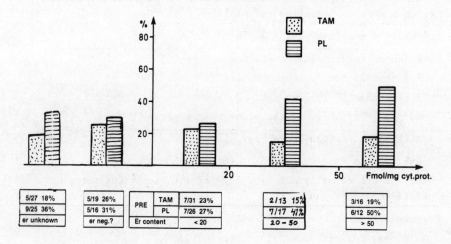

Fig. 1. Number of recurrences/number of patients and rate of recurrence (%) in premenopausal patients according to treatment and ER status (bottom). Histogram showing the rate of recurrence of tamoxifen and placebo groups in each ER category.

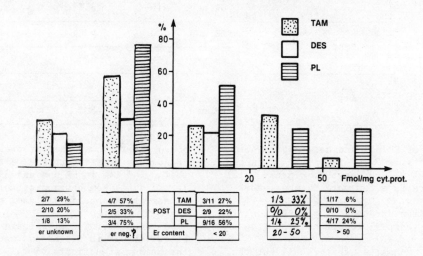

Fig. 2. Number of recurrences/number of patients and rate of recurrence (%) in postmenopausal patients according to treatment and ER status (bottom). Histogram showing the rate of recurrence of tamoxifen, DES and placebo groups in each ER category.

were observed in more than half of patients treated with tamoxifen (Table 4). Six cases of ovarian cysts were documented distributed in all treatment groups.

It was unexpected that more than 80% treated with DES had vaginal bleedings. These patients had after abrasio regular vaginal bleeding on continuous therapy by administration of medroxyprogesterone (Clinovir) 5 mg daily for 7 days every fourth week. As appears from Table 4 menostasia were induced in both the tamoxifen and placebo treated group, but only in the tamoxifen group renewed menstruation after discontinuation was observed.

DISCUSSION

These preliminary results of the Copenhagen Breast Cancer Trials indicate that both pre- and postmenopausal women with stage I-III breast cancer benefit from adjuvant additive endocrine therapy. Earlier reports of this study (7,8) have shown that only postmenopausal patients will benefit by reduced rate of recurrence and prolonged disease free interval.

Despite the limited number of patients and time of observation a marked effect of tamoxifen is observed in both pre- and postmenopausal patients and an even higher reduction of rate of recurrence is achieved with DES.

Table 4. Preliminary status of side effects in the treatment
groups.

	Tamoxifen	DES	Placebo
Hot flushes	31%	25%	19%
Nausea, vomiting	8%	26%	7%
Cyst of ovary	1%	6%	1%
Vaginal bleeding	6%	82%	0
Menstrual disturbances	53%		25%
Menostasia in 123 premenopausal pt.			
Not since operation	10% (7/67)		7% (4/56)
During adj. therapy	13% (9/67)		7% (4/56)
Renewed after discontinuation	25% (4/16)		0

These therapeutic results may retrospectively indicate the clinical level for definition of ER pos (rich) and ER neg (poor) tumors. The technique used in this study indicate that the clinical level of hormone dependency is different in pre- and postmenopausal patients (tumors) in evaluating the effect of adjuvant tamoxifen (20 fmol/mg versus 50 fmol/mg).

As observed in the placebo treated group there seems to be a better prognosis of ER neg tumors compared to ER pos tumors in the premenopausal group. This preliminary observation is not in agreement with other data, but a hypothetical explanation may include endogenous stimulation of hormone dependent tumors.

Based on these results tamoxifen should in the future be included as a treatment modality in the adjuvant situation. Adjuvant tamoxifen therapy seems to be correlated to hormone dependency of the primary tumor, and at present there is an urgent need to supply future trials with international standard definitions of hormone dependency especially if patients are stratified according to this concept. fied according to this concept.

The present study do not evaluate the effect of additive endocrine therapy according to axillary node status, but trials with adjuvant tamoxifen to node pos (high risk) patients is in progress.

In view of the results presented and the lack of toxicity tamoxifen might also serve as a adjuvant candidate to low risk patients.

ACKNOWLEDGEMENTS

The authors are grateful to the staffs of the participating departments for invaluable support and assistance. Dr. Svend-Erik Buhl Jørgensen for invaluable assistance in all gynaecological questions and treatment. Dr. Carsten Rose for constructive criticism and advice, cand. stat. Erik Kousgaard for statistical assistance, Dr. Birgitte Bruun Rasmussen for histological examination of the tumor biopsies and Mrs. Ellen Kirk for secretarial assistance.
Dr. Aage Hein Christiansen for invaluable advice and care of patients with dermatological diseases. Social advisor Mrs. Rethe Rørdam and all general practitioners of the patients for invaluable cooperation.

REFERENCES

1. W. L. McGuire, O. H. Pearson and A. Segaloff, Predicting hormone responsiveness in human breast cancer. In *Estrogen Receptors in Human Breast Cancer.* (Edited by W. L. Guire, P. P. Carbone and E. P. Volmer), p. 17. Raven Press, New York (1975).
2. R. B. J. King, Clinical relevance of steroid-receptor measurement in tumors. *Cancer Treatment Reviews* 2, 273 (1975).
3. M. P. Cole, C. T. A. Jones and I. D. H. Todd, A new anti-oestrogic agent in late breast cancer. An early appraisal of ICI 46, 474. *Br. J. Cancer* 25, 270 (1971).
4. H. T. Mouridsen, T. Palshof, J. Patterson and L. Battersby, Tamoxifen in advanced breast cancer. *Cancer Treatment Reviews* 5, 131 (1978).
5. S. G. Korenman, Radio-ligand binding assay of specific estrogens using a soluble uterine macromolecule. *J. Endocrinol. Metab.* 28, 127 (1968).
6. J. A. Katzenellenbogen, H. J. Johnson and K. E. Carlson, Studies on the uterine cytoplasmatic estrogen binding protein. Thermal stability and ligand dissociation rate. An assay of empty and filled sites by exchange. *Biochemistry* 12, 4092 (1973).
7. T. Palshof, J. L. Daehnfeldt and H. T. Mouridsen, Adjuvant endocrine therapy of breast cancer. A controlled clinical trial of estrogen and anti-estrogen. Preliminary report on The Copenhagen Breast Cancer Trials. In *Reviews on Endocrine-Related Cancer* (Edited by M. Mayer, S. Saez and B. A. Stoll) suppl. April, 168 (1978).
8. T. Palshof, H. T. Mouridsen and J. L. Daehnfeldt, Adjuvant endocrine therapy of breast cancer. A controlled clinical trial of estrogen and anti-estrogen. Preliminary results of The Copenhagen Breast Cancer Trials. *Recent Results in Cancer Research* (in press).

Adjuvant Chemotherapy, Anti-Estrogen Therapy and Immunotherapy for Stage II Breast Cancer

C. A. Hubay[1], O. H. Pearson[2], J. S. Marshall[1],
R. S. Rhodes[1], S. M. Debanne[3], E. G. Mansour[4],
R. E. Hermann[5], J. C. Jones[6], W. J. Flynn[7],
C. Eckert[8], W. L. McGuire[9], and 27 Participating

[1]Department of Surgery
[2]Department of Medicine and
[3]Department of Biometry, Case Western Reserve University, School of Medicine
and University Hospitals
[4]Cleveland Metropolitan General Hospital
[5]Cleveland Clinic
[6]St. Luke's Hospital, Cleveland, Ohio
[7]Youngstown Hospital Association, Youngstown, Ohio
[8]Albany Medical Center, Albany, New York
[9]University of Texas, San Antonio, Texas, and Akron General Medical Center,
Akron, Ohio

Participating Investigators: F. M. Barry, J. H. Berman, M. R. Bhatti, R. Bukowski,
A. M. Cooperman, D. H. Cowan, L. Deppisch, R. L. Druet, C. Esselstyn, D. Evans,
Y. S. Fu, C. Groppe, V. D. Hacker, J. S. Marshall, J. Horton, H. B. Houser,
A. Manni, A. E. Powell, R.. Reimer, B. A. Sebek, R. W. Sponzo, E. Steiger,
A. A. Stein, J. E. Trujillo, E. C. Weckesser, J. K. Weick, and R. W. Wroblewski

Correspondence to Dr. Charles A. Hubay, Department of Surgery,
2074 Abington Road, Cleveland Ohio 44106, USA

Abstract—A prospective, randomized clinical trial of three adjuvant treatment regimens, CMF, CMF + tamoxifen (CMFT) and CMFT + BCG immunotherapy in women with stage II breast cancer is reported at follow-up of 33 months postmastectomy. It was observed that stage II breast cancer patients with estrogen receptor positive (ER+) tumors had delayed recurrence when compared to patients with estrogen receptor negative (ER-) tumors (p = 0.001). Similarly, the mortality at 33 months postmastectomy was greater in the ER- patients (p = 0.0001).

The addition of the anti-estrogen drug tamoxifen to CMF chemotherapy had a significant benefit in patients with ER+ tumors, when compared to ER- patients (p = 0.0176). In ER- patients with stage II breast cancer, none of the three treatment regimens appeared superior.

With CMF treatment, premenopausal, ER- stage II breast cancer patients recur more rapidly tha ER+ premenopausal patients (p = 0.0313). This may reflect suppression of ovarian function benefiting the latter group. No effect of CMF was seen in postmenopausal patients.

At this time, no conclusions regarding the effect of BCG immunotherapy can be made, owing to the brief follow-up period.

The use of anti-estrogen therapy appears to offer a major advance in the treatment of stage II ER+ breast cancer patients. Further observation is needed to determine the duration of benefit.

INTRODUCTION

Fisher (1) has recently compiled 5 year recurrence data for women undergoing mastectomy for primary breast cancer. He points out that recurrence following surgical therapy alone is high (50-79%) and is dependent on the number of axillary nodes involved with the tumor. It has been pointed out by many investigators that breast cancer is often widespread in many women at the time of primary therapy. This has led to the adjuvant use of systemic treatments including such measures as ovarian and adrenal suppression and cytotoxic chemotherapy in an attempt to delay or prevent recurrences.

Nissen-Meyer (2,3,4) following patients treated by adjuvant ovarian irradiation has shown that such measures can delay recurrence particularly in premenopausal women. Confirmation of his data by Cole (5) and more recently by Meakin, et al. (6) using ovarian irradiation and oral prednisone to suppress adrenal function, have emphasized the role of hormonal suppression. Meakin noted that not only was recurrence delayed, but survival improved.

*Supported by Public Health Service Contract CB-43990 (CAH) and CB-23862 (WLM), Grant CA-05195-19 (OHP) from the National Cancer Institute and Grant PTD48U from the American Cancer Society (OHP).

The impetus for adjuvant cytotoxic chemotherapy was provided in 1975 by the observations of Fisher, et al. (7) and in 1976 by
Bonadonna, et al. (8) documenting delayed
recurrence in treated stage II breast cancer
patients. Subsequent follow-up of these
patients has revealed the beneficial results
to occur mainly in premenopausal patients.

This report documents the preliminary
results of a cooperative, multi-institutional
clinical trial for the treatment of primary
stage II breast cancer. The study was
designed to determine what effect a combination of adjuvant endocrine therapy, cytotoxic chemotherapy and BCG immunotherapy
would have on recurrence and survival rates
of stage II breast cancer following mastectomy. Anti-estrogen treatment was selected
for trial on the basis of the preliminary
results of Cole (9) in 1971 and others
(10,11). Engelsman, et al. (12) and Ward
(13) in 1973 demonstrated the usefulness of
these compounds in stage IV breast cancer
patients with both pre- and postmenopausal
patients benefiting by such therapy. The
selection of BCG vaccination for non-specific
stimulation of cellular immunity was based
on an animal tumor model reported by Esber,
et al. (14). Using a murine mammary carcinoma they demonstrated that a combination
of chemotherapy and an extract of tubercle
bacilli could prolong survival in animals
with metastatic spread.

With these findings as background a prospective randomized trial of cytoxan, methotrexate, 5-fluorouracil (CMF), CMF plus the
anti-estrogen drug, tamoxifen (CMFT), and
CMFT plus immunotherapy with BCG, as adjuvant
treatment in women with stage II breast
cancer was initiated in 1974.

MATERIAL AND METHODS

Women, 75 years of age or under, without
a previous history of malignancy or any
precluding medical disorder, undergoing
mastectomy for primary breast cancer were
evaluated. Pathologic staging was carried
out and those patients demonstrating one or
more axillary lymph nodes involved with
metastatic tumor were eligible for adjuvant
treatment. Estrogen receptor (ER) analysis
of the primary tumor was carried out and was
mandatory for inclusion of the study patients.
Informed consent was obtained from each
patient so selected.

To maintain uniformity of ER analysis,
most determinations (15) of ER tumor content
were performed in a single laboratory by one
of us (W. McG.). An arbitrary level of ≥ 3
femtomoles/mg (fm/mg) cytosol protein was
selected as positive (ER+) and those < 3 fm/mg
were considered negative (ER-). Seventy-four
percent of the tumors in this series were
considered ER+ and 26% were negative (ER-).

Eligible stage II breast cancer patients
were then stratified according to the above
estrogen receptor categories (ER+ or ER-)
and by the number of axillary nodes found
to contain tumor (1 - 3 or ≥ 4 positive

nodes). Patients were then randomly assigned
to one of three treatment categories:
(I) CMF, (II) CMFT and (III) CMFT + BCG.

It should be pointed out that when this
study was initiated in 1974, a control group,
treated by surgery alone, was used in place
of (I) CMF treatment above. After Bonadonna's
promising report in 1976 (8), the control
group was changed to CMF therapy. Treatment,
Fig. 1, was similar to that used by Bonadonna.
Cytoxan, 60 mg/M^2 was given orally in two
divided doses from days 1-14 for each of the
12 monthly (28 day) cycles. Methotrexate,
25 mg/M^2 and 5-fluorouracil, 400 mg/M^2 were
given intravenously on days 1 and 8 for 12
monthly cycles. Hemograms were obtained on
days of intravenous therapy and drug dosages
modified if significant myelosuppression had
occurred. The anti-estrogen drug, tamoxifen,
was given orally, 20 mg b.i.d. for one year.

BCG, vaccinations were not begun until the
second year of treatment. BCG vaccinations
were placed on the abdomen, using the Tine
technique, weekly for one month, then monthly
for eleven subsequent months, using rotating
quadrant sites.

All treatments and follow-up examinations
were performed by qualified medical oncologists. Careful physical examinations were
performed every 3 months. Routine chest
x-ray was performed biyearly and bone scans
and mammograms yearly. Other x-rays were
performed when indicated. Blood chemistry
profiles, including liver function tests
were carried out at the time of each physical
examination. The first documented recurrence
in skin, lymph nodes or distal sites was
selected as the endpoint in the study.

Subsequent therapy following recurrence
was left to the discretion of the medical
oncologist in charge of the patient.

All basic information of study patients,
including age, size, and location of the
primary tumor, number of axillary nodes
involved, tumor pathology, menopausal status
and reproductive history, ER analysis, and
other pertinent data, including drug toxicity,
recurrence data and site, have been analyzed
using computer-based statistical software.

A generalization of the Kruskal-Wallis
test was used to compare treatment effects
among three or more patient groups (16,17);
pairwise comparisons were made with a generalized Wilcoxon test (18). A series of one
way ANOVA or Chi-square tests-depending on
the form of the data - were performed to
discern whether certain patient characteristics were allocated approximately equivalently
to each treatment modality.

The results presented here are based on
the experience of 302 patients, of whom 296
have been followed for at least one month
to 4.5 years by the time of these analyses.
Of these 296 patients, 52 have had documented
recurrence and 25 have died of metastatic
breast cancer. Two additional deaths were
unrelated to breast malignancy. Twenty-nine
patients withdrew from treatment from 1 to 18
months following entry. Of these, 23 voluntarily withdrew within the first year of
treatment and 6 withdrew or refused BCG

CHEMOTHERAPY CYCLE					
	DAY				REPEAT CYCLE
	1	8	14	15-28	
5-FU — 400 mg/M²/I.v.	●	●			DAY 29 FOR 12 MONTHS
MTX — 25 mg/M²/I.v.	●	●			
CYTOXAN — 60 mg/M²/p.o. (IN TWO DIVIDED DOSES)	● ● ● ● ● ● ● ● ● ●			REST PERIOD	
TAMOXIFEN — 20 mg/b.i.d./p.o.	——————— 1 YEAR ———————				

Fig. 1. Schema of chemotherapy and anti-estrogen treatment for 12 monthly
cycles. Immunotherapy with BCG was not initiated until the second
year, following completion of chemotherapy.

vaccination during the second year. Eighty-
five mastectomy patients who were otherwise
eligible for study refused entry into treatment for various reasons. The characteristics of the treated with the eligible
untreated patients show no significant differences. All patients (withdrawal and refusal)
are being followed for recurrence.

In the statistical evaluation of results,
the patients who voluntarily withdrew from
treatment have been treated as censored
observations, their times until leaving
therapy being recorded. It was deemed
inappropriate to include as data for a given
treatment, information regarding these
patients' outcome (recurrence or nonrecur-
rence) for the following reason: once
patients leave prescribed therapy, they
cannot formally be categorized as receiving
their assigned treatment. Of 29 withdrawals,
5 patients have recurred. All 5 patients
were ER-; one was in the CMF group, one in
CMFT and 3 in CMFT + BCG; their inclusion in
the corresponding treatment group could not
weaken the inferences made.

RESULTS

Using standard statistical methods, it
was observed that the recurrence rate in
stage II breast cancer patients with ER-
tumors was more rapid than in similar
patients with ER+ tumors at 33 months post
mastectomy {ER- vs ER+ - 50.8% vs 20.3%}
(p = 0.0001). When these patients are
further subdivided into menopausal status,
Figs. 2 and 3, the results are the same with
ER- patients recurring more rapidly than
ER+ patients in both groups: pre (p = 0.0008)
and post (p = 0.0002). Patient characteristics of age, tumor size, number of positive
nodes and menopausal status were similar for
each group, although tumor size was slightly,
but significantly larger in ER- patients
{ER- (4.3 cm) vs. ER+ (3.5 cm)} (p = 0.01).

Figure 4 documents the recurrence rate of
ER+ tumors for stage II patients. It can
be noted that ER+ stage II breast cancer
patients treated with CMF alone recurred
significantly more rapid than those treated

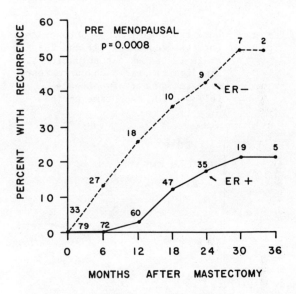

Fig. 2. Life table plot of recurrence
rates for premenopausal ER+ and
ER- stage II breast cancer
patients. The figures over each
curve represent the number of
patients followed for each time
period.

with CMFT (p = 0.0176). When both the tamoxifen treated groups (CMFT and CMFT + BCG) are
combined and compared with CMF treatment
alone, there is a decided advantage in the
tamoxifen groups (p = 0.025). When ER+
patients are divided into menopausal groups
and the three treatments compared, the tamoxifen treated patients have delayed recurrences;
premenopausal {CMFT + CMFT+BCG} vs. CMF
(p = 0.1); postmenopausal, {CMFT + CMFT+BCG}
vs. CMF (p = 0.07). The effect of tamoxifen
in these two groups is not as yet statistically significant but it is apparent that
the beneficial results are not confined to
either the pre- or postmenopausal groups of
patients.

Comparison of patient profile data show
similarity, although the average age in the
CMF group {51.3 yrs.} was slightly lower than

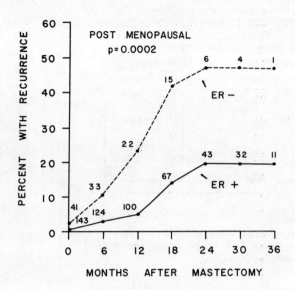

Fig. 3. Life table plot of recurrence rates
for postmenopausal ER+ and ER-
stage II breast cancer patients.
The figures over each curve represent the number of patients
followed for each time period.

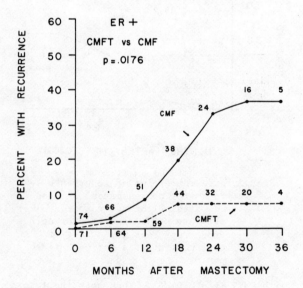

Fig. 4. Life table plot of recurrence
rates for ER+ patients in two
treatment categories CMF vs. CMFT.
The figures over each curve
represent the number of patients
followed for each time period.

that in either of the other two groups
{CMFT-55.9 yrs.; CMFT + BCG-54.5 yrs.}
(p = 0.05).

Table 1 documents the recurrence rates in
the ER negative patients among the treatment
groups. There is no significant difference
in the recurrence rates for any of the three
treatments. Comparison of patient profile
data is similar for each treatment group.
Menopausal status for ER- patients shows no

difference between pre or postmenopausal
recurrence rates.

Table 2 compares the recurrence rates for
premenopausal patients treated with CMF
alone, divided with reference to ER status.
It is apparent that the ER- patients recur
more rapidly than ER+ patients at 33 months
post mastectomy (p = 0.0313). Similar comparison of recurrence rates for postmenopausal women treated with CMF alone were not
significantly different for ER+ vs. ER-
status. These findings suggest that CMF
is exerting its benefit in premenopausal
women by suppression of ovarian function.

When recurrence data for ER+ patients
stratified by 1 - 3 or ≥ 4 positive nodes or
by menopausal status was examined, it was
found that the tamoxifen treated patients
were benefited versus the CMF alone treated
patients. The numbers of patients in each
group are still small however, and there is
no significant difference among the three
treatment regimens. For the ER- patients
similarly stratified, there was no difference
in any of the treatment categories.

Observation of the survival statistics
(Table 3) in the 25 patients dying of metastatic cancer reveals that 35.8% of the ER-
patients are dead at 33 months follow-up
vs. 8.3% of ER+ patients (p < 0.0001).
There are no significant differences in
survival among the three treatment groups at
this time.

Of the 108 premenopausal patients in this
series, the effects of treatment on the menstrual cycle can be evaluated in 93 women.
Complete cessation of menstruation occurred
in 73 women (78%) during the first year of
treatment, and resumption of menses occurred
in only 7 after treatment was completed.
Eighty-two percent of the women receiving
CMFT treatment developed amenorrhea compared
with 72% who received CMF alone. This difference is not statistically significant. In
the majority of patients who continued to
menstruate during treatment, cycles were said
to be irregular.

In the 52 patients who have documented
recurrences to date, the initial site of
recurrence was noted in skin in 9 patients,
4 in lymph nodes, 6 in lung, 14 in liver and
1 in endometrium. The remainder of the
patients had multiple sites documented at
the time of recurrence.

DISCUSSION

In the planning stage of this clinical
trial (1973) it was anticipated that optimal
forms of the three modalities of therapy
could be used. Cooper (19) had previously
shown that a 5-drug combination chemotherapy
regimen was highly effective in inducing
remission in women with advanced stage IV
breast cancer. Owing to the morbidity and
some mortality associated with the treatments,
it was deemed advisable to use a less toxic
three drug therapy.

The anti-estrogen drug, tamoxifen, had been
first used in the treatment of stage IV
breast cancer, and had shown minimal side

Table 1. Time comparison of recurrence rates for the three
treatment regimens in ER- stage II patients through
33 months post mastectomy.

Mos. post mastectomy	CMF	CMFT	CMFT+BCG
6 mos.	13.6%	16.9%	4.2%
12 mos.	28.5%	22.0%	22%
18 mos.	42.7%	42.3%	30%
24 mos.	50.9%	49.5%	30%
30 mos.	50.9%	49.5%	65%
33 mos.	50.9%	49.5%	65%

Table 2. Time comparison of recurrence rates between ER+ and
ER- premenopausal stage II patients treated by CMF
alone through 33 months postmastectomy.

Mos. post mastectomy	Premenopausal ER+	Premenopausal ER-
6 mos.	.0%	11.1%
12 mos.	7.3%	36.5%
18 mos.	15.9%	50.6%
24 mos.	28.4%	50.6%
30 mos.	36.3%	50.6%
33 mos.	36.3%	50.6%

$p = 0.0313$

Table 3. Time comparison of survival data between ER+ and
ER- stage II patients through 36 months
postmastectomy.

Mos. post mastectomy	ER+ Mortality %	ER- Mortality %
6 mos.	0.05%	0.00%
12 mos.	0.1%	12.7%
18 mos.	1.9%	21.9%
24 mos.	1.9%	31.7%
30 mos.	5.6%	35.8%
33 mos.	8.3%	35.8%

{ER+ vs. ER-} $p < 0.0001$

effects and no tumor enhancement. More
recently Manni, et al. (20) have shown that
in patients with stage IV breast cancer,
tamoxifen yielded results comparable to
surgical hypophysectomy.

BCG was empirically used for the second
year therapy for nonspecific stimulation of
cellular immunity on the basis of the studies
by Esber (14). More recently Hortobagyi,
et al. (21) have reported that BCG vaccination combined with chemotherapy can prolong
remission and survival in women with stage IV
breast cancer.

A number of important observations can be
derived from this study. Women with primary
stage II breast cancer can be subdivided
into two prognostic groups according to
estrogen receptors analysis of their tumors.
Patients with ER- tumors are shown to recur
more rapidly than patients with ER+ tumors
33 months postmastectomy (p = 0.0001).
This might be anticipated since estrogen
receptor measurements have proven to be a
useful biochemical marker of the hormone
responsiveness of human breast cancer (22,23,
24,25). In general women with ER- stage IV
breast cancer rarely, if ever, respond to
endocrine therapy. Knight, et al. (26) in
1977, reported that in women with both stage
I and II breast cancer, ER- tumors relapse

sooner than in women with ER+ tumors. They suggested that the absence of estrogen receptors in the primary tumor is an independent prognostic factor identifying a group of patient at high risk of recurrence.

Owing to the fact that a control group of ER- women treated by surgery alone was not included, the effect of CMF therapy on ER- stage II patients could not be assessed in this clinical trial. The high rate of recurrence and mortality in these patients suggests that a more effective form of chemotherapy should be sought.

The additive effect of tamoxifen to CMF therapy in stage II ER+ breast cancer patients is documented at 33 months postmastectomy. Nearly two-thirds of the patients in this series were postmenopausal suggesting that the benefit of the anti-estrogen treatment is occurring in both pre- and postmenopausal patients. Bonadonna (27) reported no difference in the recurrence rate for postmenopausal women treated with CMF, when compared with patients treated by surgery alone after three years of follow-up. Therefore we conclude that adding anti-estrogen therapy plays a major role in reducing recurrence.

It is of considerable interest that adjuvant chemotherapy with a single drug (7) or with CMF (8) significantly delays recurrence only in premenopausal women. Since it is well-known that alkylating agents profoundly suppress ovarian function as evidenced by suppression of menses in the majority of patients, it is possible that the major, if not the entire effect of CMF chemotherapy, is suppression of ovarian function. Bonadonna (27) found that in menstruating patients the incidence of relapse was not influenced by whether CMF induced amenorrhea or not. In this study (Table 2) premenopausal, ER+ patients have a significantly lower recurrence rate than ER- patients treated with CMF alone (p = 0.0313). In postmenopausal women treated with CMF alone, however, there is no significant difference in recurrence rate between ER+ and ER- patients. Thus, our study indicates that it is the ER+ premenopausal patient who benefits from CMF therapy and favors the concept that suppression of ovarian function is primarily responsible for this benefit.

At the present time there is no difference in the recurrence rates for patients treated with CMFT when compared to those treated with CMFT plus BCG. The follow-up period is brief, since BCG vaccinations were given during the second year and evaluation is now only at 33 months. Thus a further period of observation is necessary before drawing any conclusions concerning the effects of BCG vaccinations.

The treatment regimens used in this study were in general well tolerated and there was no mortaltiy related to therapy. Tamoxifen therapy was particularly devoid of side effects, although some patients had mild menopausal symptoms. Chemotherapy was well tolerated but the dose levels of the drugs had to be altered transiently in some patients because of development of leukepenia.

In no instance was the leukopenia severe and intercurrent infections were resolved without event. Alopecia was mild, rarely requiring the use of a wig. The most common complaint was a feeling of nausea and malaise for one or two days after intravenous drug administration. Tamoxifen dosages were altered in 20% of the patients. BCG vaccinations were in general well tolerated but arthritic symptoms were experienced by some women.

This study has demonstrated that women with ER- tumors respond poorly, if at all, to the adjuvant treatment used and they represent a subgroup of patients with a poor prognosis. In women with ER+ tumors, anti-estrogen treatment induced a delay in recurrence rate over and above any effect of CMF chemotherapy. A further period of observation is necessary to determine the duration of these beneficial effects.

ACKNOWLEDGEMENTS

The authors are grateful to all other surgeons whose patients were entered into this collaborative study. We also acknowledge the invaluable assistance of the following nurse clinicians: Lib Fisher, Robin France, Mary Gibbons, Ethel Gray, Ina Hardesty, Norma Jarmusch, Marge Norder and Roxia Wolfe. We are grateful to Jane Montgomery, the Administrative Coordinator; Bertha J. Adams and Theresa Courtland for secretarial assistance. Ann Merrell, Thomas George, Joan Holsinger and Jeff Crawford aided in data entry and programming. Dr. Mary Sears and other members of the Breast Cancer Task Force have been most helpful.

REFERENCES

1. B. Fisher, Biological and clinical considerations regarding the use of surgery and chemotherapy in the treatment of primary breast cancer. *Cancer* 40, 574 (1977).

2. R. Nissen-Meyer, Ovarian suppression and its supplement by additive hormonal treatment. *INSERM: Hormones and Breast Cancer*, Vol. 55, 151 (May, 1975). (Les Editions de l'Institut National de la Santé et de la Recherche Médicale).

3. R. Nissen-Meyer, Suppression of ovarian function in primary breast cancer. In *Proceedings of First Tenovus Symposium*, Cardiff, p. 139, Baltimore, Williams and Wilkins Company (1968).

4. R. Nissen-Meyer, Breast cancer management of operable cases. The Role of Adjuvant Endocrine Therapy and Chemotherapy. XI International Cancer Congress, Florence, p. 25 (New York, Excerpta Medica) (1975).

5. M. P. Cole, A clinical trial of an artificial menopause in carcinoma of the breast. *INSERM: Hormones and Breast Cancer*, Vol. 55, p. 143 (May, 1975). (Les Editions de l'Institut National de la Santé et de la Recherche Médicale).

6. J. W. Meakin, W. E. C. Allt, F. A. Beale, T. C. Brown, R. S. Bush, R. M. Clark,

P. J. Fitzpatrick, N. V. Hawkins, R. D. T. Jenkins, J. F. Pringle and W. D. Rider, Ovarian irradiation and prednisone following surgery for carcinoma of the breast. In *Adjuvant Therapy of Cancer*. (Edited by S. E. Salmon and S. E. Jones) p. 95, North-Holland Publishing Company, New York (1977).

7. B. Fisher, P. Carbone, S. G. Economou, R. Frelick, A. Glass, H. Lerner, C. Redmond, M. Zelen, P. Band, D. Katrych, N. Wolmark and E. R. Fisher, L-phenylalanine mustard (L-Pam) in the management of primary breast cancer. A report of early findings. *N. Engl. J. Med*. 292, 117 (1975).

8. G. Bonadonna, E. Brusamolino, P. Valagussa, A. Rossi, L. Brugnatelli, C. Braimbilla, M. DeLena, G. Tancini, E. Bajetta, R. Musumeci and V. Veronoesi, Combination chemotherapy as an adjuvant treatment in operable breast cancer. *N. Engl. J. Med*. 294, 405 (1976).

9. M. P. Cole, C. T. A. Jones and I. D. H. Todd, A new anti-oestrogenic agent in late breast cancer. An early appraisal of ICI 46474. *Br. J. Cancer* 25, 270 (1971).

10. E.O.R.T.C. Breast Cancer Group, Clinical trial of nafoxidine, an oestrogen antagonist in advanced breast cancer. *Europ. J. Cancer* 8, 387 (1972).

11. H. J. Tagnon, Anti-estrogens in treatment of breast cancer. *Cancer* 39, 2959 (1977).

12. E. Engelsman, J. P. Persijn, C. B. Korsten and F. J. Cleton, Oestrogen receptor in human breast cancer tissue and response to endocrine therapy. *Brit. Med. J*. 2, 750 (1973).

13. H. W. C. Ward, Anti-oestrogen therapy for breast cancer. A trial of tamoxifen at two-dose levels. *Br. Med. J*. 1, 13 (1973).

14. H. J. Esber, F. F. Menninger, Jr., D. J. Taylor and A. T. Bogden, Nonspecific stimulation of tumor-associated immunity by methanol soluble fraction of Mycobacterium butyricum. *Cancer Research* 32, 795 (1972).

15. W. L. McGuire and M. DeLaGarza, Improved sensitivity in the measurement of estrogen receptor in human breast cancer. *J. Clin. Endocrinol. Metab*. 37, 986 (1973).

16. N. Breslow, A generalized Kruskal-Wallis test for comparing K samples subject to unequal patterns of censorship. *Biometrika* 57, 579 (1970).

17. D. G. Thomas, N. Breslow and J. J. Gart, Trend and homogeneity analyses of proportions and life table data. *Computer and Biomedical Research* 10, 373 (1977).

18. E. A. Gehan, A generalized Wilcoxon test for comparing arbitrarily singly-sensored samples. *Biometrika* 52, 203 (1965).

19. R. Cooper, Combination chemotherapy in hormone resistant breast cancer. *Proc. Amer. Assoc. Cancer Res*. 10, 15 (1969).

20. A. Manni, J. E. Trujillo, J. S. Marshall, J. Brodkey and O. H. Pearson, Antihormone treatment of stage IV breast cancer. *Cancer* 43, 444 (1979).

21. G. N. Hortobagyi, J. U. Gutterman, G. R. Bluemenschein, A. Buzdar, M. A. Burgess, S. P. Richman, C. K. Tashima, M. Schwarz and E. M. Hersh, Chemoimmunotherapy of advanced breast cancer with BCG. In *Immunotherapy of Cancer: Present Status of Trials in Man*. (Edited by W. D. Terry and D. Windhorst) p. 655. Raven Press, New York (1978).

22. W. L. McGuire, O. H. Pearson and A. Segaloff, Predicting hormone responsiveness in human breast cancer. In *Estrogen Receptors in Human Breast Cancer*. (Edited by W. L. McGuire, P. P. Carbone and E. P. Vollmer) p. 17, Raven Press, New York (1975).

23. G. E. Block, R. S. Ellis, E. DeSombre and E. Jensen, Correlation of estrophilin content of primary mammary cancer to eventual endocrine treatment. *Ann Surg*. 188, 372 (1978).

24. A. J. Walt, A. Singhakowinta and S. C. Brooks, The surgical implication of estrophile protein estimations in carcinoma of the breast. *Surgery* 80, 506 (1976).

25. E. V. Jensen, E. R. DeSombre and P. W. Jungblut, Estrogen receptor in hormone-responsive tissues and tumors. In *Endogenous Factors Influencing Host-Tumor Balance*. (Edited by R. W. Wissler, T. L. Dao and S. Wood, Jr.) p. 15, Chicago, University of Chicago Press (1967).

26. W. A. Knight, III, R. B. Livingston, E. J. Gregory and W. L. McGuire, Estrogen receptor as an independent prognostic factor for early recurrence in breast cancer. *Cancer Research* 37, 4669 (1977).

27. G. Bonadonna, The value of adjunctive chemotherapy. XIIth International Cancer Congress. Panel 5, p. 103. Buenos Aires (Oct. 1978).

Cell Kinetics

Concepts for Controlling Drug-Resistant Tumor Cells*

F. M. Schabel, Jr., H. E. Skipper, M. W. Trader, W. R. Laster, Jr., T. H. Corbett and D. P. Griswold, Jr.

Chemotherapy Research Department, Southern Research Institute, Birmingham, Alabama 35205, USA

Correspondence to F. M. Schabel

Abstract—*Clinically evident and, therefore, advanced human tumors that initially regress under drug treatment commonly resume growth during continuation of the same treatment. Similar responses to treatment of advanced tumors in mice are commonly seen when using single drugs or combinations of drugs representing all of the functional classes of clinically useful anticancer drugs. With animal models in the laboratory, these treatment failures have been shown to be due to the overgrowth of drug-resistant tumor cells. Control of this problem has been accomplished by changing drugs at a time when drug-resistant tumor cells that are present in the large body burdens of initially drug-sensitive cells overgrow the drug-sensitive cells being killed by the initial drug treatment. At that point, changing the drugs being used for initial treatment to drugs active against the drug-resistant tumor cells has, at least with laboratory models, resulted in therapeutic gain, including cures. Therapeutic concepts are presented, as well as examples of their successful application, in the treatment of tumors in mice. Extensive quantitative and qualitative data on resistance, cross-resistance, and collateral sensitivity from studies with drug-sensitive and drug-resistant murine leukemias (L1210 and P388) are included. These data may be useful in planning clinical chemotherapy protocols.*

INTRODUCTION

It is commonly observed with drug treatment of both leukemias and solid tumors of man and animals that initially drug-sensitive and responsive tumors become progressively less responsive and ultimately fail to respond during continuing treatment. Studies with murine tumor models have indicated that a major reason for these treatment failures is the overgrowth of drug-resistant tumor cells during chronic treatment (1,2).

Spontaneous mutation to drug resistance is commonly observed among advanced-staged and initially drug-sensitive murine tumors, which are used as experimental models for chemotherapy trials and which were selected to represent the major histologic and organ types of human tumors. The rate of spontaneous mutation to resistance to single anticancer drugs with murine tumors appears to vary markedly, being highest to mitotic inhibitors like vincristine (VCR) (1,2), less frequent to antimetabolite drugs like 1-β-D-arabinofuranosyl-cytosine (ara-C) (1,3,4), and lowest to highly active drugs like the alkylating agents, e.g., cyclophosphamide (CPA) (1,2). However, spontaneous

mutation to resistance to all drugs, including the alkylating agents (5,6), has been observed with a total body burden of tumor cells in the mouse that is at or below the smallest body burden of all organ or histologic types of cancer in man at the time of clinical presentation.† Except for a few who are treated with surgical-adjuvant chemotherapy, most tumor patients have a body burden of tumor cells at the start of drug treatment large enough, based on observed spontaneous mutation rates to drug resistance in murine tumor models, to assure the presence of mutant cells resistant to any clinically useful anticancer drug.

Except for cross-resistance to structurally or functionally similar drugs, mutation to resistance of tumor cells to one drug usually does not result in resistance to other drugs, particularly those of other functional classes. For example, tumor cells selected for resistance in antimetabolite drugs retain full sensitivity to alkylating agents, to drugs that bind to or intercalate with DNA, or to mitotic inhibitors such as VCR. One of the logical and indicated reasons for using drug combinations is to attempt to control the overgrowth of drug-resistant

---

*Previously unpublished work reported herein was carried out under Contract N01-CM-43756 with the Division of Cancer Treatment, National Cancer Institute, National Institutes of Health, Department of Health, Education, and Welfare, USA.
†The smallest tumor cell population detectable by palpation or radiological procedures in a single site in man is estimated to be about 10^9 tumor cells (7).

mutant tumor cells by including drugs from
two or more functional classes in the drug
combination. This classical concept often
fails when applied because:
  (a) Due to additive toxicity to vital
      normal cells, usually the dose of each
      individual drug in the combination
      must be less than that when each drug
      is used alone, thus reducing the selec-
      tive cytotoxic activity for tumor
      cells of each drug.
  (b) Rapid overgrowth of tumor cell popula-
      tions resistant to some or all of the
      drugs in the combination is commonly
      seen in the laboratory (2,8,9) and
      probably also occurs in man.
  Both experimental chemotherapists and
clinical oncologists commonly treat with
initially effective single drugs or combinations of drugs until it is overtly obvious
that treatment is becoming less effective
or failing before serious consideration is
given to the use of alternate drug treatment.
Extensive experimental data indicate that
such delay in changing drug treatment, in
the face of likely overgrowth of mutant drug-
resistant tumor cell populations, is contraindicated.

REGROWTH OF ADVANCED–STAGED SOLID TUMORS IN MICE DURING CHRONIC TREATMENT WITH INITIALLY EFFECTIVE DRUG(S)

  Examples of regression and regrowth of
individual Ridgway osteogenic sarcomas (ROS)
in mice treated with actinomycin D (a DNA
binder), *cis*-DDPt (alkylating agent-like)
(10), or 5-FU (antimetabolite) and of mammary
adenocarcinoma 16/C treated with 5-FU are
shown in Fig. 1. These tumors were all
advanced-staged (100 to 3000 mg) at start
of treatment. Figure 2B shows similar
regression and regrowth under treatment of
ROS treated with 6-MP.
  Regression responses of most of these
tumors, similar to those required for
reporting objective clinical response with
solid tumors in humans (9), were seen. Many
of these initially responsive tumors regrew
under continuing treatment with the same
drug at the same dose and schedule indicating
overgrowth of drug-resistant tumor cells.
Overgrowth of ara-C-resistant colon adenocarcinoma 36 during chronic treatment of
advanced tumors that initially regressed
under ara-C treatment has also been objectively demonstrated (11).

RIDGWAY OSTEOGENIC SARCOMA

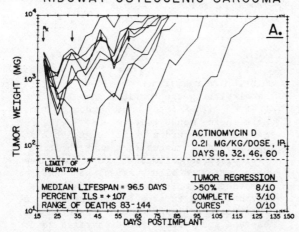

RIDGWAY OSTEOGENIC SARCOMA

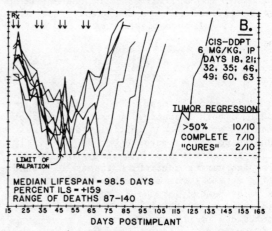

RIDGWAY OSTEOGENIC SARCOMA

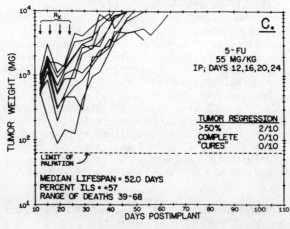

MAMMARY ADENOCARCINOMA (LINE 16/C)

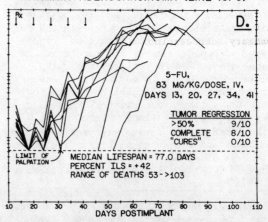

Fig. 1. Regression of advanced solid tumors in mice and regrowth during
continuing treatment with initially effective drug. Ridgway osteogenic
sarcoma treated with actinomycin D, Plot A; with *cis*-diamminedichloro-
platinum II (*cis*-DDPt), Plot B; or with 5-FU, Plot C. Mammary adenocarcinoma 16/C treated with 5-FU, Plot D.

RIDGWAY OSTEOGENIC SARCOMA

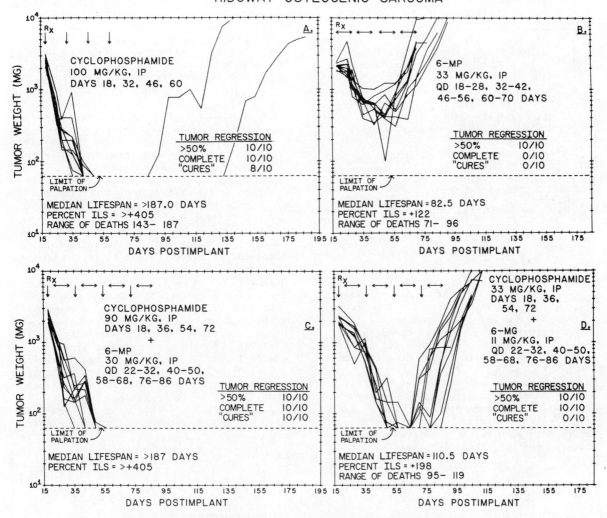

Fig. 2. Combination chemotherapy of advanced Ridgway osteogenic sarcoma with
cyclophosphamide (CPA) plus 6-MP. Individual tumor responses in
mice treated with ≤ LD_{10} doses of CPA alone, Plot A; with 6-MP alone,
Plot B; with CPA plus 6-MP at optimal doses, Plot C; and with less
than optimal doses of CPA plus 6-MP, Plot D. Note tumor regression
and regrowth during treatment with 6-MP alone (Plot B) and with low-
dose combination treatment (Plot D).

Figures 2 and 3 illustrate similar regression and regrowth responses of ROS and
mammary adenocarcinoma 16/C treated with
two-drug combinations. Figure 2C and D illustrate two important chemotherapeutic
principles:
(a) Initially regressing tumors often
    resume growth during chronic treatment
    with a drug combination at doses that
    were initially very effective. This
    is probably due to overgrowth of tumor
    cells resistant to one or both drugs
    in the combination (Figure 2D).
(b) The overgrowth of drug-resistant tumor
    cell populations is influenced, if not
    controlled, by the drug doses used.
    The combination drug doses used in
    Fig. 2C resulted in complete regression
    and cure of similarly staged advanced
    tumors that also regressed but regrew
    during continuing treatment with lower

combination drug doses (Fig. 2D).
Drug resistance of tumor cells is dose
responsive and, if reducing the body burden
of tumor cells to the lowest number possible by effective drug treatment is the goal
of cancer chemotherapy, as we believe it is,
then aggressive chemotherapy is indicated.
Figure 3 shows similar individual tumor
regression and regrowth under drug treatment
of advanced-staged mammary adenocarcinoma
16/C with 5-FU plus adriamycin (ADR). Under
chronic drug treatment, all tumors regressed
to <50% of the size at start of drug treatment, nearly 80% regressed to below palpable
size, and at least 67% regrew under continuation of the initially effective drug treatment.
The above examples indicate that overgrowth
of drug-resistant tumor cell populations,
initially showing marked and therapeutically
useful tumor cell kill by representatives of

MAMMARY ADENOCARCINOMA
(LINE 16/C)

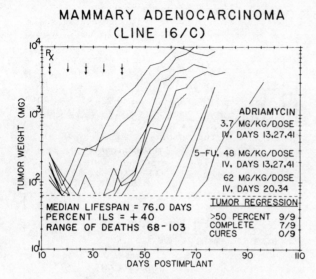

Fig. 3. Combination chemotherapy of advanced
mammary adenocarcinoma 16/C with
adriamycin plus 5-FU. Individual
tumor responses in mice treated
with $<LD_{10}$ doses of the drug combination. Note tumor regression
and regrowth during drug treatment.

all of the functional classes of clinically
useful anticancer drugs, including drug
combinations, is commonly seen with a variety
of histologic and organ types of murine solid
tumors used as possible predictive models
for drug therapy of similar human tumors

STRATEGY FOR CIRCUMVENTING THE OVERGROWTH OF DRUG-RESISTANT TUMOR CELLS

It appears to us that adding additional
numbers of the currently available anticancer
drugs to combination chemotherapy treatment
protocols is not likely to resolve this
obvious problem of overgrowth of drug-
resistant tumor cells because:

(a) Resistance to as many as six separate
drugs used in combination has been
shown to occur in drug treatment of
experimental leukemia (4).

(b) Individual drug doses usually must be
reduced as additional drugs are added
to the drug combination.

(c) Unless resistance to all drugs develops
equally in relation to both duration
of treatment and level of drug resistance, then some of the drugs in the
combination will only be providing
drug toxicity to vital normal cells
without contributing to tumor cell
kill, thus further reducing the effectiveness of the treatment.

It seems more logical to kill the maximum
number of drug-sensitive cells with limited
numbers of effective but noncurative drugs
and then to change to other drugs possessing
effective cytotoxic activity against both the
residual tumor cells that are sensitive to
the first drug treatment and also against
mutant tumor cells resistant to the first

drug treatment that are growing under its
continuing use. There are both theoretical
reasons and objective experimental data
supporting these concepts.

Murine leukemias L1210 and P388 have been
used in most experimental studies on drug
resistance because:

(a) One or more are markedly sensitive to
most of the clinically useful anticancer drugs and accurate disease
staging, at the start of drug treatment, can be controlled.

(b) Cell kill by single drugs or combinations of drugs can be quantitatively
and reliably determined (12).

(c) Sublines of tumor cells selected for
mutation to drug resistance to most
anticancer drugs are available or can
be selected with relative ease.

The murine leukemias also have historical
validity as conceptual models for improving
treatment of cancer in man since, as Holland
has said, "The leukemias and lymphomas are
a seedbed where much progress has been
attained and where many concepts have been
developed. I expect that it will continue
to be an area from which we translate to the
broad spectrum of cancer. Findings of principle in this group of diseases will make it
easier to handle the rest of the cancers in
man" (13). Holland was referring to leukemias and lymphomas of man, but we believe
that the murine leukemias and lymphomas
may be similar in regard to many fundamental
biologic and chemotherapeutic principles.

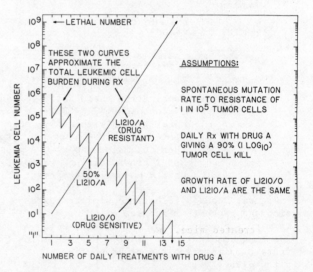

Fig. 4. Conceptual overgrowth of drug-
resistant leukemia L1210 cells
during initially effective but
noncurative treatment with drug A.

Figure 4 illustrates some concepts relating to the overgrowth of spontaneous mutation
to drug resistance in leukemia L1210.
Assuming a body burden of 10^6 L1210 cells
and a spontaneous mutation rate to resistance
to drug A of one in 10^5 tumor cells, the
following will happen under daily treatment
with a dose of drug A capable of killing 90%
of the drug-A-sensitive tumor cells:

(a) Drug-A-sensitive tumor cells surviving

drug treatment will grow at the same rate after each treatment as they did prior to any treatment (14).

(b) Tumor cells resistant to drug A have essentially the same tumor cell population growth kinetics as the parent drug-sensitive tumor cells (see Table 1).

small and the same percent of drug-A-sensitive tumor cells continues to be killed by daily treatment with drug A, but the body burden of tumor cells has reached its nadir and tumor progression under further treatment with drug A occurs.* That this actually actually happens is shown by the data

Table 1. Population doubling time of parent drug-sensitive and drug-resistnat sublines of L1210 and P388 as determined from the median life span of mice implanted intraperitoneally with Log_{10} dilutions of tumor cells ranging from 10^0 to 10^7 cells.

Leukemia subline		Doubling time (days) of IP implanted cell population in BDF1 mice
L1210/O (Parent)		0.41
L1210/CPA		0.42
L1210/BCNU		0.35
L1210/L-PAM	Drug resistant	0.44
L1210/Ara-C		0.36
L1210/6-MP		0.47
P388/O (Parent)		0.66
P388/VCR		0.63
P388/ADR		0.60
P388/Act D	Drug resistant	0.66
P388/CPA		0.72
P388/L-PAM		0.63
P388/Ara-C		0.52

The drug-resistant tumor cell lines listed were isolated and characterized by us except for the cyclophosphamide-resistant line of L1210 (L1210/CPA) isolated by DeWys (17), the ara-C-resistant line of L1210 (L1210/ara-C) isolated by Wodinsky and Kensler (18), and the 6-MP-resistant line of L1210 (L1210/6-MP) isolated by Law (19).

Since the population doubling times of the drug-sensitive and drug-resistant tumor cells are essentially the same, mixed populations will not significantly influence the life span of treated mice. We are not aware of any objectively demonstrated exceptions to the chemotherapuetic principles (a above and b) with either drug-sensitive or drug-resistant murine leukemia cells.

(c) Continuing daily treatment with drug A will show a steady reduction in total body burden of tumor cells until the ratio of drug-sensitive to drug-resistant cells in the population is about one-to-one. At that point, the total body burden of tumor cells is

in Fig. 5 that were taken from an experiment in which mice bearing intravenously implanted L1210 were treated with ara-C. Drug treatment failed to cure due to the overgrowth of L1210/ara-C under continuing treatment with ara-C (3,4).

We have attempted to control the overgrowth of naturally occurring drug-resistant L1210 and P388 tumor cells, present in body burdens of L1210/O or P388/O in excess of 10^7 at the start of effective but noncurative drug treatment, by changing the drugs being used at an interval after start of treatment at which time it was likely that overgrowth of the tumor cells resistant to the first treatment resulted in their being at or above a one-to-one ratio with the tumor cells

*Ratios of one-to-one of L1210 cells resistant to ara-C (L1210/ara-C) to parent drug-sensitive cells (L1210/O) have been shown to be unresponsive to treatment with ara-C and one-to-one ratios of L1210 cells resistant to CPA (L1210/CPA) to L1210/O have been shown to be unresponsive to treatment with CPA based on increased life span of drug-treated leukemic mice (15).

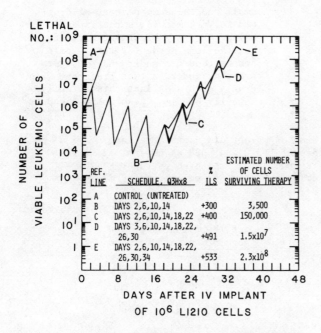

Fig. 5. Graphic idealization of the changes
in the total viable L1210 cell
population in mice under treatment
with repeated courses of ara-C.
Treatment ip at 10 mg/kg/dose on
the days indicated after iv implant
of 10^6 viable L1210 cells. All
mice died of leukemia except those
at points C and D, which were
sacrificed, and the tumor cells
that were isolated were demonstrated
to be completely resistant to
ara-C.

sensitive to the first-used drug(s).

Data presented in Table 2 were obtained
from an experiment in which mice were
implanted iv with 10^7 L1210/0 cells and
drug treatment was started 48 hours later.
Therefore, the tumor cells were widely disseminated and the disease was advanced at
start of treatment (16) with ara-C plus
6-thio-guanine (6-TG) followed by CPA plus
BCNU. We have demonstrated that treatment
with ara-C plus 6-TG of body burdens of
L1210 of the size and wide anatomical distribution used results in the overgrowth of
L1210 cell populations solidly resistant to
both ara-C and 6-TG (2). Treatment of similarly staged L1210 with CPA plus BCNU fails
to cure, probably due to overgrowth of drug-
resistant tumor cells. We know that L1210
cells resistant to each of the four drugs
used probably retain essentially full sensitivity to each of the other three drugs in
the combination (see Table 5).

Thus, the increased high cure rates seen
are consistent with the treatment strategy
outlined. Unequivocal and readily reproducible therapeutic advantage was gained
against this advanced-staged murine leukemia.

Additional similar studies were done with
leukemia P388 with which remission induction
of advanced disease can be accomplished with
either VCR or ara-C.* The mutation rate of
P388 to resistance to ara-C is similar to
that of L1210. P388 is very responsive to
treatment with VCR and the mutation rate to
resistance to VCR is probably greater than
one in 10^5 tumor cells (1).

Table 3 is a summary of available data
from experiments in which first treatment of
advanced P388 was with VCR, followed by

Table 2. Improved Cure Rates Among BDF1 Mice Implanted Intravenously with
10^7L1210 Cells. Body Burden at Start of Treatment was
$>10^8$ Tumor Cells; Optimal Dose and Schedule @ $\leq LD_{10}$.

Agent(s)	Treatment (IP) Mg/Kg/Dose	Schedule	Median Life Span in Days After R_x	Cures	Highest L1210 Burden Curable at $\geq 50\%$ Level (Approx.)
Control	None	—	5.0	0/20	—
Ara-C	10.0	Q3h x 8, Days 2,5,8	9.5	0/10	10^4
6-TG	0.5	Q3h x 8, Days 2,5,8	[-3.0	0/10]*	$<10^4$
Ara-C + 6-TG	10 + 0.5	Q3h x 8, Days 2,5,8	14.0	0/10	10^6
CPA	300.0	Day 2 only	16.0	0/10	10^6
BCNU	30.0	Day 2 only	14.0	1/10	10^6-10^7
CPA + BCNU	200 + 20	Day 2 only	14.0	0/10	10^7
Ara-C + 6-TG → CPA + BCNU	10 + 0.5 → 200 + 20	Q3h x 8, Days 2,5,8 → Day 14 only	15.0	8/10	$>10^8$

*Data obtained in a separate therapeutic trial. All other data from a single
internally controlled trial.

*The 5'-palmitate of ara-C (palmO-ara-C), a slow-release form of ara-C, was used in these
studies to avoid the necessity of short-interval repeated dosing with ara-C to obtain maximal
tumor cell kill.

Table 3. Early Substitution of Drugs to Attempt to Control Overgrowth of Drug-resistant Tumor Cells. Implant: 10^7 P388/O, IP (Tumor Cell Burden at Initiation of R_x on Day 1: $>10^7$; on Day 4: ca 10^8)

Agent(s)	Treatment @ $\leq LD_{10}$ Schedule	Mg/Kg/Dose	Percent ILS	Percent "Cures"	Approx. No. of Cells Surviving R_x
VCR	Day 1	1.5	68	0	4×10^3
MTX	Days 1,5,9	15.0	100	0	5×10^6
VCR → MTX	Day 1 → Days 3,7,11	1.5 → 15	173	0	4×10^3
VCR	Day 1	1.5	68	0	4×10^3
PalmO-ara-C	Day 1	150.0	215	0	ca 1
VCR → PalmO-ara-C	Day 1 → Day 3	1.5 → 100	257	0	ca 1
VCR	Day 4	1.5	63	0	6×10^5
PalmO-ara-C	Day 4	150.0	94	0	8×10^3
VCR → PalmO-ara-C	Day 4 → Day 6	1.5 → 100	157	0	3×10^1
VCR	Day 1	1.5	68	0	4×10^3
CPA	Day 1	200.0	136	0	ca 1
VCR → CPA	Day 1 → Day 3	1.5 → 200	278	50	<1
VCR	Day 4	1.5	63	0	6×10^5
CPA	Day 4	200.0	163	0	ca 1
VCR → CPA	Day 4 → Day 6	1.5 → 200	263	0	ca 1
VCR	Day 1	1.5	68	0	4×10^3
BCNU	Day 1	30.0	152	10	ca 1
VCR → BCNU	Day 1 → Day 3	1.5 → 30	278	30	ca 1
VCR	Day 4	1.5	63	0	6×10^5
BCNU	Day 4	30.0	210	0	ca 1
VCR → BCNU	Day 4 → Day 6	1.5 → 30	236	0	ca 1
VCR	Day 1	1.5	68	0	4×10^3
L-PAM	Day 1	12.0	115	0	7×10^0
VCR → L-PAM	Day 1 → Day 3	1.5 → 12	189	20	ca 1
VCR	Day 4	1.5	63	0	6×10^5
L-PAM	Day 4	12.0	68	0	3×10^5
VCR → L-PAM	Day 4 → Day 6	1.5 → 12	136	0	5×10^2

other drugs, all of which were known to be very active against VCR-resistant P388 (P388/VCR) (see Table 6).

The body burden of P388 cells at start of VCR treatment was $>10^7$, well in excess of the curative potential, when used alone, of any of the single drugs studied, with the possible exception of BCNU. The data in Table 3 indicate that drugs known to be active against P388/VCR, when used following remission induction with VCR and against body burdens of tumor cells assuring treatment failure with VCR alone due to overgrowth of P388/VCR, improve the therapeutic response. This is probably due to kill of P388/VCR as well as residual P388/O surviving initial treatment with VCR. Disease staging is also very important because delaying start of treatment to day 4 postimplant of 10^7 P388/O cells resulted in failure to cure any mice treated with VCR followed by CPA or L-PAM. This, of course, is to be expected. Body burden of tumor cells is probably the most critical factor in planning curative chemotherapy with effective drugs.

Table 4 lists summary data from similar experiments in which remission of advanced-staged P388 was induced by palmO-ara-C followed by treatment with other drugs known or presumed to be active against both P388/O and P388/ara-C. In relation to the principles and concepts discussed above, these data are similar and consistent with those in Table 3.

Use of drugs active against mutant tumor cells resistant to initially effective but noncurative drugs clearly increases net tumor cell kill, increases the life span of dying animals, and often results in significant cure rates in mice with very advanced disease at the start of drug treatment. Using the most active drugs in sequential treatment protocols designed to recognize the presence of and to plan the drug kill of drug-resistant mutant tumor cells, selected and growing uninhibited under initially effective drug treatment, results in markedly improved therapeutic responses including cures of very advanced-staged disease. We believe that the concepts presented are valid, the objective

Table 4. Early Substitution of Drugs to Attempt to Control Overgrowth of Drug-resistant Tumor Cells. Implant: 10^7 P388/0, IP
(Tumor Cell Burden at Initiation of R_x on Day 1: $>10^7$; on Day 4: ca 10^8)

Agent(s)	Treatment @ $\leq LD_{10}$ Schedule	Mg/Kg/Dose	Percent ILS	Percent "Cures"	Approx. No. of Cells Surviving R_x
PalmO-ara-C	Day 1	150.0	215	0	ca 1
MTX	Qd 1-9 Days	1.5	84	0	4×10^7
PalmO-ara-C → MTX	Day 1 → Qd 3-11 Days	100 → 1.5	247	60	<1
PalmO-ara-C	Day 1	150.0	215	0	ca 1
VCR	Day 1	1.5	68	0	4×10^3
PalmO-ara-C → VCR	Day 1 → Day 3	100 → 1.5	252	20	ca 1
PalmO-ara-C	Day 1	150.0	215	0	ca 1
CPA	Day 1	200.0	136	0	ca 1
PalmO-ara-C → CPA	Day 1 → Day 3	100 → 200	284 (LD_{20})	75	<1
PalmO-ara-C	Day 4	150.0	94	0	8×10^3
CPA	Day 4	200.0	163	0	ca 1
PalmO-ara-C → CPA	Day 4 → Day 6	100 → 200	257	0	ca 1
PalmO-ara-C	Day 1	150.0	215	0	ca 1
BCNU	Day 1	30.0	152	10	ca 1
PalmO-ara-C → BCNU	Day 1 → Day 3	100 → 30	~	100	<0.1
PalmO-ara-C	Day 4	150.0	94	0	8×10^3
BCNU	Day 4	30.0	210	0	ca 1
PalmO-ara-C → BCNU	Day 4 → Day 6	100 → 30	268	60	<1
PalmO-ara-C	Day 1	150.0	215	0	ca 1
L-PAM	Day 1	12.0	115	0	7×10^0
PalmO-ara-C → L-PAM	Day 1 → Day 3	100 → 12	257	60	<1
PalmO-ara-C	Day 4	150.0	94	0	8×10^3
L-PAM	Day 4	12.0	68	0	3×10^5
PalmO-ara-C → L-PAM	Day 4 → Day 6	100 → 12	205	0	ca 1
PalmO-ara-C	Day 1	150.0	215	0	ca 1
VCR	Day 1	1.5	68	0	4×10^3
CPA	Day 1	200.0	136	0	ca 1
PalmO-ara-C → VCR → CPA	Day 1 → Day 3 → Day 9	100 → 1.5 → 200	68	50	<1
PalmO-ara-C	Day 4	150.0	94	0	8×10^3
VCR	Day 4	1.5	63	0	6×10^5
CPA	Day 4	200.0	163	0	ca 1
PalmO-ara-C → VCR → CPA	Day 4 → Day 6 → Day 12	100 → 1.5 → 200	221	60	<1

experimental data presented are consistent with these concepts, and the indications for the consideration of their clinical application are clear. Therefore, drug selection for use in attempting to circumvent overgrowth of drug-resistant mutant tumor cells is of primary importance.

BASIS FOR DRUG SELECTION TO ATTEMPT TO CIRCUMVENT LIKELY OVERGROWTH OF MUTANT DRUG-RESISTANT TUMOR CELLS

There is a large and growing body of experimental data bearing on sensitivity and cross-resistance of sublines of murine leukemias selected for resistance to representatives of the major chemical and functional classes of clinically useful anti-cancer drugs. Tables 5 and 6 contain selected data from Southern Research Institute. We believe that the usefulness and likely predictive reliability of data relating to drug resistance and cross-resistance of tumor cells are, at least in part, dependent upon quantitative analysis of changes in body burden of tumor cells under drug treatment. We have described procedures by which it is possible to reliably estimate the number of viable L1210 or P388 tumor cells (either drug sensitive, drug resistant, or both) surviving drug treatment (12), and the data listed in Tables 5 and 6 were obtained by those methods. A negative $\log_{10}$ change indicates the $\log_{10}$ order of tumor cell reduction at the end of drug treatment, and a positive $\log_{10}$ change indicates $\log_{10}$ order of tumor cell increase at the end of

Table 5. Log_{10} Change[†] in L1210 Cell Populations at the End of Optimal Drug Treatment ($\leq LD_{10}$) in BDF1 or CDF1 Mice Implanted IP with 10^5 to 10^6 Leukemia Cells and Treated IP, As Indicated

Agent	NSC No.	Schedule[††]	L1210 Parent /0	/CPA	/BCNU	/L-PAM	/DDPt	/Ara-C	/6-MP
Alkylating Agents									
Cyclophosphamide	26271	A	-6	0	-6	-4	-5*	-6	
Isophosphamide	109724	A	-7	0		-5			
4-Hydroperoxyiso-phosphamide	227114	A	-7	-2*					
4-Peroxycyclophos-phamide	176986	A	-7	-1*					
Phosphoramide mustard	69945	A	-6	-5		-4			
BCNU	409962	A	-7	-7	-2	-6	0*		
CCNU	79037	A	-7	-6	-2	-7	0*		
MeCCNU	95441	A	-7	-7	-3	-7	-1*		
PCNU	95466	A	-7			-7			
Streptozotocin	85998	A	0	-1	-1	0			
Chlorozotocin	178248	A	-7	-6	-4	-6	-1*		
Nitrogen mustard	762	A	-3			-3			
Uracil mustard	34462	A	-3	-2					
L-PAM	8806	A	-6	-5	-6	-2	-5*		
Peptichemio	247516	A	-4*	-3*	-2*	0*			
Asaley	167780	A	-2			0			
Thio-TEPA	6396	A	-5	-2	-2	-2	-2*		
Dianhydrogalactitol	132313	A	-5	-5	-5	-4	-4*		
Piperazinedione	135758	A	-5	-4	-4	-5	-5*	-5*	
BIC	82196	A	-7	-6		-6	-1*		
DTIC	45388	A,D	-2*,+1		-1*	+2			
cis-DDPt	119875	A,C	-4	-5	-5	0	+3		
Mitomycin C	26980	A	-2,-5	-3*		-4			
Indicine-N-oxide	132319	A	0	+2*					
DNA Binders or Inter-calators									
Adriamycin	123127	A	-3			-3			
Actinomycin D	3053	A	-1			-2			
Mitotic Inhibitors									
Vincristine	67574	B	+4			+4			
Antimetabolites									
Palm0-ara-C	135962	A	-5	-6	-5	-6		+1	
5-FU	19893	D	+1	+1*	+2*	+1		+2	
5-FUdR	27640	D	+3	+3*	+3*				

Table 5 (Continued)

Agent	NSC No.	Schedule††	L1210 Parent /0	/CPA	/BCNU	/L-PAM	/DDPt	/Ara-C	/6-MP
Antimetabolites (Cont'd)									
3-Deazauridine	126849	D,E	+2					-6	
6-Azauridine	32074	D	+3					+4	
5-Azacytidine	102816	D	-5			-5		-2,-5	
Dihydro-5-azacyti-dine	264880	D	-2					-5	
Ara-A + 2'dCF	404241 + 218321	E	-4					-1	
2-Fluoro-ara-A	118218	D	+1					+4*	
5'-Formyl-2-fluoro-ara-A	302067	D	+5,-2					+4*	
PALA	224131	D	+4					+4	
Methotrexate	740	D	0	0	+2	+3			-5
Dichloro-methotrexate	29630	D	-1						-5*
5-Methyl-tetrahydro-homofolic acid	139490	D	+3						+2
Baker's antifol	139105	D	+4						+4
6-MP	755	A,D	+1					-2*	+4

†Log_{10} change = net log change in viable tumor cell population at the end of Rx as compared to the start of Rx; e.g., a -6 log change means that there was a 99.9999% reduction and a +3 log change means there was a 1000-fold increase in tumor burden at the end of Rx.

††Schedule: A = Single-dose treatment
　　　　　B = Treatment q4dx3
　　　　　C = Treatment qd 1-5 days
　　　　　D = Treatment qd 1-9 days
　　　　　E = Treatment q3hx8, q4dx3

*Limited data.

drug treatment.

Data shown in Tables 5 and 6 have been, except as noted, repeatedly confirmed in separate, internally controlled, and biologically acceptable experiments. Therefore, we believe that these data may be considered to be reliable, both quantitatively* and qualitatively, as indicators of drug sensitivity of the parent L1210/0 and P388/0 and also as to the resistance, cross-resistance, and collateral sensitivity** of drug-resistant tumor cells to other drugs.

The examples of drug-resistant tumor cells that are more sensitive to other drugs than are their parent drug-sensitive tumor cells should be seriously considered in selecting second drug(s). Some of these may, in fact, have been ineffective as initially useful

drugs, e.g., see L1210/0 and L1210/6-MP treated with methotrexate, L1210/0 and L1210/ara-C treated with 3-deazauridine or dihydro-5-azacytidine in Table 5, and P388/0 and P388/ara-C treated with 3-deazauridine, dihydro-5-azacytidine, PALA, or pyrazofurin in Table 6. Collateral sensitivities of drug-resistant tumor cells to other drugs have great theoretical potential for practical application.

Since no animal tumor system has been objectively demonstrated to reliably predict for the drug response of any human tumor, the reliability of the data in Tables 5 and 6, as objectively based indication(s) for their use in planning clinical treatment protocols, has not been established. However, they are the best we have outside of clinical

*The log changes in tumor cell populations listed are valid and reproducible to about one order of magnitude.
**Collateral Sensitivity: Increased sensitivity of a drug-resistant line of tumor cells to another drug over that seen in the parent drug-sensitive cells (20).

Table 6. Log_{10} Change[†] in P388 Cell Populations at the End of Optimal Drug Treatment ($\leqslant LD_{10}$) in BDF1 or CDF1 Mice Implanted IP with 10^6 to 10^7 Leukemia Cells and Treated IP, As Indicated

Agent	NSC No.	Schedule[††]	Parent /0	/VCR	/ADR	/ACT-D	/CPA	/L-PAM	/BCNU	/Ara-C	/5-FU
Alkylating Agents											
Cyclophosphamide	26271	A	-7	-7	-7	-7	0 to -3	-7	-6*	-6	
4-Hydroperoxyiso-phosphamide	227114	A	-7*				-6*				
Phosphoramide mustard	69945	A	-7				-7*	-6			
BCNU	409962	A	-7	-7	-7	-7	-7	-7	-1		
L-PAM	8806	A	-7	-7	-7	-7	-7	-1	-6*		
Peptichemio	247516	A	-6				-6*	-2			
Dianhydrogalactitol	132313	A,B	-6				-6	-3	-6*		
Piperazinedione	135758	A	-6	-6	-6	-5	-6	-3			
BIC	82196	A	-6				-6	-6*			
cis-DDPt	119875	B,C	-6	-4	-6	-6	-6	+2	-6*		
Mitomycin C	26980	A	-3				-4*	-2			
Indicine-N-oxide	132319	D	+3				0				
DNA Binders or Inter-calators											
Adriamycin	123127	A	-6	-4	-2	-5	-6	-:			
AD-32	246131	C	-6	-6							
Daunomycin	82151	A	-6	0	-1*						
Rubidazone	164011	A	-6*		0*						
Aclacinomycin A	208734	B	0*		+3*						
Carminomycin	180024	B	+2*		+3*						
Marcellomycin	265211	B	+2*		+3*						
Nogamycin	265450	B	+2*		+3*						
Anthracenedione	196473	D	-6		+2						
Anthracenedione, diacetate	287513	D	-6		+2						
Anthracenedione, dihyroxyl	279836	A,D	-7		+1*(D)		-7*(A)				
Actinomycin D	3053	A	-5	-3	-1	-2	-6	-2			
Azetomycin I	244392	B	-6*		+1*						
Azetomycin II	244393	B	-6*		+1*						
AMSA (Cain's acridine)	249992	B	-6		+2		-6				
Mitotic Inhibitors											
Vincristine	67574	B	-6	+2	+3	+3	-6	0			
Vinblastine	49842	B	-3	0							
Vindesine	245467	B	-6	+2							
Bis(N-Ethylidene vindesine)disulfide, disulfate	277096	B	-4	-1							
VP-16-213	141540	B	-7	-6	+1	-5	-7	-7			
Maytansine	153858	E	-6*	-2*							
Antimetabolites											
PalmO-ara-C	135962	A	-6	-6	-6	-6	-6			-1	-7
5-FU	19893	D	-5	-3	-4	-3	-1*			-6	+2
5-FUdR	27640	D	0	-3	-1*	-2*					
3-Deazauridine	126849	D	+3							-1	+3
5-Azacytidine	102816	D	-6							-6	
Dihydro-5-azacyti-dine	264880	D	-1							-6	

Table 6 (Continued)

Agent	NSC No.	Schedule[††]	Parent /0	/VCR	/ADR	/ACT-D	/CPA	/L-PAM	/BCNU	/Ara-C	/5-FU
Antimetabolites (Cont'd)											
Ara-A + 2'dCF	404241 + 218321	D	-6							-6	
PALA	224131	D	+2				+3*			-3	0
Pyrazofurin	143095	D	+3							-2	+2
Methotrexate	740	D	-3	-4	-2	-3					
Bruceantin**	165563	D	-2		+1*			-1*			

[†]Log$_{10}$ change = net log change in viable tumor cell population at the end of Rx as compared to the start of Rx; e.g., a -6 log change means that there was a 99.9999% reduction and a +3 log change means there was a 1000-fold increase in tumor burden at the end of Rx.

[††]Schedule: A = Single dose treatment
        B = Treatment q4dx3
        C = Treatment qd 1-5 days (or qd 1-4)
        D = Treatment qd 1-9 days
        E = Treatment q3hx8, q4dx3

*Limited data.

**Selectively inhibits protein synthesis; inhibits DNA synthesis also, and prevents the elongation of polypeptide chains.

experience. The reliability and utility of such data, and the therapeutic concepts we believe they support, can only be established by their use in carefully planned and conducted cancer chemotherapy trials in man. We believe that, in planning clinical trials to test the therapeutic concepts we have presented, the laboratory data obtained in murine tumor systems included here may be useful.

REFERENCES

1. H. E. Skipper, *Cancer Chemotherapy - Volume 1: Reasons for Success and Failure in Treatment of Murine Leukemias with the Drugs Now Employed in Treating Human Leukemias*, 166 pp. University Microfilms International, Ann Arbor, Michigan (1978).
2. Unpublished data from Southern Research Institute.
3. R. W. Brockman, Circumvention of resistance. In *Pharmacological Basis of Cancer Chemotherapy* (27th Annual Symposium on Fundamental Cancer Research, The University of Texas M.D. Anderson Hospital and Tumor Institute, Houston, 1974) p. 691. The Williams and Wilkins Co., Baltimore (1975).
4. F. M. Schabel, Jr. and L. Simpson-Herren, Some variables in experimental tumor systems which complicate interpretation of data from in vivo kinetic and pharmacologic studies with anticancer drugs.
In *Antibiotics and Chemotherapy, Volume 23, Fundamentals in Cancer Chemotherapy*. (Edited by F. M. Schabel, Jr.) p. 113. S. Karger, Basel (1978).
5. F. M. Schabel, Jr., Nitrosoureas: A review of experimental antitumor activity. *Cancer Treat. Rep.* 60, 665 (1976).
6. F. M. Schabel, Jr., M. W. Trader, W. R. Laster, Jr., G. P. Wheeler, and M. H. Witt, Patterns of resistance and therapeutic synergism among alkylating agents. In *Antibiotics and Chemotherapy, Volume 23, Fundamentals in Cancer Chemotherapy*. (Edited by F. M. Schabel, Jr.) p. 200. S. Karger, Basel (1978).
7. V. T. DeVita, R. C. Young, and G. P. Canellos, Combination versus single agent chemotherapy: Review of basis for selection of drug treatment of cancer. *Cancer* 35, 98 (1975).
8. F. A. Schmid, D. J. Hutchison, G. M. Otter, and C. C. Stock, Development of resistance to combinations of six antimetabolites in mice with L1210 leukemia. *Cancer Treat. Rep.* 60, 23 (1976).
9. F. M. Schabel, Jr., D. P. Griswold, Jr., T. H. Corbett, W. R. Laster, Jr., J. G. Mayo, and H. H. Lloyd, Testing therapeutic hypotheses in mice and man: Observations on the therapeutic activity against advanced solid tumors of mice treated with anticancer drugs that have demonstrated or potential clinical utility for treatment of advanced solid tumors of man. In *Cancer Drug Development,*

Part B. Methods in Cancer Research.
(Edited by H. Busch and V. DeVita, Jr.)
Vol. 17, p. 3. Academic Press, New York
(1979).

10. F. M. Schabel, Jr., M. W. Trader, W. R.
    Laster, Jr., T. H. Corbett, and D. P.
    Griswold, Jr., *cis*-Diamminedichloroplati-
    num II: Combination chemotherapy and
    cross-resistance studies with tumors of
    mice. *Cancer Treat. Rep.*, in press.
11. F. M. Schabel, Jr., Test systems for
    evaluating the antitumor activity of
    nucleoside analogues. (Proceedings of
    NATO Advanced Study Institute on
    *Nucleoside Analogues: Chemistry, Biology,
    and Medical Applications*). Plenum Press,
    New York (1979).
12. F. M. Schabel, Jr., D. P. Griswold, Jr.,
    W. R. Laster, Jr., T. H. Corbett, and
    H. H. Lloyd, Quantitative evaluation of
    anticancer agent activity in experimental
    animals. *Pharmacol. Ther. Part A* 1, 411
    (1977).
13. J. F. Holland, Future prospects in
    lymphoma and leukemia. *Cancer* 42, 1035
    (1978).
14. F. M. Schabel, Jr., In vivo leukemic
    cell kill kinetics and "curability" in
    experimental systems. In *The Prolifera-
    tion and Spread of Neoplastic Cells*
    (21st Annual Symposium on Fundamental
    Cancer Research, The University of
    Texas M. D. Anderson Hospital and Tumor
    Institute, Houston, 1967) p. 379. The
    Williams and Wilkins Co., Baltimore
    (1968).

15. H. E. Skipper, F. M. Schabel, Jr., and
    H. H. Lloyd, Experimental therapeutics
    and kinetics: Selection and overgrowth
    of specifically and permanently drug-
    resistant tumor cells. *Semin. Hematol.*
    15, 107 (1978).
16. F. M. Schabel, Jr., H. E. Skipper, W. R.
    Laster, Jr., M. W. Trader, and S. A.
    Thompson, Experimental evaluation of
    potential anticancer agents. XX.
    Development of immunity to leukemia
    L1210 in BDF1 mice and effects of
    therapy. *Cancer Chemother. Rep.* 50,
    55 (1966).
17. W. D. DeWys, A dose-response study of
    resistance of leukemia L1210 to cyclo-
    phosphamide. *J. Natl. Cancer Inst.* 50,
    783 (1973).
18. I. Wodinsky and C. J. Kensler, Activity
    of cytosine arabinoside (NSC-63878) in
    a spectrum of rodent tumors. *Cancer
    Chemother. Rep.* 47, 65 (1965).
19. L. W. Law, V. Taormina, and P. J. Boyle,
    Response of acute lymphocytic leukemias
    to the purine antagonist 6-mercaptopurine.
    Ann. N.Y. Acad. Sci. 60, 244 (1954).
20. D. J. Hutchison, Cross resistance and
    collateral sensitivity studies in cancer
    chemotherapy. In *Advances in Cancer
    Research* (Edited by A. Haddow and
    S. Weinhouse) Vol. 7, p. 235. Academic
    Press, New York (1963).

The Relevance of Cell Kinetics for Human Cancer

H. Bush

CRC Department of Medical Oncology, Christie Hospital and Holt Radium Institute,
Wilmslow Road, Withington, Manchester M20 9BX, U.K.

Correspondence to H. Bush

Abstract—*In this review models of the cell cycle are assessed with respect
to data obtained from human tumours and proliferating normal cell populations.
The validity of the methods available for determining cell kinetic parameters
are assessed and their applicability in the human tumour situation evaluated.*
*Newer techniques allowing less laborious analysis to be made are discussed
and the applications of cell kinetics to clinical cancer is reviewed. Finally,
approachs to the synchronisation of normal proliferating cell populations,
which is described, an area of neglected cell kinetic research, but one which
offers the prospect of decreasing the toxicity of cancer therapy whilst
enhancing the therapuetic index.*

INTRODUCTION

The discovery that mitosis was not the only
discrete phase identifiable in the cell cycle
was made in 1953 when the incorporation of
tritiated thymidine into DNA, signifying DNA
synthesis, was found to occur in a discrete
phase of the cell cycle (1). Since that time
a variety of different models of the cell
cycle have emerged (2,3,4,5).

Although the experimental limitations of
many of these models has been closely evaluated, their use by clinicians has often been
arbitrary and may have been applied to the
study of widely differing populations of
cells inappropriately. Since 1953 many techniques for further evaluating the behaviour
of proliferating cells have been developed
and have been reviewed elsewhere (6,7).

This brief review examines four aspects of
cell kinetics in man; the available methods
and their limitations; the practical requirements for measuring cell kinetic parameters
in human solid tumours; the present and
future applications in man and the evaluation
of newer methodologies.

MODELS OF THE CELL CYCLE

Before attempting to define experimentally
the behaviour of a proliferating cell it is
important to recognise that there may be
several different patterns of replication.
Some of these may be evident between normal
(self renewing) populations of cells and
their malignant counterparts. Much attention
has been paid to cells that are apparently
not "in cycle" but it should be remembered
that the concept of the "Go phase" was
derived from careful studies with normal
mouse haemopoietic cells. Although there is

good evidence for the presence of stem cells
in other self renewing normal populations
such as the gastro-intestinal tract, the
evidence in man that malignant populations
in solid tumours exhibit the same pattern
of proliferative behaviour is not available.
Often the simple assumption is made that
because S phase cannot be defined in human
solid tumours by the available methods that
malignant cells are not proliferating.
However, there is good in vitro evidence
that malignant cells may grow at widely
differing rates. It has also been shown
that these differences in growth rates may
be explained by an expansion of the phase of
the cell cycle prior to DNA replication (4,8).

Other models propose that malignant cells
growing at widely differing rates may exhibit
a cell cycle expanded in all its phases
(Fig. 1), (9). This cycle expansion may not
be a simple function of limited nutrient
supply but that identifiable differences in
the regulation of DNA synthesis may occur
(9). Detailed consideration of the different
patterns of proliferative behaviour between
normal and malignant cells and within malignant cell populations is necessary when considering the relevance of "cell kinetics"
to human cancer.

METHODS AVAILABLE

Some of the available methods will be
evaluated here, Table 1. Table 2 summarizes
some of the requirements for evaluating cell
kinetic parameters in human solid tumours.
The mitotic index of tumours has been assessed
by Pathologists for many years, but there
are difficulties in evaluating the number of
mitoses in quantitative terms. In a situation in which the mitotic index may not rise

The Cell Cycle

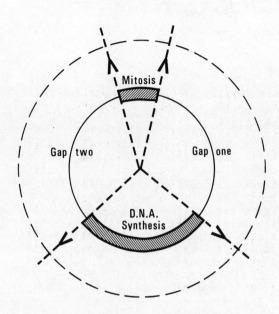

Fig. 1. Representation of the cell cycle
expanded in all its phases. A
model to describe variations in
rates of growth of malignant cells.

above a few percent it is necessary to count
many thousands of cells before accurate and
reproducable mitotic indices can be obtained.
In addition there are many sources of sampling error in any human solid tumour.
Recently methods have become available for
assessing mitotic indices quantatively in
experimental animal tumours but these require
further development before they can be used
in man.   The ^{3}H thymidine labelling index
has been used for many years, both by in vivo
methods and in vitro methods. ^{3}H thymidine
may be used in three common ways for evaluating cell cycle kinetic parameters, autogra-
diography allows the assessment of the percentage of cells in S phase whilst grain
counts and quantitative assessment of counts
incorporated into acid insoluble material
may give some assessment of the rate of DNA
synthesis.   More recently double labelling
techniques using both ^{3}H thymidine and 14C -
thymidine have been used to elegantly demonstrate the length of the cell cycle and its
various phases by extrapolation.

There are however, several technical and
biological reasons for variation in thymidine
labelling indices and these are summarised
in Table 3.

The use of the fraction labelled mitosis
curve (Fig. 2) has been a major experimental
tool for determining the length of the

Table 1. Methods available for measuring cell kinetic parameters
in human tumours.

Thymidine Labelling Index (TI)

Mitotic Index

Fraction Labelled mitosis curves (FLM)

Tumour doubling time/Growth Fraction

Cell generation time (double labelling technique)

S-Phase length measurements, Rates of DNA synthesis

Cytofluorimetry

Primer-dependant DNA polymerase activity/Growth Fraction

Anti nucleoside antibody techniques

Specific molecular markers for tumour cells (eg. CEA, HCG,M-Protein)

Table 2. Practical requirements for evaluating cell kinetic
parameters in human solid tumours

Repeatedly accessible material (biopsy, cytology etc.)

Applicable techniques for human tumour sections

    3HTdR

    PDP

    Anti nucleoside antibody

Viable, dissociated cells recognisable as malignant

    3HTdR

    PDP

    Cytofluorimetry

Table 3. Difficulties of thymidine labelling techniques

Thymidine availability to individual cells

Uptake variation

Variation in intra cellular nucloside pool size

Requires the presence of intra cellular thymidine kinase

Competition with other nucleotide precursors

Only evaluates cells in S

Problems of unscheduled DNA synthesis

    i) DNA repair

    ii) Mitochondrial DNA synthesis

Interference of competing cytotoxic drugs and metabolites

Mis-estimates due to impending cell death

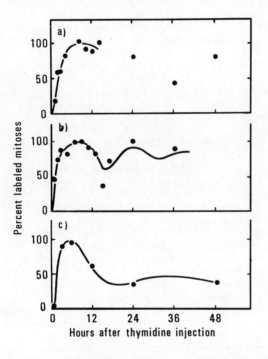

Fig. 2. Examples of fraction labelled
mitosis curves in normal human bone
marrow (a, c) and in a patient with
polycythaemia.

various phases of the cell cycle in proliferating cells. Even in the experimental
situation, however, the methods are extremely
time consuming and largely because of the
quantitative difficulties of evaluating the
mitotic index in human solid tumours, it is
unlikely that at the present time this
method will be routinely available. However,
several authors have accurately delineated
the cell cycle phases of human haemopoietic
stem cells using this method and with the
appropriate laboratory facilities it remains
one of the most sensitive tools available.
Whole tumour doubling time and the problems
of identifying the growth fraction have been
recently reviewed and will not be dealt with
further here (10).

The use of flow-cytometry has allowed a

number of important developments particularly
in relation to cell kinetics in human solid
tumours. Rapid evaluation is possible of
the distribution of cells in the cell cycle
in whole cell populations. In addition the
rapid identification of different populations
of cells with respect to their cell cycle
distribution may be made and more recently
methods have been developed to identify
specific malignant cell populations from
hetrogeneous mixtures of normal and malignant
cells. Many major technical and biological
difficulties still remain particularly in the
study of solid tumours rather than tumours
of haematological origin. These are summarised in Table 4.

NEWER METHODS

With the availability of more sophisticated
and computerised analysis of the cell cycle,
it is possible to obtain three dimensional
plots of the distribution of cells in the
cell cycle using flow-cytometry (Blackledge
and Swindell; unpublished observations).
This technology allows easy identification
of the heterogeneity of tumour cell populations with respect to their proliferative
behaviour, and may also allow rapid identification of distinct sub-populations of tumour
cells with widely differing proliferative
characteristics.

Many of the older methods identify only
cells that are already in S phase but there
is good evidence that closer correlation of
cellular growth and subsequent response to
therapy may be made by identifying the growth
fraction (that is those cells committed to
replicate). A number of methods are available
for this. Of these methods that of Schiffer,
(primer-dependent DNA polymerase activity)
is an elegant and simple method of identifying not only the cells in S phase but also
those cells in G1 that are committed to DNA
synthesis (11). Simply this method identifies
the intracellular activity of primer-
dependent, DNA polymerase by the use of
labelled exogenous nuclotides using an
autoradiographic technique. Confirmation
of the reproducibility of this technique

Table 4. Cytofluorimetry of cells from solid tumours

Requirement for single cell suspension

Difficulties of tissue disaggregation and cell viability

Identification of tumour cells in a heterogeneous population

Aneuploidy/Polyploidy

will be required before it becomes generally accepted. More recently Chang et al. (12) has developed a technique for rapidly identifying the number of cells in S phase using an anti-nucleotide antibody technique on cryostat preparations of human solid tumour material. During DNA synthesis the double stranded alpha helix is unwound and single stranded DNA exposed as a template for further replication. Using antibodies to a specific nuclotide, a simple immunoperoxidase technique has allowed identification of the single stranded regions of DNA exposed during replication. This apparently correlates well with thymidine labelling index studies but again this technique requires confirmation in other laboratories before it is generally accepted.

Many of the major problems associated with the measurement of cell kinetic parameters in human tumours lie within the area of identification of specific malignant cell populations. The use of tissue sections overcomes this difficulty but if more rapid and sophisticated methods such as flow-cytometry are required, then the additional use of specific molecular markers for tumour cells will be required. This has now been achieved for multiple myeloma and the potential exists in a number of solid tumours for extending these techniques. In relation to breast cancer it may subsequently be possible to use specific malignant cell markers proteins such as CEA, alpha HCG, lactalbumin. With the availability of fluorescent markers for both DNA content and also for cell-surface specific proteins, sub-populations of malignant cells may be rapidly identified by flow-cytometry and certain cell kinetics parameters evaluated.

APPLICATIONS IN MAN

In a number of human tumours a simple correlation between the number of cells in S phase (flow-cytometry, ^{3}H thymidine labelling index) has been made with correlations between both initial response to treatment and the completeness of that response. In acute myelogenous leukaemia, acute lymphoblastic leukaemia, and certain non-Hodgkin lymphomas, correlation has also been made between labelling index and remission duration. Elegant studies in multiple myeloma have demonstrated a close correlation between tumour mass, labelling index, response to therapy and remission duration. In neuroblastoma of childhood ^{3}H thymidine labelling index has also shown to correlate with body tumour burden and in some instances with response to therapy. Other relevant areas of the application of cell kinetic principles

and measurements to man are summarised in Table 5.

Much emphasis has been made in the literature of the Bruce model for cellular proliferation in human tumours. In many instances the experimental animal data is excellent but the simplistic extrapolation from animal studies to man particularly in relation to drug scheduling has been of little value. Despite the theoretical rationalisation of much cancer chemotherapy very little measurement of the kinetics of human tumours has been undertaken, in a way that will allow either description of the proliferative behaviour of the cells under study or the clinical prediction of response. The lack of relevance of cell kinetics at the present time to human cancer (apart from certain well defined diseases, such as multiple myeloma), is a function of a number of important variables. These are summarised in Table 6.

Insufficient, inaccurate and non-reproducible measurement is often a cause of failure. The availability of tissue for multiple measurements also imposes restrictions as to the type of disease and the type of patient available for study. Many studies reporting cell kinetic parameters have not been carried out in the context of a prospective clinical study and thus estimates of prognosis and evaluation of response have not allowed accurate clinical correlation. Little data is availabe on the perturbation of cell kinetic parameters by individual cytotoxic drugs and the influence of pharmacological and pharmaco-kinetic measurements on drug handling in relation to perturbations of the cell cycle is an important area for future study. Tannock (13) has rightly emphasised the importance of a simultaneous evaluation of normal tissue cell kinetics particularly in bone marrow.

Prospects for the future advances in the technology of flow-cytometry may soon allow identification of sub-population of malignant cells within human tumours, and the use of specific markers, lectins, CEA, alpha HCG, myeloma protein, may further allow evaluation of specific malignant clones of cells in relation to their cell kinetic parameters. The newer techniques of primary dependant DNA polymerase activity as a measurement of growth fraction and the technique of anti-nucleotide antibody labelling, may allow more accurate and more rapid identification of certain aspects of malignant cell growth. Important in assessing the relevance of cell kinetic for human cancer is the correlation of accurate and reproduciable methods of estimating cell kinetic parameters in the context of well controlled prospective

Table 5. Applications in man

Prognostic Index (LI) e.g.	ALL
	Non Hodgkins lymphoma
	Neuroblastoma
Scheduling	Phase specificity
	Interval between therapies
	Drug synergism in cell cycle
	Tumour size and cell proliferation rate
Extrapolation from animal studies	
Exploitation of differences between normal and malignant cells	
- differential synchronisation	
- selective protection of normal cells	
- selective killing of malignant cells	

Table 6. Relevance of cell kinetics for human tumours depends on:

Available tissue (multiple measurements)

Easily applicable and accurate techniques

Accurate clinical evaluation

      estimate of prognosis

      evaluation of response

      parallel pharmacokinetic studies in perturbation studies

Evaluation of normal tissue cell kinetics (bone marrow, gut) if therapeutic
   index is to be improved using cell kinetic alone

Synchronisation of normal and malignant cells

clinical studies. The possibility of differential synchronisation of normal and malignant cells exists but has yet to be fully exploited in human tumours. For this purpose simultaneous evaluation of the cell kinetics of normal tissues is required and so far has rarely been undertaken in man.

DISCUSSION

The use of cell kinetic markers in human cancer at the present time has been both limited and disappointing. Methods of evaluation have proved to be one of the limitations for solid tumours in humans but with the advent of newer methods, these difficulties may be resolved in part. The theoretical extrapolation from animal experimental systems has proved to be a clinical abstraction. Future studies demand more accurate, reproducible and repeated measurements using a combination of the available methods in the context of prospective and accurately defined clinical studies. In addition evaluation of tissue handling of individual cytotoxic drugs in relation to cell kinetic changes is also needed together with simultaneous measurement of the changes taking place in normal tissues such as bone marrow and gastro-intestinal tract. The possibility of selectively synchronising normal and malignant cell populations exists and is an

important area for further study.

Although isolated cell kinetic measurements may be used empirically as prognostic indices, the most exciting area in which cell kinetic measurement may be used with relevance in man is the exploitation and improvement of the therapeutic index. Clear differences exist in the proliferative pattern of normal and malignant cells in man. The first requirement is to identify and measure these differences in order to allow their subsequent exploitation in therapy.

ACKNOWLEDGEMENTS

I would like to thank Janet Widd for typing the manuscript, and the Cancer Research Campaign for support.

REFERENCES

1. A. Howard and S. E. Pelc, Synthesis of DNA in normal and irradiated cells and its relation to chromosonal breakage. *Heredity (Suppl)* 6, 261 (1953).
2. L. G. Lajtha, On the concept of the cell cycle. *J. Cell Comp. Physiol.* 69, 143 (1963).
3. W. R. Bruce, B. E. Mecker and F. A. Valeriote, Comparison of the sensitivity of normal and haematopoietic and lymphoma

colony forming cells to chemotherapeutic agents administered in vivo. *J. Natl. Cancer Inst.*, 37, 233 (1966).

4. J. A. Smith and L. Martin, Do cells cycle? *Proc. Natl. Acad. Sci. (US)*, 70, 1263 (1973).

5. H. Bush and M. Shodell, Cell cycle changes in transformed cells in the presence and absence of serum. *J. Cell. Physiol*. 90, 573 (1977).

6. J. M. Mitchinson, *The Biology of the cell cycle*, Cambridge Univ. Press (1971).

7. G. G. Steel, *Growth kinetics of tumours*, Clarendon Press (1977).

8. M. L. Mendelson, Autoradiographic analysis of cell proliferation in spontaneous breast cancer of C3H mouse. *J. Nat. Cancer Inst*. 25, 477 (1960).

9. H. Bush and M. Shodell, Uptake of molecular weight substances by SV40 transformed to 3T3 cells is invariant with growth rate in the presence and absence of serum. *Extp. Cell. Res*. 114, 27 (1978).

10. S. E. Shackney, W. McCormack and G. J. Cuchural, Growth rate patterns of solid tumours and their relation to therapy. *Ann. Int. Med*. 29, 107 (1978).

11. L. M. Schiffer, A. M. Markoe and J. S. R. Nelson, Estimation of tumour growth fraction in murine tumours by the primer-available DNA-dependent DNA polymerase activity. *Cancer Res*. 36, 2415 (1976).

12. T. H. Chang, D. Leibskind, F. Elequin, M. Janis and R. Bases, Labelling index in clinical specimens by the anti-nucleoside anti-body technique. *Cancer Res*. 38, 1012 (1978).

13. I. Tannock, Cell kinetics and chemotherapy. A critical review. *Cancer Treat. Rep*. 62, 1117 (1978).

Psychological Aspects of Breast Cancer

Psycho-Physiologic Aspects of Breast Cancer

B. A. Stoll

Departments of Oncology, St. Thomas' Hospital and Royal Free Hospital, London, United Kingdom

Correspondence to B. A. Stoll, Department of Oncology, St. Thomas' Hospital, London SE7 7EH, U.K.

Abstract—*A correlation has been suggested between the rate of growth of breast cancer on the one hand, and personality, emotional stress or affective disorders in the patient, on the other. Endocrine mechanisms could be involved in such a relationship and the hypothalamus may mediate it. Long continued stress could lead to high circulating levels of prolactin, growth hormone, thyrotrophin, oestrogen and corticosteroids, some of which might affect the growth of breast cancer.*

There have been reports suggesting that the prognosis may be worse in breast cancer patients who are overanxious. It is possible that mental factors could activate the tumour or else that the toxic effects of a more active tumour could cause specific mental effects. There are also firm clinical impressions that giving-up can shorten a patient's life expectancy, that optimism will improve the quality of life and that faith can cause placebo effects. None of these benefits need necessarily involve an effect on tumour growth, and the fact that a mechanism can be postulated for an effect by stress on tumour growth, does not prove that it occurs.

There is now considerable evidence that emotion can influence the release of anterior pituitary hormones. Emotional impulses are thought to originate either in the cerebral cortex or in the limbic system, of which the amygdala especially is thought to determine emotional reactions. These impulses affect the median eminence of the hypothalamus and from there, specific releasing factors pass through the portal plexus to the anterior pituitary gland where they stimulate the secretion and release of the appropriate hormone.

But emotional stimuli originating in the frontal lobes can also affect the posterior hypothalamus, leading to the release of epinephrine or norepinephrine through the sympathetic nervous system. It is believed that, whereas acute stress of the "fight or flight" variety stimulates release of epinephrine, more sustained stress such as that associated with mourning, separation, stress or anxiety, stimulates particularly the release of ACTH. It may also stimulate the release of growth hormone, prolactin and thyroid hormone while at the same time inhibiting the release of gonadotrophin. But individuals differ. The amount of cortisol released by stress varies widely from person to person and the release of one stress hormone may be independent of the release of another.

Some of these endocrine effects of stress may exert a direct effect on the growth of breast cancer. The raised prolactin level may interact with oestrogen in promoting tumour growth, and the increased ACTH levels may stimulate the secretion of oestrogen precursors from the adrenal cortex.

There is evidence also that stress can cause depression of the patient's immunological competence, and this again could increase the growth of breast cancer. While cortisol is probably the major factor in depressing the immune response, both epinephrine and prostaglandins are also able to depress lymphocyte and macrophage activity. Growth hormone and thyroid hormone also may be involved in modulating the immune response and are said to stimulate the growth of lymphoid tissue.

Clinical evidence linking emotional stress and depression with the patient's immune function has recently been published by Bartrop in Australia (1). He showed that bereavement caused marked increase in the lymphocyte response for the first 12 months after the death of a spouse.

But apart from all these theoretical considerations, what is the clinical evidence of an effect by stress on the growth of breast cancer? There are three possible areas where such evidence may be looked for; an effect on the patient's susceptibility to breast cancer; an effect in triggering the manifestation of either the primary tumour or of recurrence; an effect on the prognosis of the established disease.

With regard to an effect increasing the incidence of breast cancer, there are several reports that patients presenting with the disease give a history of highly traumatic events in their lives, or show an abnormally anxious or inhibited personality. It has been shown that patients with evidence of high corticosteroid and low androgen excretion levels are more likely to develop breast cancer, while experimental animals which are stressed in various ways show an increased incidence of mammary cancer.

Other reports suggest that stress can trigger off clinical activity in a tumour. Thus, a history of recent bereavement or depression has been noted in an abnormally high proportion of patients just before the appearance of a primary tumour. It has also been repeated by several authorities that after a long dormant interval, the experience of severe stress seems to trigger off recurrence.

Several reports have suggested that neuroleptic agents such as phenothiazine and antihypertensive agents of the Rauwolfia group may increase the incidence of breast cancer, possibly by stimulating prolactin release. This has not been confirmed in later reports.

The third area in which stress may affect cancer growth is by an influence on the mortality from the disease. There are various reports that the patient showing an overanxious or inhibited personality at the time of diagnosis, will have a poorer prognosis. Similarly death seems to follow sooner in patients who show a poor coping reaction after treatment. But an alternative explanation for these observations is that the mental changes may be the result of the more advanced disease and not the cause of the more rapidly growing tumour. To clarify this point, I have looked for a history of treatment for an anxiety state in the 10 years before diagnosis in 250 patients with breast cancer. I found that more of the patients with the poorest prognosis had a significant history of anxiety than did the patients who remained recurrence-free for 5 years.

Let us sum up. There is some evidence that mental factors may be associated either with increased incidence of cancer, increased activity of cancer or decreased life expectancy. It is possible that mental factors could be activating cancer, or else that the toxic effects of a more active cancer process cause certain mental effects. A third possibility is that both the breast cancer and the mental symptoms are being stimulated by the same factor. For example, increased MAO levels in the brain could be associated with depression, while in the hypothalamus it could cause abnormal hormone release.

There is little other scientific evidence on the relationship between mind and cancer but there are some firm clinical impressions. They are that "giving-up" can shorten a patient's life expectancy, optimism will improve the quality of life and faith may cause placebo effects. There is therefore only anecdotal evidence that the mental attitude of the patient can inhibit cancer growth or prolong life. The mere fact that a mechanism can be postulated for such an effect does not prove it occurs.

REFERENCE

1. R. W. Bartrop, E. Luckhurst, L. Lazarus, L. G. Kilch, and R. Penny, Depressed lymphocyte function after bereavement. *Lancet* 1, 834 (1977).

A Comparison of Subjective Responses in a Trial Comparing Endocrine with Cytotoxic Treatment in Advanced Carcinoma of the Breast

M. Baum*, T. Priestman**, R. R. West*** and E. M. Jones*

*Department of Surgery, Welsh National Medical School, Cardiff, U.K.
**Velindre Hospital, Cardiff, U.K.
***Department of Medical Statistics, Welsh National Medical School, Cardiff, U.K.

Correspondence to M. Baum, Department of Surgery, King's College Hospital
Medical School, Denmark Hill, London SE5, U.K.

Abstract—*Linear analogue self assessment (LASA) has been used to evaluate the quality of life in women entering a prospectively randomised trial comparing endocrine and cytotoxic therapy in advanced breast cancer. Although patients receiving cytotoxic therapy had a significantly greater incidence of alopecia, nausea, vomiting and constipation, scores for well-being were consistently and at one point significantly (p < 0.05) higher than for the endocrine treated group. The objective response rate was significantly higher in the cytotoxic group (p < 0.02) but patients who failed to respond to cytotoxic therapy rapidly showed a deterioration in LASA scoring compared to responders. These results indicate that even relatively severe side effects are well tolerated if there is objective regression of disease. If such remission is not rapidly apparent however, treatment should be terminated or ammended in order to avoid undue distress.*

INTRODUCTION

In previous publications the response rates and survival data from a prospectively randomised study comparing endocrine and cytotoxic drug therapy, in women with advanced breast cancer, were reported (1,2). This paper gives details of the subjective effects of treatment on patients entering the trial.

MATERIALS AND METHODS

One hundred women with locally advanced or metastatic adenocarcinoma of the breast were randomly allocated to receive either appropriate endocrine therapy or combination cytotoxic therapy. The treatment regimes employed are summarised in Table 1. The rationale for their choice has been discussed previously (1).

Subjective response was assessed by means of the Linear Analogue Self Assessment Technique (LASA). The application of this method of monitoring the quality of life in women with advanced breast cancer was found reliable in a pilot study at the Cardiff Breast Clinic (3). In the present trial the patient was provided with a chart which measured 25 subjective parameters. There were 10 for symptoms and side-effects (pain, dyspnoea, fatigue, anorexia, nausea, vomiting, constipation, diarrhoea, alopecia and "other"). There were five categories relating to anxiety and depression (irritability, apprehension, depression, insomnia and well being). Five aspects of personal relations were examined

(getting on with husbands, getting on with other people, sexual relationships, social relationships and decision making, and finally, five aspects of physical performance (ability to perform housework, chores, employment, hobbies and shopping). The charts were filled in before treatment and then at 1,2,3,7,11, and 15 weeks after the commencement of treatment. The patients filled in the charts at home and were asked to assess how they felt over the week previous to the time of scoring.

The scores from the LASA charts were analysed as follows: The mean and standard error for each subjective variable at each interval of time were plotted, so that patterns of response could be studied rather than individual scores. In addition to comparing the endocrine with the chemotherapy group, a further analysis was performed to compare those responding to chemotherapy with those failing on chemotherapy. As a crude initial method of statistical analysis the graphs were studied with a view to picking out separations of the standard errors for a given variable with a persistant trend in the same direction over a period of observation. For a more formal analysis a two tailed t test was carried out for the variables that seemed to demonstrate this separation in the comparison of cytotoxic and endocrine treated patients. For the comparison of cytotoxic responders and non-responders a one tailed t test was used, because we were only interested in showing that responders were not worse than non-responders. Previous workers using LASA have carried out a logarithmic transformation

Table 1. Treatment regimens used in study

Subgroup	Endocrine	Cytotoxic
Premenopausal .. .. Postmenopausal with soft- tissue disease .. Postmenopausal with secon- dary deposits in bone Postmenopausal with secon- dary deposits in lung par- enchyma .. .. .. Postmenopausal with liver involvement or lymphang- itis carcinomatosa ..	Ovarian ablation Tamoxifen 20 mg twice daily Methyltestosterone 5 mg thrice daily + nandro- lone phenylpropionate 50 mg intramuscularly once weekly Striboestrol 5 mg thrice daily Prednisone 10 mg thrice daily	Doxorubicin 60 mg plus cyclophosphamide 750 mg plus fluorouracil 750 mg plus vincristine 2 mg by intravenous injection day one every three weeks

of the data prior to analysis because of the skew distribution of the patients' mark along the lines of the chart (4). Further analysis of the present data following logarithmic transformation did not, however, alter the results. Finally a factor analysis was carried out using B.M.D. computer programmes (5).

RESULTS

Evaluation of objective parameters of response showed a significantly higher response rate to cytotoxic therapy with similar remission durations for cytotoxic and endocrine responders. The sequence in which the two forms of treatment were given however, did not appear to influence survival, except possibly in women with rapidly progressing disease, when cytotoxic therapy was to be preferred (2). Ninety-two patients were available for objective assessment but of these only 51 completed LASA proformas. Of these there were initially 25 women in the endocrine group and 26 in the chemotherapy group. Only those patients who completed score sheets for more than six weeks were considered evaluable and as a result there was a large fallout in the endocrine group only 14 being available for the final analysis.

In the overall comparison of cytotoxic and endocrine treatment, five parameters showed a significant variation, (Table 2). Nausea, vomiting and constipation were more apparent in cytotoxic treated patients. In addition, all patients receiving chemotherapy developed alopecia, but this was not reflected by deterioration in scores for mood, personal relations or physical performance. Indeed there was a constant trend for a higher score for well being in the cytotoxic group although this only reached significance at 11 weeks.

In the comparison of cytotoxic responders and non-responders a significant difference in five subjective appeared after only one course of chemotherapy (Table 3). Furthermore after 3-5 courses of chemotherapy there was a significant fall in 9 scores in the non-responders. An example of the later deterioration in the non-responders is the score for depression (Fig. 1).

Factor analysis did not prove to be useful, merely demonstrating the expected congruance of the scores for nausea and vomiting and the somewhat unstable grouping of symptoms, social and performance indices.

DISCUSSION

In the treatment of advanced breast cancer, aggressive cytotoxic therapy is generally

Table 2. Levels of significance in subjective variables showing
apparent differences comparing endocrine with
chemotherapy

Weeks of treatment	0	1	2	3	7	11	15
Nausea	NS	NS	NS	NS	<.05	NS	NS
Vomiting	NS	<.05	NS	NS	<.05	<.05	NS
Constipation	NS	NS	NS	NS	<.01	NS	NS
Well being	NS	NS	NS	NS	NS	<.05*	NS

*In favour chemotherapy.

Table 3. Levels of significance in subjective variables showing
apparent differences comparing patients responding to
chemotherapy to those failing on chemotherapy

Weeks of treatment	0	1	2	3	7	11	15
Pain	NS	NS	NS	<.05	NS	NS	NS
Dyspnoea	NS	NS	NS	NS	NS	NS	<.01
Anorexia	NS	NS	NS	NS	NS	<.05	<.05
Depression	NS	NS	NS	NS	NS	<.01	<.01
Insomnia	NS	NS	NS	<.05	NS	NS	<.01
Well being	NS	NS	NS	NS	NS	<.01	<.001
Housework	NS	NS	NS	<.01	NS	<.05	<.001
Chores	NS	NS	NS	<.01	NS	<.05	<.001
Shopping	NS	NS	NS	<.05	NS	<.01	<.001
Socializing	NS	NS	NS	NS	NS	<.05	<.001

All significant differences favour responders.

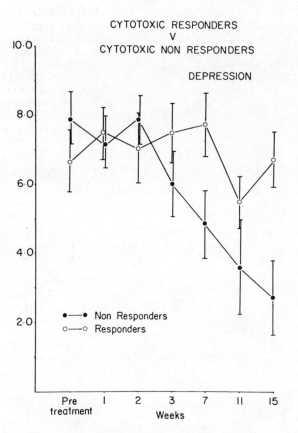

CYTOTOXIC RESPONDERS
V
CYTOTOXIC NON RESPONDERS

DEPRESSION

•—• Non Responders
o—o Responders

Pre
treatment   Weeks

Fig. 1. LASA scores (mean ± s.e.) for
depression comparing cytotoxic
responders with cytotoxic non-
responders.

associated with much greater toxicity than
endocrine manipulation. We therefore considered it important that, in addition to
measuring response rate and survival, we
should also attempt to assess the effect of
the two forms of treatment on the patients'
quality of life.

The results described above indicate that
overall, although patients in the cytotoxic
treatment group had a significantly higher
incidence of certain side effects (alopecia,
nausea, vomiting and constipation) their
quality of life, as indicated by the score
for wellbeing, was better than in the endocrine group. The observations that the
response rate was significantly higher in
patients given cytotoxics (p < 0.02) and
that women responding to chemotherapy showed
higher scores than those who failed on
similar treatment, suggest that the higher
incidence of side effects with chemotherapy
is more than offset by the greater incidence
of response. Furthermore the rapidity with
which the scores for cytotoxic responders
and non-responders diverge indicates that if
an objective response is not apparent after
two or three courses of chemotherapy, treatment should be changed to avoid undue distress
to the patient.

Apart from these specific findings the
results of this study indicate that the
LASA technique is a reliable tool for measuring the subjective effects of different forms
of anti-cancer treatment. In the past,
subjective toxicity in oncological studies
has been ignored or monitored by grading scales
based solely on the patients' physical performance (6,7). We feel that the LASA technique,
whilst retaining simplicity and reliability,
offers a more comprehensive evaluation of the
impact of treatment on the patients' quality of
life.

ACKNOWLEDGEMENTS

Miss Griffiths and Miss Speary, Nursing
Officers at Velindre Hospital gave enormous
help in launching this project.
Dr. Peter Maguire helped in the development and initial trial of the LASA charts
and Professor Hubert Camppell advised on
their mathematical interpretation. This
work was generously supported by a grant from
the Cancer Research Campaign.

REFERENCES

1. T. Priestman, M. Baum, V. Jones and
   J. Forbes, Comparative trial of endocrine
   versus cytotoxic treatment in advanced
   breast cancer. *Br. Med. J.* 1, 1248 (1977).
2. T. Priestman, M. Baum, V. Jones and
   J. Forbes, Treatment and survival in
   advanced breast cancer. *Br. Med. J.* 2,
   1673 (1978).
3. T. Priestman and M. Baum, Evaluation of
   quality of life in patients receiving
   treatment for advanced breast cancer.
   Lancet 1, 899 (1976).
4. A. Bond and M. H. Lader, The use of
   analogue scales in rating subjective
   feelings. *Br. J. Med. Psychol.* 47, 211
   (1974).
5. D. A. Karnofsky and J. H. Burchenal,
   The clinical evaluation of chemotherapeutic agents in cancer. In *Evaluation of
   chemotherapeutic agents*. (Edited by C. M.
   MacLeod) p. 191. Columbia University
   Press, New York (1948).
6. P. S. Burg, T. A. Prankerd, J. D. Richards,
   M. Sare, D. S. Thompson and P. Wright,
   Quality and quantity of survival in acute
   myeloid leukaemia. *Lancia* 2, 621 (1965).

Quality of Survival of Patients Following Mastectomy

R. G. Wilson*, J. R. Farnon** and A. Hutchinson***

*Department of Surgery, Newcastle General Hospital, Newcastle upon Tyne, U.K.
**Department of Surgery, Royal Victoria Infirmary, Newcastle upon Tyne, U.K.
***Department of Psychiatry, Royal Victoria Infirmary, Newcastle upon Tyne, U.K.

Correspondence to R. G. Wilson

Correspondance to: R. G. Wilson, Department of Surgery, Newcastle General
Hospital, Newcastle Upon Tyne, United Kingdom

Abstract—*Significant levels of anxiety, depression and sexual problems have been reported in patients one year after mastectomy. Using an interview, a questionnaire and the Eysenck Personality Inventory, the physical, social and emotional problems in a group of women 2-6 months after mastectomy, were compared with a group of women undergoing biopsy for benign breast disease. Mastectomised patients desire further pre and post-operative information and support from the hospital, and are more likely than benign breast disease patients to experience sexual problems and "disability" as a result of the operation. Some women would have preferred confirmatory biopsy to the traditional frozen section with immediate mastectomy.*

INTRODUCTION

Since Halsted first advocated radical mastectomy for the treatment of primary breast cancer in 1894, women have had to face the psychological impact of both the disease and its treatment.

As radical surgery has been shown not to confer any improved survival, there has been a step-wise reduction of the extent of the tissue removed, but the breast itself is still removed. Only recently and slowly have clinicians begun to wonder *how* these patients survive and fulfill their role in the family, socially and at work.

It is clear that the cancer patient, including those who are theoretically cured, has to adapt psychologically and physiologically to an altered state. This will include the ability to deal with the presence of a potentially life-threatening disease and the ability to adapt and cope with the surgical loss and perhaps the local and widespread effects of radiotherapy and chemotherapy.

In assessing the success of therapy for cancer, and other chronic diseases, recently greater attention has been given to the "quality of survival". Unfortunately a major hinderance to many of these efforts has been the lack of clarity and consistancy in the definition of quality of survival and how to assess it.

Some studies have focused on purely functional indices where the patient provides information on their ability to resume and carry out "normal" functions in the family and the community - such as employment tasks and everyday household activities (1).

The Linear Analogue Self Assessment method (L.A.S.A.) is a simple test in which the patient scores her self for a number of parameters. This method has been used in patients with breast cancer (2).

Other studies have attempted to include more "global" indices such as attitude and interpersonal relationships (3). Many of the previous studies have not employed systematic measurement or standardised techniques.

MATERIALS AND METHODS

A prospective and controlled study was designed that endeavoured to do this. Patients who attended a surgical out-patients with a breast lump were to be studied pre- and post-operatively. After the diagnosis had been confirmed pairing was to be carried out for age, marital status, menopausal status, social class and verbal I.Q. Assessment of the patients was to be by interview, a questionaire and the Eysenck Personality Inventory, a standardised psychological test. Unfortunately the study in its original form had to be abandoned because of its unexpected publicity in the local press, and the immediate effect this had on the response of women who were undergoing investigations of breast pathology.

Subsequently it was only possible to carry out a retrospective pilot study to investigate whether mastectomised patients experience an inferior quality of life post-operatively and to test the methods.

The questionaire was based on information from existing studies on this subject. The questionaire and the Eysenck Personality Inventory were to be administered to both mastectomised and benign breast disease patients two months after surgery. The questionaire was administered verbally and a score given for each answer. The patient was given a copy of the part that required a choice of response. The Eysenck Personality Inventory was self administered.

It was hoped to gain information regarding the needs of these patients with details about any further help and support that they required as a prelude to carrying out the fuller study.

RESULTS

There was no difference between the two groups in marital status, social class or verbal I.Q. With regard to the differences between the two groups some of the variables that remain significant once the effects of age and menopause are taken into account will be presented.

There was a significant difference between the two groups in the Total Self-Care Activity Score (p = 0.01) and the Total Residual Disability Score (p < 0.01).

The Total Self-Care Activity Score includes items such as the ability to brush hair, to dress, to bath etc.

The Total Residual Disability Score includes the presence of swelling of the arm, weakness of the arm, unexpected pains and sensations, etc.

It is unclear from this study whether the disability is primarily of a physical nature or a combination of physical and psychological factors. Collection of objective medical data as originally planned would have clarified this point, e.g. an objective measure of arm range of movement could have been compared with the subjective report of such physical disability. However, there would still have been some variables, such as pain, that have no comparable medical measurement.

The rating of the information received in hospital was significantly different for the two groups (p < 0.01). Mastectomised patients rated the information as "lees good" than benign breast disease patients. There was a significant difference between the two groups with regard to requiring further support from the hospital (p = 0.05). All the mastecto-mised patients referred to the postoperative period, many patients saying that they felt "lost and alone" after their discharge from hospital and that they were unsure of the things that they should or should not do.

Many of the mastectomised patients expressed a wish for further information regarding the nature and prognostic pattern of their lump and the effect on their appearance of mastectomy. Here a difference between the two surgical units participating in the study became apparent. One used the traditional frozen section/mastectomy technique, while the other obtained a pre-operative diagnosis by out patient needle biopsy. This latter method permits more extensive pre-operative discussion with the patient.

Post-operatively, anxiety regarding recurrence and concern whether all of the cancer had been removed were particularly noticeable.

DISCUSSION

The most important facts to emerge from this pilot study were that mastectomised patients desire much more pre- and post-operative information and support from the hospital; and more information regarding diagnosis and prognosis as well as post-operative guidance and reassurance.

Clearly more detailed investigation is required in the area of communication pre-operatively. It may be that frozen section is a surgical convenience and is not the best way of achieving the definitive diagnosis from the women's point of view.

The design of this pilot study does not account for any pre-existing psychological differences between the two groups and so the results obtained must be viewed in this light. We hope that a prospective study, as originally planned, will take into account these levels and including comparison of frozen section and pre-operative biopsy will help us offer women an improvement in their quality of life after mastectomy.

REFERENCES

1. D. Schottenfeld and G. F. Robbins, Quality of survival among patients who have had a radical mastectomy. *Cancer* 26, 650 (1970).
2. T. J. Priestman and M. Baum, Measurement of the quality of life during treatment for advanced breast cancer. *Clin. Oncol.* 3, 308 (1976).
3. F. Ch. Izsak and J. H. Medalie, Comprehensive follow up of carcinoma patients. *J. Chron. Dis.* 24, 179 (1972).

Life with Cytostatic Drugs

F. S. A. Van Dam*,**, A. C. G. Linssen*,**, E. Engelsman*, J. van Benthem** and G. J. F. P. Hanewald**

*Antoni van Leeuwenhoek Hospital, The Netherlands Cancer Institute, Amsterdam
**Laboratory of Psychology, University of Amsterdam, Department of Clinical
Psychology, Amsterdam

Correspondence to F. S. A. M. van Dam, Antoni van Leeuwenhoek Hospital,
The Netherlands Cancer Institute, Plesmanlaan 121, Amsterdam, The Netherlands

Abstract—This research examined consequences of a treatment with cytostatic
drugs in patients with breast cancer. For that purpose three groups were
involved in the research: a group of patients with metastasis receiving
palliative chemotherapy, a second group receiving adjuvant chemotherapy, and
a third (control) group who in the past had been radically treated for breast
cancer by mastectomy and/or radiotherapy.

In the treatment with cytostatic drugs a salient consequence is the feeling
of general malaise. There are additional complaints such as nausea and
vomiting after administering injections. The patients receiving palliative
treatment appeared to be considerably disturbed in their daily activities,
in contrast to patients receiving the adjuvant treatment.

The group being treated with cytostatic drugs state, somewhat paradoxically,
that they feel reasonably well, despite the considerable number of complaints.
(An average of 5 to 6).

The control group had fewer complaints; however, a considerable number
stated that they were tired and nervous.

INTRODUCTION

Cytostatic drugs are being used increasingly
in the past few years in the treatment of
cancer. These drugs are known to have
numerous side effects. The side effects
are mainly described in biochemical and physiological terms and seldom in behavioral
terms. To what extent treatment interferes
with a patients daily life, which complaints
they have (including 'psychological' ones),
how they feel and whether they ever considered refusing treatment are all issues that
are hardly mentioned in the literature.

Cytostatic therapy is usually palliative,
that is to say that the aim of treatment is
to prolong life or to reduce complaints and
not to cure the disease. One should con-
stantly therefore raise the question whether
the possibility of remission counterbalances
the trouble therapy causes for the patient.
But even when the goal of cytostatic therapy
is curative, it is highly necessary to find
out what the consequences of this therapy
are in the daily life of the patient.

Patients with breast cancer were selected
for this research of the pattern of complaints
and the consequences of chemotherapy in
daily life. One out of every fifteen to
twenty women gets breast cancer and approximately half of them will die of the disease.
This therefore concerns quite a large group
of patients. The majority of patients with
metastasis will, in due time, be treated
rather uniformly, as outpatients, with
cytostatic drugs. Cytostatic drugs are
being used for breast cancer in two different
ways: firstly, for patients with manifest
metastasis causing complaints, and secondly,
for those patients where it is obvious
during primary treatment that there is a
high risk of recurrence. This last group
does not have any metastasis causing disturbances. In using this group, receiving the
so-called adjuvant treatment, it is possible
to differentiate between those complaints
due to metastasis and those due to cytostatic
drugs. The experiences of both groups
treated are analyzed in comparison to those
of a group of patients with breast cancer
who previously had an amputation, in some
cases followed by radiotherapy.

MATERIALS AND METHODS

1. The Patients

This research involved 120 women who were
being or had been treated for breast cancer
at the Antoni van Leeuwenhoek Hospital.
- 41 patients with advanced breast cancer
  treated as outpatients with a combination
  of cytostatic drugs. The average age
  of this group, which we will call the
  'Meta' group, is 53 years (sd: 11 years).

- 39 patients with breast cancer with a
  high risk of recurrence treated addi-
  tionally with a combination of cytostatic
  drugs. This group, which we will call the
  'Adjuvant' group, had no complaints or
  irregularities due to metastasis. The
  average age is 50 years (sd: 10 years).
- 40 patients treated for breast cancer by
  means of amputation and/or radiotherapy
  at least one year ago. Primary therapy
  seems successful; they come to the poli-
  clinic for a check-up once every three or
  six months. The average age of this
  group, which we will call the *'Control'*
  group, is 56 years (sd: 11 years).

The Control group is significantly older
than the Adjuvant group (p < 0.5).

2. The Therapies

A. Primary therapy. Table 1 shows, as
expected, that the Adjuvant group has been
treated more recently than both other groups.

3. The Instruments of Measure

The patients were asked to complete a
complaint calendar (taken from K.v.d. Woude
(1) once a week for a month. Hereby data
were obtained on five different times. The
complaint calendar consist of four sections:
A. The checklist of complaints. (Example:
Were you bothered today by fatigue, spiritlessness, dizzyness etc., with a scale of
four possible answers: a lot, moderate, a
bit, none). The items on the checklist of
complaints were arrived at in collaboration
with the specialists for internal diseases.
B. Use of medicine. Here the patient was
to state the use that day of sleeping pills
and tranquilizers, painkillers and 'other
medicine'. C. Rest - day and night. The
number of hours of rest per day and per night
was computed from this section. D. Well-
being. In medical practice it is not
uncommon to ask: 'how are you feeling today?'
We also put this question to the patients
in this investigation, providing them with

Table 1. Primary therapy.

		Meta group n = 41	Adjuvant group n = 39	Control group n = 40
Primary therapy	Mastectomy and/or Radiotherapy	34	39	40
	'Miscellaneous'	7	0	0
Average number of months since primary therapy		28 Sd = 14,3 months	8 Sd = 7,4 months	35 Sd = 8,3 months

'Miscellaneous' = ovariectomy or immediate chemotherapy.

B. Chemotherapy. Patients in the Meta and
Adjuvant group were treated with a combination of cytostatic drugs. The cytostatic
drugs were administered according to two
schedules: CMF-schedule (cyclophosphamide
100 mg/m^2 p.o. day 1-14, methotrexate
40 mg/m^2 i.v. day 1 and 8, 5-fluorouracil
600 mg/m^2 i.v. day 1 and 8, 1 cycle is 28
days) and AV-schedule (adriamycin 40-500
mg/m^2 i.v. day 1, vincristin 1.4 mg/m^2 (max.
2 mg) day 1 and (often) day 8, one cycle is
21 days or 28 days when vincristin is given
on day 8). Some patients were treated alter-
nately on the CMF and AV schedules.
Uniformity of dose was aimed at, but often
had to be varied for several reasons. In
the investigation two specialists for internal diseases, independently of each other,
rated the doses by weight, on a two point
scale (light and heavy). They agreed on
88% of the doses.
The doses on which no agreement was
reached, were rated by a third specialist
for internal diseases. The weight of the
dose is important because 'heavy injections'
may cause more complaints. For that matter,
there was no systematic difference in the
weight of the doses between both groups.

a scale of five possible answers: very
poorly, somewhat poorly, not poorly but not
well either, reasonably well, well.

4. The Interview

A list of daily activities (DAL) was rated
during a short interview. This list gives
an impression of the degree to which patients
are restricted in the performance of a number of daily activities pertaining to self
care, mobility and housekeeping. Finally
the patients were asked the question: 'Have
you ever considered refusing an injection?'

RESULTS

The number of complaints within the
groups treated with cytostatic drugs was
twice as high as in the Control group:
the Meta group listed an average of 6,5
complaints a day during a month, the Adjuvant group had an average of 5 complaints
a day and the Control group had an average
of 3 complaints a day during a month. The
difference between the Meta and the Adjuvant group is not significant, but there
is a significant difference between these

Table 2. Percentages of incidence of complaints per group

Complaint	Meta-group N = 32		Adjuvant-group N = 35		Control-group N = 36	
	injection week	rest week	injection week	rest week	week 3	week 5
fatigue	88%[a]	71%[a]	73%[b]	53%	44%[ab]	39%[a]
spiritlessness	79%[d]	53%[a]	54%[d]	36%	15%[d]	17%[a]
lack of appetite	56%[d]	32%[ac]	24%[d]	11%[c]	5%[d]	3%[a]
nausea	53%[a]	14%	41%[b]	15%	--[ab]	--
nervousness	47%	41%	32%	33%	39%	28%
worrying	32%	15%	19%	19%	31%	17%
shortness of breath	29%[a]	29%[a]	30%[b]	28%[b]	5%[ab]	6%[ab]
shivering	32%[a]	15%	35%[b]	22%	8%[ab]	8%
other pain	29%	47%[ac]	30%	19%[c]	18%	17%[a]
depression	24%	24%	35%	19%	21%	14%
insomnia	24%	38%	30%	33%	31%	25%
muscular spasms	24%	18%	30%	31%	31%	11%
oral/swallowing pain	21%	3%	16%	6%	3%	8%
headache	18%	15%	24%	25%	18%	6%
tingling in hands/feet	21%	21%	--	11%	--	6%
heartburn	24%	6%	16%	11%	10%	6%
stomach ache	21%[a]	9%	8%	--	3%[a]	3%
constipation	21%[a]	18%[a]	8%	8%	3%[a]	--[a]
itch	8%	12%	22%	19%	18%	11%
other complaint	18%	35%	27%	22%	8%	14%
dizzyness	15%	21%	24%	11%	5%	3%
vomiting	15%[a]	9%	11%	6%	--[a]	--
crying fits	9%	9%	5%	11%	8%	3%

a = Meta group significantly more troubled by complaint than Control group.
b = Adjuvant group significantly more than Control group.
c = Meta group significantly more than Adjuvant group.
d = The three groups differ significantly: Meta > Adjuvant > Control.
Method: Chi-square, computed for rough frequencies. Degrees of freedom: 1 ($p < .05$).

two groups and the Control group ($p < .01$).

The most frequently occuring complaint was fatigue (Table 2), as was the case in earlier research of patients treated wth cytostatic drugs for a advanced testicular cancer (2) or advanced breast cancer (1).

During a one month period an average of 78% of the patients in the Meta group and 63% of the patients in the Adjuvant group indicated that they were troubled by fatigue. An average of more than 40% of the patients in the Control group also listed this complaint. Therefore one cannot speak of a complaint caused solely by the treatment. The time both groups treated, rest during the day concurs with this result. This was 2 hours and 20 minutes for the Meta group, 1 hour and 18 minutes for the Adjuvant group, and an average of 18 minutes a day for the Control group. The difference between the groups is significant ($p < .01$). The time the Control group rests during the day is the same as that for a comparable group of Dutch women (3).

In both groups treated a positive correlation was found between the total number of complaints and the number of hours of rest during the day (Meta group r = .55, Adjuvant group r = .58; $p < .001$). The more complaints, the more one rested; this did not apply to the Control group.

In addition to complaints about fatigue, during treatment, other common complaints are spiritlessness and lack of appetite. Contrary to expectation there was no difference between the three groups in the occurrence of nervousness and depression.

The complaints of patients being treated with cytostatic drugs can best be described as a 'general feeling of malaise'. This general feeling of malaise however, also seems to be present for a considerable part of the Control group.

The groups being treated with cytostatic drugs had also short-term complaints such as nausea and vomiting following the

injections. There seemed some increase in
the general feeling of malaise on the days
the injections were given, and it seemed to
be present for more patients (see Fig. 1).

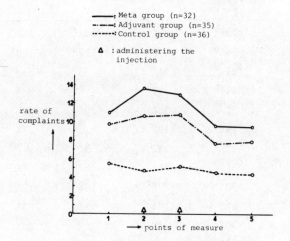

Fig. 1. Mean rate of complaints per group
per point of measure.

There was a discrepancy between the high
level of complaints and the measure of well
being rated by the patients. Patients
hardly stated that they felt poorly, despite
the large number of complaints.

Generally patients did not rate lower than
the middle of the five point scale, running
from well to very poorly, that is to say,
not lower than 'not poorly but not well
either'. Here again there is a significant
difference between both groups being treated
with cytostatic drugs and the Control group
(p < .05).

The most striking finding on the rating on
the list of daily activities is the fact that
the patients of the Meta group can perform
their household activities only with difficulty or need assistance (see Fig. 2).

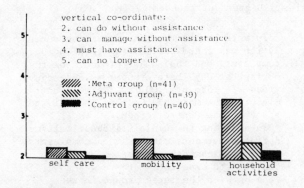

Fig. 2. Daily activities: mean rate per
group per category.

In general the patients of the Meta group
are somewhat less mobile than the patients
of the Adjuvant group.

Both, the Adjuvant and the Control group,
differ significantly from the Meta group in
mobility and household activities (p < .05).
It is not surprising that there is no

significant difference in the degree of self
care between the groups. In most cases,
patients who can not care for themselves
will be hospitalized. Since their illness,
patients in the groups treated had household
help more often than patients in the Control
group. This indicates that household help
should be organised before starting a treatment with cytostatic drugs. Further, about
75% of the women in the Meta and Adjuvant
group have stopped working; this is much
less in the Control group (30%). Apparently
this treatment with cytostatic drugs is not
compatible with maintaining a job.

DISCUSSION

Giel (2) remarks, referring to an investigation of patients with advanced testicular
cancer treated with Actinomycin D,: 'that
in general they tolerate reasonably well a
terrible treatment like that of cytostatic
drugs, and are even content with what is
offered'. On the basis of the favourable
answers of patients in our research on the
question of how they are feeling, one could
draw this conclusion as well. If such a
favourable answer is viewed as reflecting
her adaptibility then the value a single
answer is perhaps justifiable. But other
interpretations are possible. In the first
place there may be a strong response tendency.
Numerous research demonstrates that people
tend to answer favourably to questions such
as 'how do you feel' and rate accordingly
on scales devised by psychologists - the
so-called 'hello-goodbye effect'. Another
interpretation may be that standards people
have about health change in chronic illness
so that they adapt more easily to their new
situation. Another possibility may be that
at one time an answer given by a patient is
based on a successful adaptation and at
another time it is based on response tendency.

It is important to stress that one must
realise exactly what one is asking the
patient. It is not surprising that a lot
of confusion arises when the doctor at one
time asks how the patient feels and at
another time what complaints she has. This
makes it all the more speculative to talk
about quality of life without specifying
what is meant.

Furthermore patients were asked whether
they had ever considered refusing an injection. It appears that more than 25% of the
patients has considered stopping or inter-
rupting treatment on their own initiative.
30% of the patients who have never considered
refusing an injection say that, in fact,
they have no choice (!).

Those patients who have refused chemotherapy from the start (± 5%) are, of course,
not included in this research.

It is striking that only clear difference
between the two groups being treated is that
in daily activities. No differences were
found in complaint scores and on the question
of well being (see above).

Apparently the two groups treated with
cytostatic drugs only differentiate on items

pertaining to mobility and household activities of the list of daily activities. One
may conclude that chemotherapy determines
many of the complaints, while daily activities are mainly influenced by the fact of
advanced breast cancer.

In clinical investigations on the effectiveness of cytostatic drugs we would like to
urge obtaining more systematically, psychological and social data. The differences in
this area may help determine the choice
between two otherwise equivalent drugs.

It is still an open question whether our
method is useful in decisions concerning
individual patients. Further research shall
determine how much weight must be given to
the various psychological and social factors.

REFERENCES

1. K. van de Woude, *Ervaringen van patienten
   die met cytostatica behandeld worden*,
   p. 122. MA Thesis, University of
   Amsterdam (1977).
2. R. Giel, W. Frankenberg, J. Oldhoff,
   B. Otten, E. van der Ploeg, E. Schraffordt
   Koops, and H. Vermey, De chirurg-oncoloog
   en de kwaliteit van het leven van zijn
   patienten. *Ned. Tijdschrift Geneesk*. 121,
   1315 (1977).
3. W. P. Knuist, Een week tijd. In *S.C.P.-
   Cahier* No. 10, p. 180. Staatsuitgeverij,
   's-Gravenhage (1977).

New Aspects of Primary Treatment

Selection of Local Therapy for Primary Breast Cancer by Lower Axillary Node Histology

A. P. M. Forrest*, M. M. Roberts* and H. J. Stewart**

*Department of Clinical Surgery, University of Edinburgh
**Department of Radiation Oncology, Western General Hospital, Edinburgh

Correspondence to A. P. M. Forrest, Dept. of Clinical Surgery, The Royal Infirmary,
Edinburgh EH3 9YW, U.K.

Abstract—*Two controlled randomized trials have been carried out to test a policy of treatment for primary breast cancer consisting of simple mastectomy and axillary node biopsy supplemented by postoperative radiotherapy should the lower axillary (pectoral or axillary tail) nodes prove to be involved. In Cardiff we compared this policy with a routine radical surgical approach, supplemented by radical radiotherapy, in patients with positive axillary nodes. In Edinburgh simple mastectomy and node biopsy was adopted as standard primary treatment; patients with positive nodes were included in trials of adjuvant systemic therapy; those with negative (or non-identified) nodes were randomized either for no further treatment or for postoperative radical radiotherapy.*

The results indicate that a selective policy of local treatment, the extent of which is based on node histology, gives equal survival and dissemination rates to a routine radical approach. Loco-regional recurrence is also controlled provided that in node positive patients simple mastectomy is supplemented by radiotherapy which includes the chest wall. Identification of the lower axillary nodes for histology is an essential prerequisite to the safe conservation of the axillary nodes.

INTRODUCTION

The policy of management which we put to the test of controlled randomised trials in Cardiff and in Edinburgh was designed to avoid the potential morbidity of unnecessary treatment by dissection or radiotherapy to the axillary lymph nodes when these were not involved by tumour (1). The primary operation was a simple (total) mastectomy, at which the lowermost group of pectoral lymph nodes which are in-continuity with the nodes lying in the axillary tail of Spence were sampled for histological examination. It was suggested that the need for further local treatment, by radiotherapy could be determined by the histology of these nodes. If this indicated involvement by tumour, post-operation radiotherapy was advised; if there was no evidence of involvement, no further immediate treatment was planned.

MATERIALS AND METHODS

1. Technique of Node Sampling

This has been under continuous review (2). Initially, we were primarily concerned with sampling those nodes of the pectoral group which lie above and medial to the apex of the axillary tail at its junction with the lower axillary fat. A detailed study was then carried out which indicated that the relevant nodes formed a continuous chain from breast to axilla and that good sampling included a careful and complete dissection of the axillary tail of the breast; as well as a search by the surgeon for those nodes which lie outside the substance of the axillary tail in the pectoral region; and careful palpation and dissection of the tail by the pathologist for nodes within its substance (3). On average, 5 nodes lie within the axillary tail of the breast; and nodes can be identified in the tail of the breast and pectoral region in over 90% of cases. Should obvious nodes not be found in these lower regions we now do not hesitate to perform a more formal dissection of the lower axilla, but preserving those tissues which lie immediately surrounding the axillary vein.

TRIALS OF POLICY OF SIMPLE MASTECTOMY AND SELECTIVE RADIOTHERAPY

1. Cardiff

In the Cardiff trial, started in 1967, the conservative policy of treatment outlined above was compared with a routine radical approach. Patients with primary breast cancer of UICC stages I and II (T_1 T_2, N_0 N_1, M_0) were admitted to the trial. They were stratified according to the clinical stage of the tumour, the palpability of nodes, and menstrual status. Random allocation for conservative or radical treatment was within these stratified groups (4).

In the *conservative* (simple mastectomy) group, patients with *involved* pectoral nodes received immediate postoperative radiotherapy, only to the axilla. This consisted of 4,000 rads delivered from a cobalt source in 10 fractions over three weeks. If there was no evidence of spread to the axillary nodes, no further treatment was given, the patient thus treated by simple mastectomy alone. In the *radical* group, the surgeon performed a radical mastectomy by the technique of his choice provided full clearance of axillary nodes was included. In the event, most patients had a modified operation with preservation of pectoral muscles. If the axillary nodes were histologically involved, this was followed by radical postoperative radiotherapy consisting of 4,000 rads to the chest wall, 3,500 rads to the supraclavicular and internal mammary region, and 4,000 rads to the axilla given in 10 fractions over four weeks. If the axillary nodes were free of tumour no radiotherapy was given. Therefore in both the conservative and radical treatment groups there were two subgroups depending on node histology treated by (i) simple mastectomy and (ii) simple mastectomy plus axillary radiotherapy in the conservative group; (i) radical mastectomy and (ii) radical mastectomy plus radiotherapy in the radical group.

From October 1967 to June 1973 200 patients were admitted to the trial. Their allocation to treatment groups is shown in Table 1.

Patients have been regularly followed-up, and in April 1978 all trial records and individual case notes were reviewed. At that time one of us (H. J. Stewart) acted as an external reviewer.

2. Edinburgh Trial

The Edinburgh trials were initiated in 1974, at which time the general policy of treatment for all cases of primary cancer was simple mastectomy and radical postoperative radiotherapy (5). They were designed to answer two questions. The first trial was complementary to the Cardiff Trial and was designed to determine whether, when histological examination of those nodes sampled at simple mastectomy showed no evidence of invasion of tumour, immediate radical radiotherapy conveyed any advantage over a watching policy. The second was designed to determine whether, in patients in whom examination of the pectoral nodes indicated metastatic disease, adjuvant chemotherapy improved the survival rates achieved by conventional local treatment alone. Notes on the protocols of these trials have been reported (6).

Only the first is relevant to this report. It included patients of UICC stages I and II cancer in whom histological examination of a pectoral node or nodes taken at the time of simple mastectomy showed no evidence of metastases; or in whom no node was identified by surgeon or pathologist. Patients were stratified according to the size of tumour, its site and menstrual status and after operation were randomly

Table 1. Cardiff trial: allocation of patients to treatment groups. These allow comparisons between simple and radical mastectomy in 130 node negative patients and between simple mastectomy with axillary radiotherapy and radical mastectomy with radical radiotherapy in 70 patients with proven node involvement.

	Node status	Treatment	Number of patients
Conservative policy			103
	pectoral node negative	simple mastectomy alone	64
	pectoral node positive	simple mastectomy + radical radiotherapy	39
Radical policy			97
	axillary nodes negative	radical mastectomy alone	66
	axillary nodes positive	radical mastectomy + radical radiotherapy	31

allocated within groups for (i) radical
radiotherapy (4,250-4,500 rads to max to
chest wall and node areas) given in 10
fractions over 4 weeks, or (ii) for a watching policy. In patients included in the
watched group, the enlargement of previous
palpable nodes or the appearance of new nodes
has not been regarded as a treatment failure.
Provided histological confirmation of metastatic disease was obtained, it indicated
the need for further treatment by radical
radiotherapy or radical radiotherapy and
chemotherapy.

1. Survival

The percentage of patients surviving each
year after treatment in the Cardiff Trial is
shown in Fig. 1.

Analysis by the log rank test (8) has confirmed that there are no significant differences between those treated by the conservative policy and those treated by the radical
policy; or between the patients included in
the two treatment subgroups (Fig. 2).

Thus patients with negative or non-identified pectoral lymph nodes treated by simple

Table 2. Edinburgh trials: allocation of patients to 31st March
1979.

	Number of patients
Node 'negative' patients	313
simple mastectomy alone	155
simple mastectomy plus radical postoperative radiotherapy	158
Node positive and operable stage III patients	334
simple mastectomy plus radical postoperative radiotherapy	166
simple mastectomy plus radical postoperative radiotherapy plus systemic 5 Flouro-uracil for 12 months	168

Six hundred and forty-seven patients have
been admitted to the Edinburgh studies, of
whom 313 with negative or non-identified
nodes have been admitted to Trial 1 (Table
2). One hundred and fifty-eight of these
received radical postoperative radiotherapy;
155 were allocated to the watched group. In
each case a careful record has been kept of
the success of node identification.

These 647 patients admitted to these trials
have been regularly reviewed; no detailed
analysis of the results have yet been made.

RESULTS

In presenting the results of the Cardiff
trial we have adhered to the original allocated treatment groups irrespective of whether
the patient was correctly allocated, or had
received the treatment expected (Table 1).
On review it was evidence that two patients
who had negative nodes had been wrongly
allocated to the positive node group and
received radiotherapy to the axilla; and that
5 patients with positive nodes either were
allocated to the negative node group and did
not receive radiotherapy, or were correctly
allocated but failed to attend for it (7).
External review of the Edinburgh Trial has
not yet been carried out, but frequent cross-
checks have been made to ensure that correct
allocation and treatment policies have been
adhered to.

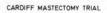
CARDIFF MASTECTOMY TRIAL

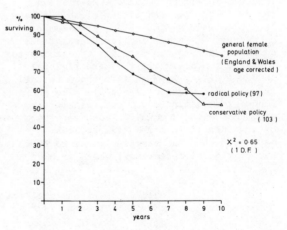

Fig. 1. Cumulative survival curves of
patients in Cardiff trial treated
by conservative (simple mastectomy
± axillary radiotherapy) and
radical policies (radical mastectomy ± radical radiotherapy).

mastectomy alone have fared as well as those
treated by radical mastectomy alone; patients
with positive nodes treated by simple mastectomy and axillary radiotherapy have fared as
well as those treated by radical mastectomy
and radical radiotherapy. Although there is
some divergence of the curves in Fig. 2 to

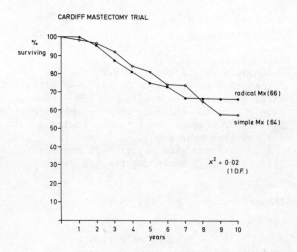

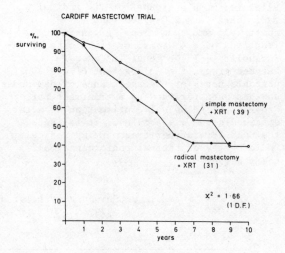

Fig. 2. Cumulative survival curves of: (a) patients with negative or non-
identified lymph nodes treated by simple or radical mastectomy; and
(b) patients with involved lymph nodes treated by simple mastectomy
and axillary radiotherapy or radical mastectomy and radical radiotherapy.

the advantage of those treated by simpler
surgery and not receiving radical radiotherapy, this is not statistically significant. At 10 years the survival rates are
identical.

2. Recurrent disease

Comparisons of the *total* recurrence rates,
i.e. the total incidence of progressive
residual systemic and loco-regional disease
have been made as follows: (a) Disseminated
Metastatic Disease. The incidence of disseminated disease in patients treated by the
conservative policy in the Cardiff Trial
does not differ from that in those in the
radical policy group (Table 3). The incidence of disseminated disease within the
subgroups also is equal. Those with negative
or non-identified nodes treated by simple
mastectomy had the same incidence to those
having radical mastectomy; those with

positive nodes treated by simple mastectomy
and axillary radiotherapy had the same
incidence as those treated by radical mastectomy and radical radiotherapy. Those results
agree with the survival statistics in Figs.
1 and 2.

(b) Loco regional Disease. Even with radical methods of treatment loco-regional
recurrence rates leave much to be desired.
In Table 4 we have listed reported rates of
loco-regional recurrence in controlled trials
of radical surgery and radiotherapy.

The incidence of loco-regional recurrence
in the Cardiff trial shown in Table 5 is
high, possibly because only 10% of all cases
admitted to it had tumours of less than 2 cms
in diameter. Noteworthy is the 19% incidence
of axillary recurrence in those patients
with negative or non-identified nodes treated
by simple mastectomy alone; and the 28%
incidence of scar recurrence in those patients
with positive axillary nodes who were treated
by simple mastectomy and axillary radiotherapy.

Table 3. Total incidence of disseminated disease observed to
1st April 1978 in the Cardiff trial.

	Number allocated to treatment group	Number (%) with dissemination
Nodes 'negative'		
simple mastectomy	64	21 (33%)
radical mastectomy	66	19 (29%)
Nodes positive		
simple mastectomy and radiotherapy	39	18 (46%)
radical mastectomy and radical radiotherapy	31	17 (55%)

Table 4. Reported 5 year rate of loco-regional recurrence following
radical treatment in Stage I and II cases in the Manchester
(9) and Guys (10) trials.

	loco-regional recurrence
Stage I	
Radical mastectomy alone	
+ 2700 rad postoperatively	15%
+ 4000 rad postoperatively	10%
Stage II	
Radical mastectomy alone	42%
+ 2700 rad postoperatively	35%
+ 4000 rad postoperatively	25%

Table 5. Total incidence of loco-regional recurrence observed
to 1st April 1978 in Cardiff trial.

		number (%) with loco-regional recurrence		
		scar	axilla	total
Nodes 'negative'				
simple mastectomy	64	9 (13%)	12 (19%)	18 (28%)
radical mastectomy	66	10 (15%)	1 (2%)	15 (23%)
Nodes positive				
simple mastectomy and axillary radiotherapy	39	11 (28%)	1 (3%)	13 (33%)
radical mastectomy and radical radiotherapy	31	1 (3%)	2 (6%)	4 (13%)

Unlike those in the radical mastectomy group
who had a scar recurrence rate of 3% these
patients did not receive radiotherapy to the
chest wall.

The axillary recurrence rate of 19% in
patients with negative or non-identified
nodes treated by simple mastectomy alone
reflects the accuracy of node sampling.
However, in 6 patients this was associated
with, or shortly preceded, the appearance
of disseminated disease; and in 1 patient
node histology had been positive but the
patient allocated wrongly to the watched
group; and only in 3 patients (5%) was the
axillary recurrence the sole manifestation
of recurrent disease. Following radiotherapy
all three patients are well 1-5 years after
initial treatment.

3. Node Identification

In setting up the trials in Edinburgh and
in Cardiff we did not know whether failure
by either the surgeon or pathologist to
identify a node or nodes was important;
patients with proven negative nodes have been
grouped with those with non-identified nodes
as a single 'negative' group.

Twenty-eight of 103 patients (27%) in the
Cardiff Trial and 119 of 313 (38%) patients
in the Edinburgh Trial who were regarded as
node 'negative' had not had nodes identified
for histological examination. This event
has proved to be more common in those operations carried out by trainee surgeons than
by consultants.

The relevance of non-identification of
nodes can be defined from the incidence of
loco-regional recurrence in those patients
treated by simple mastectomy alone. In the
Edinburgh Trial loco-regional recurrence rates
in those patients who have not had nodes
identified for histological examination have
proved to be higher than that in those with
proven negative nodes (Table 6).

DISCUSSION

These findings suggest that simple mastectomy and node biopsy, supported by additional
local postoperative radiotherapy if the pectoral lymph nodes prove to be involved, is a
safe method of treatment and that the survival
of patients treated by this policy of management is equal to that in those treated by
radical mastectomy. Our findings also suggest

Table 6. Observed loco-regional recurrence in patients treated
by simple mastectomy alone in the Cardiff and Edinburgh
trials according to whether nodes were identified for
histology or not. (One patient in the allocated
treatment group in the Cardiff trial had a positive
node). (χ^2 - Cardiff 0.330; Edinburgh 11.833).

		Number (%) with loco-regional recurrence
Cardiff		
Node identified and proven negative	37	9 (24%)
Node not identified	26	8 (31%)
Edinburgh		
Node identified and proven negative	95	10 (11%)
Node not identified by surgeon or pathologist	60	19 (32%)

that the state of the axillary nodes will
indicate the likelihood of local recurrence
and can be used to select the extent of local
treatment. However, the axilla should be
left untreated only if nodes have been identified for histological examination and if
this proves their non-involvement by tumour.
In most patients this can be ascertained from
axillary tail and pectoral node histology,
but this demands careful surgery and a meti-
culous examination of the resected specimen
(2,3). We now believe that the surgeon must
take responsibility for defining and submit-
ting nodes and if in doubt not hesitate to
perform a formal lower axillary dissection.

The demonstration of involvement of the
axillary nodes, even at a low level, is
associated with a high incidence of loco-
regional recurrence, particularly in the skin
of the chest wall. This can be largely prevented by postoperative radiotherapy, which
causes less morbidity when given in conjunction with a simple surgical approach.
Radical mastectomy followed by radical radiotherapy is morbid local treatment, particularly when the Halsted operation is used.

We suggest that the choice and extent of
local treatment as well as systemic treatment
for primary breast cancer, may be influenced
by the state of the lower axillary nodes; and
that irrespective of the type of definitive
local treatment, axillary node biopsy is a
rational development in the management of the
disease.

REFERENCES

1. A. P. M. Forrest, E. N. Gleave, M. M.
   Roberts, J. M. Henk and I. H. Gravelle,
   A controlled trial of conservative treatment for early breast cancer. *Proc. R.
   Soc. Med.*, 63, 107 (1970).
2. A. P. M. Forrest, M. M. Roberts, E. L.
   Cant and A. A. Shivas, Simple mastectomy
   and pectoral node biopsy. *Brit. J. Surg.*
   63, 569 (1976).
3. E. L. Cant, A. A. Shivas and A. P. M.
   Forrest, Lymph-node biopsy during simple
   mastectomy. *Lancet* 1, 995 (1975).
4. M. M. Roberts, A. P. M. Forrest, L. H.
   Blumgart et al, Simple versus radical
   mastectomy. Preliminary report of the
   Cardiff breast trial. *Lancet* 1, 1073
   (1973).
5. R. McWhirter, The value of simple mastectomy and radiotherapy in the treatment
   of cancer of the breast. *Brit. J.
   Radiol.*, 21, 599 (1948).
6. W. Duncan, A. P. M. Forrest, N. Gray,
   T. Hamilton, A. O. Langlands, R. J.
   Prescott, A. A. Shivas and H. J. Stewart,
   New Edinburgh primary breast cancer
   trials. *Brit. J. Cancer*, 32, 629 (1975).
7. M. M. Roberts, The Cardiff mastectomy
   trial. In *Proceedings of Symposium:
   Trials in Early Breast Cancer*. (Edited
   by H. Scheurlen and D. Leibrand, Heidelberg). In press (1979).
8. R. Peto and M. C. Pike, Conservatism of
   the approximation $\Sigma(O-E)^2/E$ in logrank
   test for survival data in tumour incidence data. *Biometrics*, 29, 579 (1973).
9. E. C. Easson, Postoperative radiotherapy
   in breast cancer. In *Prognostic factors
   in breast cancer* (Edited by A. P. M.
   Forrest, P. B. Kunkler), p. 118, Living-
   stone, London (1968).
10. J. L. Hayward, The Guy's trial of treat-
    ments of 'early' breast cancer. *World J.
    Surg.*, 1, 314 (1977).

A Reappraisal of Radiotherapy in the Treatment of Operable Breast Cancer. The New Light on the Internal Mammary Chain Role

M. Tubiana and D. Sarrazin

Institut Gustave-Roussy, 94800 Villejuif, France

Correspondence to M. Tubiana

Abstract—*Two criteria should be used for the evaluation of a cancer treatment: survival and quality of survival, the latter in the case of breast cancer means in particular cosmetic results.*

For small tumors (2 to 3 cm) tumorectomy + irradiation of the breast and the lymph nodes areas give good cosmetic results and a survival rate that is similar to that obtained with radical mastectomy.

For larger tumors, all data indicate that pre or post operative radiotherapy significantly reduce the incidence of local and regional recurrences. Furthermore the most recent studies (Norwegian Radium Hospital, Stockholm trial, M.D. Anderson-Houston and Gustave-Roussy-Villejuif) show a small increase in survival, statistically significant or at the borderline of significance, in particular for those patients with poor prognostic indicators and for tumors of the medial quadrants.

Moreover in non irradiated series a higher proportion of patients with coincident regional and distant metastases is observed. These data suggest that viable cancer cells in the regional lymphatics are a likely nidus for further dissemination in a small but not negligible proportion of patients. It is worthwhile to note that the data of the surgical trial which show for patients with tumor of the inner quadrants a small but significant increase in survival rate obtained after internal mammary dissection support this conclusion. If this is so, radiotherapy of regional lymphatics and in particular of the internal mammary chain is deserved as this procedure is less mutilating than supraradical surgery.

In 1979 two questions remain to be solved: 1) to what extent local radiotherapy interferes with adjuvant chemotherapy? 2) is it possible to reduce the side effects of radiotherapy without diminishing its effectiveness?

INTRODUCTION

For over 40 years it has been known through Baclesses's studies (1) that treatment of breast cancer by irradiation solely can achieve long term cures. However high doses are required and there is considerable incidence of side effects. The indications for this technique are therefore not frequent and radiotherapy is mostly used in combination with surgery.

During the past decade the usefulness of preoperative or postoperative radiotherapy has been much debated and Sijernswärd in 1974 (2) even claimed it could be detrimental.

A reappraisal of the role of radiotherapy in the treatment of breast cancer might therefore be useful in the light of the new data brought about by recent studies. Firstly we shall discuss the conservative treatment of small tumors by tumorectomy and irradiation and secondly the rationale of postoperative radiotherapy for larger, but still operable, tumors.

CONSERVATIVE TREATMENT OF SMALL TUMORS

The aim of research in cancer treatment is to increase long term survival rates but also to improve the quality of survival, the latter in the case of breast cancer means in particular cosmetic results.

Since 1954 a few authors have reported their experiences with conservative treatment (3-10) in patients with T_1, T_2, N_0-N_1 tumors. All claimed that radical mastectomy was not necessary to control the primary tumors and Vera Peters (5), comparing patients treated by lumpectomy plus irradiation to 3 separate series of control chosen by an individual matching process, found that the survivals were equivalent up to a follow-up of 30 years. However Atkins et al. (11) were the first to confirm this premice in a controlled clinical trial; no survival differences were found up to 10 years.

In another paper we report the results obtained at Villejuif with this technique (10). Tumorectomy was followed by irradiation of the breast at 4,500 rads and of the tumor bed at 6,000 rads. For T_1, T_2

($<$ 2,5 cm) - N_0, N_1 - M_0 tumors the 5 year-survival rate is 87%; the cosmetic results are either excellent or good in about 90% of the cases. The incidence of local recurrence is small.

For tumors larger than 3 cm the cosmetic results are less satisfactory due to the necessity of a larger excision; furthermore the incidence of local recurrence is higher. However most of these can be controlled either by mastectomy or in a small percentage of cases by a more limited resection. For example in Calle's series out of 13 recurrences, 12 were operated on and 8 are living without any evidence of disease after a 10 year follow-up; in 2 of these patients a limited resection was possible and sufficient (8).

Most authors consider that conservative treatment is indicated only for patients with no suspicious palpable axillary lymph node (N_0 or N_{1a}). Atkins et al. (11) reported a high incidence of axillary recurrence in patients with palpable lymph nodes (N_{1b}); however the doses delivered to the axilla were low, judged by present standards, only 2,500-2,700 rads in 3 weeks. It is now well known that much higher doses (6,000 to 7,000 rads) are required when the axillary nodes appear to be involved (N_{1b}) at palpation. However the cosmetic results would not be as good after such high doses and if the aim of conservative treatment is to keep the breast and thorax of nearly normal appearance this goal would not be fulfilled.

Furthermore many feel that it is important to know the number of axillary lymph nodes involved because this represents prognostic indicator of high significance, in particular in view of a possible adjuvant chemotherapy. This is why in many series an axillary dissection is carried out systematically when palpable nodes are present (N_{1b}). In other groups low axillary dissection is performed even in cases without palpable nodes (N_0 - N_{1a}). When the frozen section studies of the lymph nodes is positive, an axillary dissection is performed. If no involved lymph node is found, the irradiation of the axillary and other lymph node areas is deleted.

These conservative methods are now widely accepted and constitute one of the greatest advances in cancer treatment of these decades.

RATIONALE AND INDICATIONS OF POST OPERATIVE RADIOTHERAPY

Prior to any assessment of the results obtained by radiotherapy, it should be stressed that radiotherapy is a technical act and that its effectiveness depends upon the quality with which it is performed. In fact this quality has improved considerably during the past two decades.

In particular it is now known that an effective treatment of subclinical disease requires doses as high as 4,500 to 5,000 rads in 4 to 5 weeks (12). In the past the doses delivered have often been too low and such studies are difficult to evaluate.

Moreover the target volumes have to be properly delineated. Progress has also been accomplished in this respect. For example the internal mammary lymph nodes were more precisely located through the use of lympho-scintigraphy. It was then shown that although the average lateral displacement from the mid-sternal line is 2.5 cm, the actual distances range from 0 to 5.3 cm. Similarly the depth from the skin ranges from 0.7 to 5 cm. With many of the formerly standard techniques, such as the opposed tangential chest wall fields, a noticeable proportion of the patients had some of their internal mammary lymph nodes underdosed because they were located at the margin or out of the field (13).

Another advance is the use of computer dosimetry which enables the study of dose distribution not only in the plane located at the level of the center of the target volume but also in other parallel planes. It was then found that irradiation in some of these planes was inadequate. For example in some cases due to changes in the contours of the thorax the internal mammary nodes located a few centimeters above the mid-plane were grossly underdosed.

Taking into account these technical considerations we shall now briefly review some of the recent data. In all the trials which have compared surgery versus surgery plus irradiation, a marked reduction in the incidence of loco-regional recurrences was observed (10, 19-21).

The contribution of radiotherapy to local control of the disease is unquestioned and appears to be of some clinical benefit. Nevertheless in many of the controlled clinical trials there is no concomitant improvement in survival rate. This has often been explained in the following way: 1) the local recurrences are easy to control by secondary radiotherapy and 2) they do not metastasize.

By combining results from five different controlled trials, Stjernswärd (2) concluded that post-operative radiotherapy decreases survival and yet in none of these studies taken individually did radiotherapy change significantly the survival rates (Table 1). Stjernswärd's statistical methods and conclusions have been seriously criticized (12,14,15); furthermore in the Edinburgh trial quoted by Stjernswärd the 5-year survival rate differences of 76% versus 66% came from a preliminary analysis (16). This difference in a later paper was narrowed to 74% versus 72% (17). There was no difference in survival in the Copenhagen trial which was also quoted (18). Concerning the NSABP trial if one compares failure rate instead of survival rate, at 5 years 49.4% of patients receiving post-operative radiotherapy had recurrent disease versus 50.4% of the patients treated by surgery alone (21). Therefore of the five trials pooled by Stjernswärd, only the Manchester data remain (19) and in these rather old studies the crucial lymphatics of the internal mammary chain and the medial supraclavicular fossa have received an uncertain dosage (12,20). Moreover, Stjernswärd interpreted his

Table 1. Comparison of results in patients treated with surgery
alone or surgery and irradiation (Stjernswärd (2)).

Study	Years post-op.	Survival Rates		Increased mortality in irradiated groups (%)	Comments
		Survival rate (%)			
		Surgery + irradiation	Surgery only		
Manchester (19) "Quadrate" technique, radical mastectomy with or without post-operative irradiation	5	55.0	56.5	1.5	uncertain dosage to
	10	42.7	44.0	1.3	internal mammary and
"Peripheral" technique. Radical mastectomy with or without post-operative irradiation.	5	56.5	61.0	4.5	supraclavicular fossa
	10	44.2	47.5	3.3	
Copenhagen (18) Extended radical mastectomy versus simple mastectomy and irradiation.	5	66.0	67.0	1.0	
Edinburgh (16,17) Radical mastectomy versus simple mastectomy and irradiation	5	66.0 (72%)	76.0 (74%)	10.0 (16) (3%) (17)	difference not confirmed by more recent data
NSABP 1970 (21) Radical mastectomy with post-operative irradiation or placebo	5	56.0	62.0	6.0	(17)
Frequency of disease by 5 yeasrs		49.4	50.4		

alleged finding by the hypothesis that radiotherapy impairs the immune response against
cancer cells and thereby enhances the growth
of micrometastases (2,22). This hypothesis
has been questioned by many immunologists
(15,23) and is not supported by experimental
evidence.

However, Stjernswärd's challenge has not
been unuseful and has led radiotherapists
to critically evaluate their own methods.

In fact the main question is: does post-
operative radiotherapy help to cure some
patients? and if so which is or are the
subgroups of patients who benefit from it?
Obviously post-operative radiotherapy is not
equally effective for all patients. Pooling
all of them might interfere with the identification of the subgroup, or subgroups, in
which radiotherapy is worthwhile.

We shall now concentrate on four recent
sets of data which may provide answers to
these questions.

Høst and Brennhovd (24) reported in 1977
the results of a controlled randomized trial
which compared, with 1,090 patients, radical
mastectomy followed or not by radiotherapy.
During the first years of the trial the
patients were irradiated with 200 kV X-rays,
but, in the period 1968-1972, telecobal-
therapy was used. This allowed an increase
of the dosage and a more uniform dose distribution within the target volumes. No effect
of irradiation was demonstrated in stage I
patients, regarding survival, local recurrences or metastases. In stage II, 200 kV
irradiation reduced the incidence of local
recurrences and local metastases but did
not affect the survival; cobalt caused a
similar reduction in local and regional
relapses but in addition increased significantly the survival. This was due to a
significantly lower number of patients with
coincident regional and distant metastases
whereas the incidence of other types of

Table 2. Norwegian Radium Hospital trial (24).

	Local rec. (4 years)	Regional rec. (4 years)	Distant metast. (≤ 36 mo)	Both local or regional and distant	Survival rate (5 years)
200 kV	7%	4.6%	28.4%	10.1%	72%
Control	12%	16.3%	28.3%	28.2%	70%
Co-60	5%	4.2%	16.8%	7.3%	86%
Control	8.7%	13%	28.2%	19.6%	70%

metastases was the same in control and irradiated patients (Table 2).

Comparison of the 2 irradiation techniques helps to interpret this observation. Patients treated by kilovoltage X-rays had a sufficient dose to the chest wall, the supraclavicular area and the axilla whereas the dose to the internal mammary nodes was low. With telecobalt the dose to the internal mammary chain was higher. It seems to us that the possible role of irradiation of the parasternal lymph nodes is substantiated by the fact that survival was not increased for tumors of the outer quadrants whereas it was improved for medial tumors. Similarly survival was not influenced by radiotherapy for patients without axillary lymph node involvement, whereas it was influenced in patients with 4 or more lymph node metastases, that is in patients with a high probability of parasternal lymph node involvement.

Wallgren et al. in 1978 (25) reported the results of a randomized trial comparing, with 900 patients, radical mastectomy solely versus either pre-operative or post-operative adjuvant radiotherapy. Pre-operative radiotherapy reduced the incidence of local and regional recurrences and of distant metastases, and also the mortality as compared with the surgery-only group. Post-operative radiotherapy as given in the trial gave equal reduction of local and regional recurrences but did not diminish the incidence of distant metastases nor the mortality (Table 3).

more positive axillary lymph nodes (Table 4).

Despite the absence of randomization, this comparison is particularly instructive because the patients treated by surgery only were essentially patients with tumors of the outer quadrants whereas the patients treated by post-operative radiotherapy were essentially patients with tumors of the medial or inner quadrants whose prognosis is normally poorer (26), probably due to the frequent involvement of the internal mammary chain. In this study pre-operative irradiation does not appear to be more effective than post-operative and, if anything, is less effective.

The results of what we shall call now the Villejuif studies made these three sets of data easier to interpret. In 1963 an international group initiated a cooperative study with Villejuif acting as the coordinating center. The aim of this trial was to find out whether the theoretical advantages of internal mammary dissection were borne out by an increase in the survival rate. 1,580 cases of breast cancer were included and the five-year results have recently been published by J. Lacour et al. (26). Briefly it was shown that the extended mastectomy improved the results in only one subgroup: patients with T_1 or T_2 tumors of inner or medial quadrants with histologically positive axillary lymph nodes (Table 5).

In this subgroup 31% of the patients had their internal mammary nodes involved. This

Table 3. Stockholm breast cancer trial (25).

	No patients	Local + regional recurrences	Rec.	Metast.	All relapses	Deaths
Pre-op. irrad.	316	15		51	55	29
Post-op. irrad.	323	18		67	69	46
No irradiation	321	55		66	89	49

There are two possible explanations for this finding: either pre-operative irradiation reduces the shedding of viable cancer cells when the tumor is manipulated at operation, or it delivers more adequate irradiation to the crucial areas.

In fact Wallgren et al. (25) note that the post-operative technique may have resulted in less adequate irradiation of the internal mammary nodes whereas the dose to the other areas was satisfactory.

In a recent study Fletcher (20) compared the 10-year survival rates for patients treated with radical mastectomy alone, radical mastectomy followed by post-operative peripheral lymphatic irradiation or 4,000 rads of pre-operative irradiation followed by radical mastectomy. For those patients with histological positive axillary lymph nodes, the 5-year survival rate is significantly higher for patients having received post-operative irradiation. The improvement of survival is striking for patients with 4 or

incidence is much higher than in other $T_1 + T_2$ subgroups (Table 5). Incidentally it should be noticed that for cancer of the outer quadrants without axillary involvement the survival rate is significantly lower in the extended mastectomy series. This suggests that the removal of non-involved lymph nodes might be detrimental.

In this trial no patient had been irradiated but through the use of a matching process, a comparison was carried out between the Villejuif patients included in this trial with matched patients having received post-operative irradiation and treated during the same period at Villejuif. The results are summarized in Fig. 1 and shall be published in detail. Four groups of patients were compared, in all 431 patients with tumors T_1, T_2 or T_3 of a size less than 7 cm, and all with histologically positive axillary lymph nodes. Two groups were treated by surgery alone (radical mastectomy or radical mastectomy plus internal mammary dissection).

Table 4. 5- and 10-year survival rates[*] - M.D. Anderson Hospital - 1959-1972.

Treatment modality	Histologically negative axillary nodes			Histologically positive axillary nodes		
	Number of patients	Survival rates		Number of patients	Survival rates	
		5 yr.	10 yr.		5 yr.	10 yr.
Radical mastectomy alone (essentially outer quadrants)	265	76%	58%[+]	(Total 36) 48%[++] 1-3 N+ - 19 64% ≥ 4 N+ - 17 31%		33% 42% 0%
Radical mastectomy followed by peripheral lymphatic irradiation (essentially central or inner quadrants) (5000 rads in 4 weeks to the supraclavicular area and internal mammary chain through straight-on portals)	134	87%	76%[+]	(Total 234) 67%[++] 1-3 N+ - 140 77% ≥ 4 N+ - 94 52%		47% 54% 36%
Preoperative irradiation (4000 rads in 4 weeks to the supraclavicular area and axilla and 5000 rads in 5 weeks to the internal mammary chain; some of the patients had this chain partially irradiated with the tangential field)	312[†]	81%	68%	(Total 130)[††] 49% 1-3 N+ - 98 53% ≥ 4 N+ - 32 38%		31% 35% 20%

[*]Berkson-Gage, not age adjusted.
[+]p < 0.0005
[++]p < 0.05
[†]The patients who would have had histologically positive axillary nodes, had it not been for the preoperative irradiation, are in this group.
[††]These patients had a heavy tumor burden in the axillary nodes since the disease was not sterilized.

From Fletcher, *Textbook of Radiotherapy*, 3rd Ed., (20).

Table 5. Breast cancer - internal mammary dissection trial (26).

		No of patients	% int. mam. involv.	Survival RM	RM + IMD	
Axill. T$_1$ + T$_2$	N- Outer Quad.	239	4%	87%	78%	p = 0.05
	Inn. Quad.	214	11%	89	88	
Axill. T$_1$ + T$_2$	N+ Outer Quad.	297	17%	63	68	
	Inn. Quad.	192	32%	52	71	p = 0.01

RM = radical mastectomy
IMD = internal mammary dissection.

The two others had the same two types of surgery followed by post-operative radiotherapy which delivered 4,500 rads to the internal mammary chain, the supraclavicular fossa, the axillary and the chest wall.

In brief for patients who had internal mammary dissection, post-operative radiotherapy did not improve the relapse-free survival rate nor the survival rate (Fig. 2).

Conversely, these survival rates were significantly improved by post-operative radiotherapy for patients having had radical mastectomy. A more detailed analysis showed that this was especially true for patients with tumors of the inner or medial quadrants (Fig. 3), whereas for tumors of the outer quadrants there was no difference.

Nor is there a difference between patients treated either by radical mastectomy plus irradiation or extended radical mastectomy

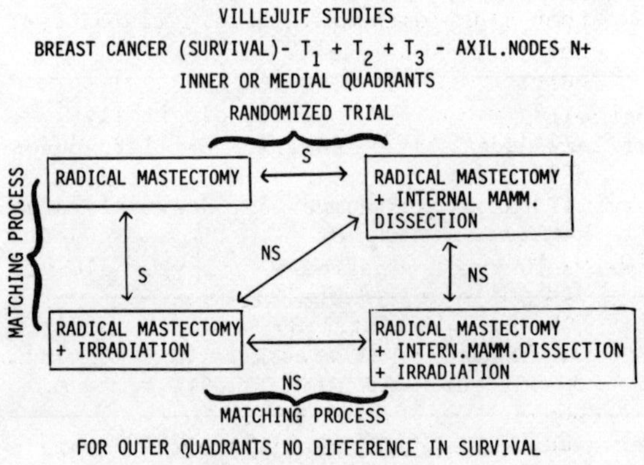

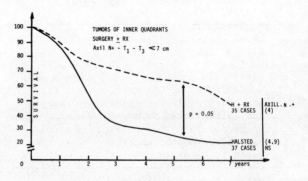

VILLEJUIF STUDIES
BREAST CANCER (SURVIVAL)- $T_1 + T_2 + T_3$ - AXIL.NODES N+
INNER OR MEDIAL QUADRANTS
RANDOMIZED TRIAL

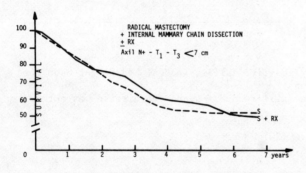

FOR OUTER QUADRANTS NO DIFFERENCE IN SURVIVAL

Fig. 1. Schematic representation of the
comparison carried out at Villejuif
between four groups of patients
treated by surgery alone or by
surgery followed by post-operative
radiotherapy (see text).
S means significant difference
in the 5-year survival rates.
NS means difference in 5-year
survival rates non significant.

Fig. 2. Comparison of the survival rates
in patients with histologically positive axillary nodes treated at
Villejuif by radical mastectomy
and internal mammary dissection
alone (S) or followed by post-
operative radiotherapy (S + RX).
The 2 survival curves are identical.

whether or not this procedure was followed
by radiotherapy (Fig. 1).

All these Villejuif data converge to
demonstrate that the internal mammary chain
is a crucial area for tumors of the inner
quadrants. Hence analysis of all the recent
studies strongly suggest that these lymph
nodes when involved are a likely nidus for
further dissemination either by local invasion
of the pleura and the lung or through the
blood and/or the lymphatic vessels. This
would be in accordance with the so-called
multistep dissemination process (27). In
this context it is worth mentioning that in
Hayward's randomized study (28) the incidence
of distant metastases was higher in patients
whose axillae were treated by a relatively
low dose irradiation which left some axillary
nodes uncontrolled, than in patients treated

Fig. 3. Comparison of the survival rates of
patients with tumors of the inner
quadrants and with histologically
positive axillary nodes treated at
Villejuif by radical mastectomy
without internal mammary dissection
(Halsted) with (H + RX) or without
(H) post operative radiotherapy.
The difference between the 2 curves
is statistically significant.

by surgery in whom no axillary recurrences
occured.

In conclusion post-operative irradiation
does not appear to improve the survival
rates for patients without axillary lymph
node involvement or for patients with tumors
of the outer quadrants; but in all the recent
studies an improvement of the survival rate
is observed for tumors of the inner or medial
quadrants when the internal mammary chain
receive 4,500 to 5,000 rads. This very important observation may have been, till now,
hidden by two facts: 1) in many studies the
internal mammary chain had not been adequately
irradiated, 2) often all patients were pooled
without considering the location of the tumor
or its size. Obviously when the tumors are
too small or too large, irradiation of the
regional lymphatics is of little use either
because they are not involved or because the
cancer is already disseminated. This irradiation is useful only for the small, but far
from being negligible, intermediary group.

REFERENCES

1. F. Baclesse, Five years results in 431
   breast cancer treated solely by Roentgen
   Rays. *Ann. Surg.* 161, 103 (1965).
2. J. Stjernswärd, Decreased survival
   related to irradiation postoperatively
   in early operable breast cancer. *Lancet*
   2, 1285 (1974).
3. S. Mustakallio, Treatment of breast
   cancer by tumour exstirpation and roentgen
   therapy instead of radical operation.
   J. Fac. Radiolog. 6, 23 (1954).
4. P. M. Rissanen, A comparison of conservative and radical surgery combined with
   radiotherapy in the treatment of Stage I
   carcinoma of the breast. *Br. J. Radiol.*
   42, 423 (1969).
5. V. Peters, Wedge resection with or without

radiation in early breast cancer. *Int. J. Radiat. Oncol. Biol. Phys.* 2, 1151 (1977).

6. L. Wise, A. Y. Mason, and L. V. Ackerman, Local excision and irradiation: an alternative method for the treatment of early mammary cancer. *Ann. Surg.* 174, 392 (1971).

7. R. Calle, F. H. Fletcher, and B. Pierquin, Les bases de la radiotherapie curative des epitheliomas mammaires. *J. Radiol. Electrol.* 54, 929 (1973).

8. R. Calle, P. Schlienger, J. R. Vilcoq, Place et limites des therapeutiques á visee conservatrice des epitheliomas mammaires. Resultat a lo ans. *Bull. Cancer* 64, 633 (1977).

9. B. Pierquin, F. Baillet, and J. F. Wilson, Radiation therapy in the management of primary breast cancer. *Amer. J. Roentgenol.* 127, 645 (1976).

10. D. Sarrazin, F. Fontaine, M. Le, and H. Mouriesse, Donnees actuelles sur la radiotherapie du cancer du sein. *Bull. Cancer* 62, 373 (1975).

11. H. Atkins, J. L. Hayward, D. J. Klugman, and A. B. Wayte, Treatment of early breast cancer: a report after 10 years of a clinical trial. *Br. Med. J.* 2, 423 (1972).

12. G. H. Fletcher, Reflections on breast cancer. *Int. J. Radiat. Oncol. Biol. Phys.* 1, 769 (1976).

13. C. M. Rose, W. D. Kaplan, and A. Marck, Lymphoscintigraphy of the internal mammary lymph nodes. *Int. J. Radiat. Oncol. Biol. Phys.* 2, 102 (1977).

14. S. H. Levitt, R. B. McHuch, and C. W. Song, Radiotherapy in the postoperative treatment of operable cancer of the breast. II - A re-examination of Stjernswärd's application of the Mantel-Haenszel statistical method. Evaluation of the effect of the radiation on the immune response and suggestions for post-operative radiotherapy. *Cancer* 39, 933 (1976).

15. P. Alexander, The bogey of the immunosuppressive adtion of local radiotherapy. *Int. J. Radiat. Oncol. Biol. Phys.* 1, 369 (1976).

16. J. Bruce, The enigma of breast cancer. *Cancer* 24, 1314 (1969).

17. T. Hamilton, A. O. Langlands, and R. J. Prescott, The treatment of operable cancer of the breast: a clinical trial in the South-East region of Scotland. *Brit. J. Surg.* 61, 758 (1974).

18. S. Kaae and H. Johansen, Simple mastectomy plus postoperative irradiation by the method of McWhirter for mammary carcinoma. *Ann. Surg.* 170, 895 (1969).

19. R. Paterson and M. H. Russel, Clinical trials in malignant disease. Part III - Breast cancer: evaluation of post-operative radiotherapy. *Clin. Radiol.* 10, 175 (1959).

20. G. H. Fletcher, *Textbook of radiotherapy.* 3rd edit. (to be published), Lea & Febiger (1980).

21. B. Fisher, N. H. Slack, P. J. Cavanaugh, B. Gardner, and R. G. Ravdin (and Cooperating Investigators), Postoperative radiotherapy in the treatment of breast cancer: results of the NSABP Clinical Trial. *Ann. Surg.* 172, 711 (1970).

22. J. Stjernswärd, F. Vanky, M. Jondal, H. Wigzell, and R. Sealy, Lymphopenia and change in distribution of human B and T lymphocytes in peripheral blood induced by irradiation for mammary carcinoma. *Lancet* 1, 1352 (1972).

23. H. Blomgren, Lymphopenia and breast metastasis. *Int. J. Radiat. Oncol. Biol. Phys.* 2, 1177 (1977).

24. H. Høst and I. O. Brennhovd, The effect of post-operative radiotherapy in breast cancer. *Int. J. Radiat. Oncol. Biol. Phys.* 2, 1061 (1977).

25. A. Wallgren, O. Arner, J. Bergström, B. Blomstedt, P. O. Granberg, L. Karnström, L. Räf, and C. Silfversvärd, Preoperative radiotherapy in operable breast cancer. Results in the Stockholm breast cancer trial. *Cancer* 42, 1120 (1978).

26. J. LaCour, P. Bucalossi, E. Caceres, G. Jacobelli, T. Koszarowski, M. Le, C. Rumeau-Rouquette, and U. Veronesi, Radical mastectomy versus radical mastectomy plus internal mammary dissection. Five-year results of an international cooperative study. *Cancer* 37, 206 (1976).

27. E. Viadana, I. D. Bross, and J. W. Pickren, Cascade spread of blood-borne metastases in solid and non solid cancers of humans. In *Pulmonary metastasis* (Edited by L. Weiss and H. A. Gilbert) G. K. Hall & Co., Boston (1978).

28. J. Hayward, The conservative treatment of early breast cancer. *Cancer (Philad.)* 33, 593 (1974).

Conservative Treatment of Minimal
Breast Cancer

D. Sarrazin*, M. Tubiana*, M. Le**, F. Fontaine* and
R. Arriagada*

*Radiation Department, Institut Gustave-Roussy, Villejuif, France
**Statistics Department, Institut Gustave-Roussy, Villejuif, France

Correspondence to Daniele Sarrazin, Radiation Department, Institut Gustave-Roussy,
94800 Villejuif, France

Abstract—Two hundred and twenty-eight cases of stage I breast cancer were
treated at the Institut Gustave-Roussy by a conservative treatment associating
a large tumor excision and external irradiation by Co 60.
The whole breast received 45 Gy and a boost of 15 Gy was given to the tumor
bed. The lymphatic draining areas were irradiated only when the low axillary
nodes were found to be involved. All patients (except 36) had a complete
axillary dissection when the extemporaneous section studies of the low
axillary nodes have been positive. Satisfactory cosmetic results have been
obtained in 92% of cases and the sequelae are minimal. The actuarial overall
survival and relapse-free survival rates, at 6 years, are respectively 86%
and 80%.
These results are confirmed by those of the W.H.O. therapeutic trial which
shows no difference, for N- or N+ cases, between the patients treated either
by mastectomy or by conservative therapy.

INTRODUCTION

The aim of research in cancer treatment is
not only to increase long term survival rates
but also to improve the quality of survival
which, in the case of breast cancer, particularly concerns cosmetic results.

Few authors, since 1954, have reported
their experience in conservative treatment
in patients with T_1, T_2, N_0, N_1 tumors:
Mustakallio (1), Baclesse (2), Atkins and
Hayward (3,4), Peters (5), Calle (6),
Pierquin (7), Sarrazin (8). All claimed that
a radical mastectomy was not necessary to
control the primary tumor. Vera Peters (5),
comparing patients treated by lumpectomy
plus irradiation to three separate series of
controls chosen by an individual matching
process, found that the survival was equivalent in the four groups with a follow-up of
30 years. However, Atkins et al. (3) were
the first to confirm this premice in a
controlled clinical trial. No difference in
survival has been found up to 10 years.

MATERIALS AND METHODS

Two hundred and twenty eight breast cancer
patients with T_1 tumor, as staged by mammography (i.e. clinical T_1 or small T_2), N_0/N_1,
M_0 were treated at the Institut Gustave-Roussy
from 1963 to 1978 using a conservative treatment which combined tumorectomy with a large
safety margin and external irradiation. An
axillary dissection was performed on some of
these patients. Since 1972 approximately 30
new cases a year were treated using this

protocol; whereas there had been only 10
patients treated in this manner before 1972.

The mean age of this population is 50.6
years. Two patients had bilateral breast
cancer and 13% of the patients had serious
intercurrent disease affecting their survival.

Pathological studies of mastectomies of
identical stages performed at our hospital
proved that intra-mammary dissemination is
found in 19% of breast cancer patients for
tumors of less than 1 centimeter and in 36%
for 2 centimeter tumors. In 38% of the cases
the axillary lymph nodes were found to be
involved.

The treatment protocol includes:

a) For the breast, tumor excision with a
wide margin for the new patients. For
patients who already had a lumpectomy before
coming to IGR and only when the tumor size
is ≤ 2 cm on the mammography and the pathological specimen, a second excision of the
tumor bed is carried out. When the tumor is
larger a mammectomy is performed.

b) A low axillary dissection is done for
an extemporaneous section examination. When
this is positive, the axillary dissection
is completed.

The irradiation is performed with Cobalt
and includes the breast and the chest wall
(45 Gy). The lymphatic draining areas
(axillary, supra clavicular and internal
mammary nodes) are included either when the
axillary nodes are N^+ or when the low axillary
dissection has been contraindicated. The
tumor bed receives a boost of 15 Gy.

101 low axillary dissections and 91 complete axillary dissections were performed.
Lymph node irradiation was carried out for

104 cases or 46%, out of them 36 were without histological information.

Low axillary dissection is the surgical act limited to the first lymphatic relays of the axilla and is correlated with the removal of about 8 nodes. Complete axillary dissection implies a surgical procedure extended to all the anatomic relays of the axilla and is correlated with the removal of 20 to 30 nodes.

RESULTS

One hundred and eight patients have had a 3 year follow-up and 43 a 5 year follow-up.

1. Functional Results

The conservative treatment of breast cancer would not be desirable unless satisfactory results were obtained from a cosmetic point of view with no serious sequelae.

The preliminary results are encouraging. The cosmetic results were excellent in 52% of cases and good in 40%, the breast being slightly elevated and a little smaller (Figs. 1, A and B). Only 8% of cases had poor cosmetic results, half of these resulted from a bulky surgery. The cosmetic results were comparatively estimated by both the patient and the physician.

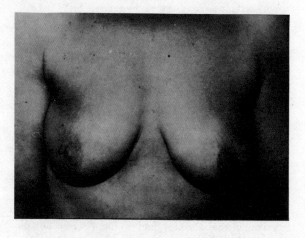

Fig. 1A. Patient, 65 years old, treated in 1973 for a right breast tumor (Tl No Mo). Perfect cosmetic result at 6 year follow-up.

We have observed a few sequelae. Only 3% of the cases had serious edema of the arm, 1 after axillary irradiation at 80 Gy, the others after a radio-surgical association.

A few other side effects were due to the irradiation: shoulder stiffness (6%) which is often temporary, temporary functional respiratory disturbance (2%) and one case of sensory-motor disturbance which disappeared after neurolysis of the brachial plexus.

2. Survival and Disease Free Survival Rates

The actuarial rates of the survival and of

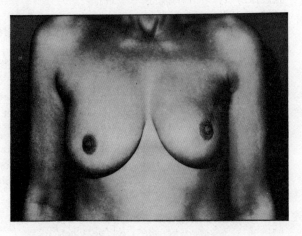

Fig. 1b. Female, 52 years old, treated in 1974 for a left breast cancer by wide excision and radiotherapy. Mean cosmetic result at 5 year follow-up

the disease-free survival at 6 years are respectively 86% and 80%, i.e. identical to those of radical mastectomy (9). It should be noticed that 15% of patients had from the onset a poor prognosis due to either a second cancer of a different site (thyroid, uterine cervix or corpus uteri) or of anther serious disease (hypertension, cardiac disease, diabetes) contraindicating anesthesia.

We have observed 6 local recurrences (i.e. 3%) all in the breast. We have not seen any lymphatic recurrence between the first and the fifth year. Metastases occurred in 17 patients (i.e. 7%).

Similar encouraging results were also observed in the randomized W.H.O. trial which started at Villejuif during 1972 and will be published soon. This on-going trial compares - for the treatment of the breast - mastectomy versus tumor excision and external irradiation (Fig. 2). An axillary dissection is always carried out. Thereafter, when

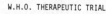

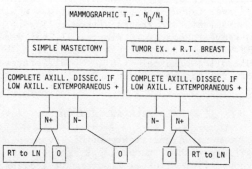

W.H.O. THERAPEUTIC TRIAL

MAMMOGRAPHIC $T_1 - N_0/N_1$

Tumor ex = tumor excision
R.T. breast = radiotherapy to the breast
R.T. to LN = radiotherapy to lymph nodes.

Fig. 2. The WHO therapeutic trial.

axillary lymph nodes are found to be involved half of the patients are allocated to lymph node irradiation by a second randomization.

The aim of this second part of the trial is to evaluate the role of post-operative irradiation.

180 patients have been included in the trial during the past seven years and no statistically significant difference has been observed both for overall survival and relapse free survival, neither among N- patients, nor between the two N+ groups. However in the group of patients treated by mastectomy, the recurrence rate is slightly higher though the difference is not significant.

A sufficient number of N- patients will be attained during 1979, representing 65% of the patients in the trial. Consequently, the results of this part of the trial will be published. The number of N+ patients required to evaluate the role of post-operative irradiation is too elevated and the trial will probably be stopped.

DISCUSSION

In breast cancer, as in cancer of other sites, the trend, for the past few years, has been to correlate the heaviness of treatment to the prognostic factors.

The conservative treatment of minimal breast cancer (T_1, small T_2, N_0/N_1, M_0) by tumor excision plus axillary dissection and external irradiation gives the same survival rates as by radical mastectomy (9). This has been demonstrated by Peters (5), most European authors (1,2,3,6,7) and by the preliminary results of two controlled trials: Milano (10) and the W.H.O.

The low axillary dissection is justified to reveal the pathological status of the nodes. Actually, the results of the randomized trial on the treatment of the internal mammary chain shows that surgery or radiotherapy to normal lymph nodes may render the prognosis poorer (9).

The rate of sequelae due to conservative treatment is low. Cosmetic results, in our series, are good or excellent in 90% of the cases; they are evaluated by both the patient and the physician.

Conservative treatment of these cases does not improve the prognosis but it certainly improves the quality of survival avoiding a mutilating treatment. Moreover, this local approach does not prevent the indication of general treatment such as systemic chemotherapy in patients presenting poor prognostic factors (N+ > 3 or Bloom grading III).

REFERENCES

1. S. Mustakallio, Conservative treatment of breast carcinoma. Review of 25 years follow-up. *Clin. Radiol.* 23, 110 (1972).
2. F. Baclesse, A. Ennuyer and J. Cheguillaume, Est-on autorisé à pratiquer une tumorectomie simple suivie de radiothérapie en cas de tumeurs mammaires ? *J. Radiol. Electrol. Med. Nucl.* 41, 137 (1960).
3. H. Atkins, J. L. Hayward, D. J. Klugman and A. B. Wayte, Treatment of early breast cancer: a report after ten years of a clinical trial. *Brit. Med. J.* 2, 423 (1972).
4. J. Hayward, The conservative treatment of early breast cancer. *Cancer (Philad.)* 83, 593 (1974).
5. M. V. Peters, *Cutting the "Gordian Knot" in early breast cancer*. Annals of the Royal College of Physicians and Surgeons of Canada, 186 (1975).
6. R. Calle, *The role of radiation therapy in the loco-regional treatment of breast cancer*. Recent Results in Cancer Research, 57, 164. Springer Verlag Ed. Berlin, Heidelberg (1976).
7. B. Pierquin, W. Mueller, F. Baillet, Maylinc, M. Raynal and Y. Otmezguine, Radical radiation therapy for cancer of the breast. The experience of Créteil. *Front. Radiat. Ther. Onc.* 12, 150. Karger, Basel (1978).
8. D. Sarrazin, F. Fontaine, P. Lasser and J. Rouesse, Le traitement conservateur du cancer du sein. *Rev. Prat. (Paris)* 28, 963 (1978).
9. J. Lacour, P. Bucalossi, E. Caceres, G. Jacobelli, T. Koszarowski, M. Le, C. Rumeau-Rouquette and U. Veronesi, Radical mastectomy versus radical mastectomy plus internal mammary dissection. *Cancer (Philad.)* 37, 206 (1976).
10. U. Veronesi, A. Banfi, R. Saccozi, B. Salvadori, M. Greco, A. Luini, G. Muscolino, F. Rilke, C. Clemente and L. Sultan, *Conservative treatment of breast cancer*. XII International Cancer Congress. Abstracts 3, 74. Buenos-Aires (1978).

Chemotherapy before Mastectomy may be a More Effective Therapeutic Sequence than Its Reverse in Primary Operable Breast Cancer

A. N. Papaioannou

Surgical Unit, Evangelismos Medical Center, Athens

Correspondence to A. N. Papaioannou, 24 Ravine St., Athens 140, Greece

Abstract—*Breast cancer (B.C.) appears to be a systemic disease in many instances at the time of diagnosis. It is suggested that in the traditional management of B.C., the primary tumor is resected, but various tumor-enhancing perioperative events may facilitate growth of micrometastases, reducing the chances for response to systemic treatment after operation. Chemotherapy before operation however, may prevent enhancement of the systemic component of B.C. perioperatively, by (a) avoiding treatment delay (b) suppressing or eliminating existing micrometastases, and (c) reducing growth potential of cells in the primary destined to form metastases. Preoperative chemotherapy may also be exploited as means of non-specific immunostimulation, if mastectomy is performed during the period of the rebound of immunity observed after the initial phase of immunosuppression associated with chemotherapy. Available experimental and clinical evidence in addition to the theoretical arguments introduced, suggest that this proposed reversal of the current policy is safe and promising and should be further explorated.*

INTRODUCTION

Although it has been repeatedly emphasized, it is not generally appreciated that if all breast cancer (B.C.) patients are followed to death, 88% will ultimately succumb to it regardless of the type of treatment (1). Nearly all these patients die of systemic metastases and the majority without local recurrence. Even in Stage III B.C., only one half of the patients who die will have persistent local disease (2). Despite this knowledge, we apparently fail to perceive the true magnitude and lethal potential of the systemic component of this disease.

Micrometastases may contain anything from one to 10^8 cells and their overall mass may be as great or in fact exceed that of the primary tumor itself (3). These microscopic foci may become so entrenched as a result of various tumor-enhancing factors present in the perioperative period, that the likelihood for response to any postoperative therapeutic modality might be reduced (4). These factors have been amply documented in many clinical and animal studies indicating that (a) substantial immunosuppression exists after operation as a result of trauma, anesthesia and the use of various drugs or blood transfusions (b) increased coagulability known to develop post-operatively added to the already existing hypercoagulability of the neoplastic state may enhance "takes" of the new micrometastases resulting from operative manipulations and (c) the preoperative anxiety and post-operative depression leads to a substantial degree of endogenous stress which may also promote tumor growth. The possibility for enhancement of micrometastases under these conditions is obvious.

THEORETICAL CONSIDERATIONS

1. The likelihood to eliminate the systemic component of the disease increases with length of time before onset of systemic treatment because microscopic foci presumably divide more actively and are here by more vulnerable to cell-cycle-specific drugs (5). It may also constitute a homogeneous cell-population, less likely to have reduced oxygen supply, and no accumulated metabolites capable of inhibiting the effects of chemotherapeutic agents (5).

2. With an average doubling time of B.C. at the time of diagnosis of about 90 days (6), the usual current delay of about one month until post-operative systemic treatment begins, may increase the tumor burden by about 30%. In view of the immunosuppressive effects of anesthesia (7), operation (8,9), and of radiotherapy (10) which may accelerate neoplastic growth and since micrometastases may in fact grow faster after removal of the primary (11,12), it is reasonable to estimate that by the end of the post-operative and radiotherapeutic periods, the micrometastatic burden could at least be doubled.

3. Early systemic therapy may suppress tumor-elaborated mechanisms which allow tumors to escape immune destruction by the shedding of antigenic determinants from the

tumor cell surface (13,14), tumor-promoting
properties such as the tumor angiogenesis
factor (15) or elaborate other substances
suppressing macrophage migration (16) and
function (17).

4. Cell-variants that are capable of forming metastases preexist in the primary (18).
If these cells are forced into the circulation at operation with intact potential, they
are likely to establish new micrometastases.
A 50% reduction in the size of the primary
tumor which we have consistently observed in
B.C. patients with one course of pre-operative polychemotherapy (Unpublished observations), will decrease clonogenic cells by
more than 99% (19). In theory, if chemotherapy is given before operation, surgery
is performed at the lowest point of clono-
genic-cell survival, and the tumor might be
"sterile" of cells with the potential to form
metastases. Invisible cells in the periphery
of the primary tumor may also be "sterilized"
with much greater ease by chemotherapy before
operation when their blood supply is intact
and adequate concentrations of cytotoxic
agents can be achieved.

5. The immunosuppressive effects of cytotoxic agents are not an obstacle for their
use before operation. After a short intensive course of chemotherapy, in vitro lymphocyte reactivity becomes depressed but if
treatment is discontinued, immunity gradually
recovers and ultimately "rebounds" to higher
than the pretreatment levels of function (20).
Peripheral T and B lymphocyte counts also
become depressed and later rebound in
parallel with their functional activity (21).
The speed of immunological recovery varies
with the type and intensity of the regimen
but might return to the prechemotherapy level
before the end of the second week and beyond
it for another week (21). If operation is
performed during this latter week, chemotherapy can be exploited as a non-specific
immunostimulant which may partly offset the
immunosuppressive effects of surgery.

EXPERIMENTAL DATA

The first experiment supporting the view
that systemic treatment may indeed be more
effective if begun before rather than after
operation or in the perioperative period, was
done by Brock in 1959 (22) in a 100% lethal
tumor system of the rat. In this model
surgery alone would cure 15% and cyclophosphamide alone 28% of the animals. Perioperative chemotherapy increased curability to 50%
whereas preoperative chemotherapy achieved
90% survival.

Subsequently experiments by Karrer et al.
(23) using the Lewis lung tumor showed a
linear dose response curve when chemotherapy
was initiated two days before amputation of
the tumor-bearing extremity and continued
every fifth day. Only 20% of the control
animals survived, treated with amputation on
the 12th postimplantation day without any
chemotherapy. If treated with adjuvant,
300 mg/kg of cyclophosphamide, 100% of the
animals survived; with 225 mg/kg, 78%; with

168 mg/kg, 56%; and with 122 mg/kg, 22% of
the animals survived. Chemotherapy alone
failed to increase the survival or the median
survival time. Conversely, post-operative
chemotherapy at day 4, 7 and 10 days after
amputation that was performed on the 12th
post inoculation day increased the average
survival time at each dose level but reduced
the number of surviving animals in all but
one group compared with animals subjected to
amputation alone.

More recently, Bogden et al. (24) using a
spontaneously metastasizing adenocarcinoma
in Fisher rats which is 100% lethal if
treated by surgery alone, showed that chemotherapy on the day of surgery or 10 days
before surgery cured 70-80% of the animals.
If immunotherapy was added postoperatively,
the cure rate increased up to 100%. The same
combination of a single course of chemotherapy preceding surgery and followed by
immunotherapy was also more successful than
any other regimens in the treatment of B16
melanoma in C57Bl mice (25). Likewise, in
a mouse model with simulated metastases,
there was an advantage to delaying the
removal of the primary tumor in order to
treat the "metastatic" disease first, by
various chemoimmunotherapy regimens (26).

Preoperative systemic chemotherapy was
also studied in a spontaneous mammary adenocarcinoma transplanted in C57Bl male mice
(27). Although this is a non-metastasizing
model and hence a less relevant one to the
human situation, the efficacy of preoperative
chemotherapy was again documented. Preoperative cyclophosphamide tested in two dose
levels (225 mg or 150 mg/kg) was given at
day 8 and 1 before surgical excision performed either on day 1, 4, 7, 10, 14, 18 or
22 after tumor implantation. Preoperative
chemotherapy when compared with surgery alone
or chemotherapy alone was effective particularly in the groups at highest risk. In
moribund animals 26 days after implantation
expected to have 100% surgical mortality,
preoperative chemotherapy markedly reduced
operative deaths and improved mean survival
time. In fact, among those animals escaping
mortality from surgery or chemotherapeutic
toxicity, 4 of 5 in the high dose and 5 of
5 animals in the moderate dose schedule were
cured.

CLINICAL DATA

Two clinical trials support the value of
perioperative systemic treatment in B.C.:
In an analysis of the first surgical adjuvant
study in the U.S., ten years after it was
begun, perioperative chemotherapy benefited
the sub-group with the worst prognosis (4 or
more positive lymph nodes) but this effect
was restricted to premenopausal patients
(28). Niseen-Meyer (29) on the other hand
showed in his Scandinavian trial, using
a 6-day course of cyclophosphamide intravenously beginning at day of mastectomy,
a statistically significant reduction of
recurrence rate and an equally significant
increase in survival of all patients on

chemotherapy. Only in one participating institution, a radiotherapy clinic, to which patients were referred after mastectomy for radiotherapy, chemotherapy was given 2-4 weeks after operation, and this treatment delay cancelled out completely the effect of chemotherapy. The failure of treatment in this latter group not only underscores the importance of chemotherapy administration in the perioperative period, but also strongly suggests that an effective agent is rendered impotent, if given nearly 2 or more weeks after operation. The differences in benefit were more pronounced in patients with more advanced disease and were sustained 12 years later (30).

Our prospectively randomized studies testing the principle of preoperative systemic therapy began in October, 1976. Shrinkage of the tumor was consistently observed often more than 50%, resulting in improved operability and decreased blood loss. Adverse postoperative sequellae from the chest wound were not observed. Systemic post-operative complications were unimpressive. Thus the feasibility and safety of preoperative chemotherapy is certain, but it is too early to assess efficacy in terms of survival. A cooperative trial testing this idea in Stage II breast cancer patients was begun by the Hellenic Breast Study Group under the auspieces of the Hellenic Society of Chemotherapy in the summer of 1978.

REFERENCES

1. C. B. Mueller, F. Ames and G. D. Anderson, Breast cancer in 3558 women: Age as a significant determinant in the rate of dying and causes of death. *Surgery* 83, 123 (1978).

2. S. V. Whitaker and C. Batterby, The dilemma of stage III breast cancer: A study of preoperative radiotherapy. *Austr. NZ J. Surg.* 47, 684 (1977).

3. F. M. Schabel Jr., Rationale for adjuvant chemotherapy. *Cancer* 39, 2875 (1977).

4. A. N. Papaioannou, Preoperative chemotherapy in the management of solid tumors. A proposal. Submitted for publication (1979).

5. E. Frei III, Rationale for combined therapy. *Cancer* 40, 569 (1977).

6. G. G. Steel, *Growth Kinetics of Tumors.* Clarendon Press, Oxford (1977).

7. J. Lundy, E. J. Lovett III, S. Hamilton and P. Conran, Halothane, surgery, immunosuppression and artificial pulmonary metastases. *Cancer* 41, 827 (1978).

8. T. G. Antikatzides and T. M. Saba, Decreased resistance to intravenous tumor cell challenge during periods of R.E. depression following surgery. *Brit. J. Cancer* 34, 381 (1976).

9. I. Han, Postoperative immunosuppression in patients with breast cancer. *Lancet* I, 742 (1972).

10. J. Stjernswärd, Decreased survival related to irradiation post-operatively in early operable breast cancer. *Lancet* II, 1285 (1974).

11. W. D. DeWys, Studies correlating the growth rate of a tumor and its metastases and providing evidence for tumor-related systemic growth-retarding factors. *Cancer Res.* 32, 374 (1972).

12. E. Gorelik, S. Segal and M. Feldman, Growth of a local tumor exerts a specific inhibitory effect on progression of lung metastases. *Int. J. Cancer* 21, 617 (1978).

13. G. A. Currie and P. Alexander, Spontaneous shedding of TSTA by viable sarcoma cells: Its possible role in facilitating metastatic spread. *Brit. J. Cancer* 29, 72 (1974).

14. D. M. P. Thomson, S. Eccles and P. Alexander, Antibodies and soluble tumor-specific antigens in blood and lymph of rats with chemorally induced sarcomata. *Brit. J. Cancer* 28, 6 (1973).

15. J. Folkman and R. Cotran, Relation of vascular proliferation to tumor growth. *Int. Rev. Exp. Pathol.* 16, 207 (1976).

16. R. J. North, D. P. Kirstein and R. L. Tuttle, Subversion of host defense mechanisms by murine tumors. I. A circulating factor that suppresses macrophage-mediated resistence to infection. *J. Exp. Med.* 143, 559 (1976).

17. M. C. Pike and R. Snyderman, Depression of macrophage function by a factor produced by neoplasms: A mechanism for abrogation in immune surveillance. *J. Immunol.* 117, 1243 (1976).

18. I. J. Fidler and M. L. Kripke, Metastasis results from pre-existing variant cells within a malignant tumor. *Science* 197, 893 (1977).

19. B. Fisher, Biological and clinical considerations regarding the use of surgery and chemotherapy in the treatment of primary breast cancer. *Cancer* 40, 574 (1977).

20. J. B. Hersh, Jr. and J. J. Oppenheim, Inhibition of in vitro lymphocyte transformation during chemotherapy in man. *Cancer Res.* 27, 98 (1976).

21. J. Harris, D. Senger, T. Stewart and D. Hyslop, The effects of immunosuppressive chemotherapy on immune function in patients with malignant disease. *Cancer* 37, 1058 (1976).

22. N. Brock, Neue experimentelle ergebnisse mit N-lost-phosphamidestern. *Strahlentherapie* 41, 347 (1959).

23. K. Karrer, S. R. Humphreys and A. Goldin, An experimental model for studying factors which influence metastases of malignant tumors. *Int. J. Cancer* 2, 213 (1967).

24. A. E. Bogden, H. J. Esher, D. J. Taylor and J. H. Gray, Comparative study on the effects of surgery, chemotherapy and immunotherapy alone and in combination on metastases of the 13762 mammary adenocarcinoma. *Cancer Res.* 34, 1627 (1974).

25. W. J. Pendergrast, Jr., W. P. Drake and M. R. Mardiney, Jr., A proper sequence for the treatment of B16 melanoma: Chemotherapy, surgery and immunotherapy. *J. Nat. Cancer Inst.* 57, 539 (1976).

26. B. Fisher, M. Gebbardt and E. Saffer,
    Further observations on the inhibition
    of tumor growth by C. Parvum with cyclo-
    phosphamide: VII Effect of treatment
    prior to primary tumor removal on the
    growth of distant tumor. *Cancer* 43, 451
    (1979).

27. M. J. Straus, V. Sege and S. C. Choi,
    The effect of surgery and pretreatment
    or post-treatment adjuvant chemotherapy
    on primary tumor growth in an animal
    model. *J. Surg. Oncol.* 7, 487 (1975).

28. B. Fisher, R. G. Ravdin, R. K. Ausman,
    N. H. Slack, G. E. Moore and R. J. Noer
    (and cooperating investigators), Surgical
    adjuvant chemotherapy in cancer of the
    breast: Results of a decade of coopera-
    tive investigations. *Ann. Surg.* 168, 337
    (1968).

29. R. Nissen-Meyer, K. Kjellgren, K. Malmiok,
    B. Mansson and T. Norin, Surgical adju-
    vant chemotherapy. Results with one
    short course with cyclophosphamide after
    mastectomy for breast cancer. *Cancer* 41,
    2088 (1978).

30. R. Nissen-Meyer, K. Kjellgren, K. Malmiok,
    B. Mansson and T. Norin, Surgical adju-
    vant chemotherapy with one single six-day
    cyclophosphamide course: 12-year follow-up
    results. XII International Cancer
    Congress, Abstract W47, No. 8, Buenos
    Aires (1978).

Primary Breast Cancer Treatments:
A Locoregional Recurrence Review

W. H. Mattheiem and G. Andry

Department of Surgery, Institut Jules Bordet, Brussels University Tumor Center
Correspondence to W. H. Mattheiem, Institut Jules Bordet, 1, rue Héger-Bordet,
1000 Bruxelles, Belgium

Abstract—*Three treatment regimens for breast cancer applied in Institut Jules Bordet are reviewed as to their loco-regional recurrence rates.*
The regimen with the lesser loco-regional recurrence rate gives no better cure or survival results than less mutilating or agressive regimens.
Local recurrence in absence of generalised disease does not compromise ultimate cure.
Prevention of disseminated disease by systemic treatment is more important than prevention of loco-regional recurrence alone by agressive or mutilating loco-regional treatments.

INTRODUCTION

Surgery, radiotherapy or a combination of both are able to cure breast cancer patients according to the stage of the actual disease.

Prevention of development of disseminated metastasis is out of reach of a loco-regional therapeutic procedure and can only depend on systemic measures.

An optimal loco-regional therapy should combine the lesser possible functional and cosmetic disability and a good rate of definitive loco-regional cure.

These are the factors that we want to analyse in this brief presentation with a review of our experience at the Institut Jules Bordet, Brussels University Tumor Center.

MATERIAL AND METHODS

Three successive treatment regimens were analysed in our Institute from 1954 to 1976.

1. In 1971, Barkay (1) reported a comparison between two treatments then used in our Center from 1954 to 1969 in a non randomized distribution:
- radical mastectomy associated with tangential irradiation (3.500 rads) and
- simple mastectomy with McWhirter radiotherapy (4.500 rads).

2. In 1969, we abandoned both procedures and a modified radical mastectomy became our standard procedure, consisting in a total mastectomy including the pectoralis major fascia and a en-bloc total axillary dissection.

Node negative patients received no further treatment.

Node positive patients received postoperative radiation on the chest, axillary, supra-sternal and para-sternal areas.

Operable stage III cases only received preoperative radiotherapy. The results including 319 consecutive patients treated from 1969 till early 1976 were reported by Mendes da Costa in 1977 (2).

3. In 1973, we started to use chemotherapy as an adjuvant in primary breast cancer treatment, first on patients not refered for a specific form of therapy and later systematically to all patients eligible to current E.O.R.T.C. protocols.

The standard surgical procedure is still a modified radical mastectomy.

Node negative patients receive no further treatment.

Node positive patients receive radiation (4.500 rads) to the internal mammary chain only (homolateral) and systemic chemotherapy during one year.

Operable stage III patients receive preoperative radiation and chemotherapy at reduced dosage, and later full dosage chemotherapy after surgical recovery.

Andry (3) is currently reviewing that cohort of 390 patients treated from the end of 1973 till early 1977.

RESULTS

Table 1 shows the recurrence rates in our oldest series. With a median time of observation of more than 8 years it demonstrates a remarkably low rate of loco-regional recurrences when the loco-regional treatment is very aggressive, but no superiority was demonstrable for one of the regimens regarding cure or survival rate.

Table 2 shows the figures for the second therapeutic regimen. Here the median time of observation is much shorter, 4 years, but the given figures are highly indicative in our opinion because up to now, more than

W. H. Mattheiem and G. Andry

Table 1. Primary breast cancer treatments. Loco-regional
recurrences 1954–1969: 181 patients.

Radical mastectomy + radiation (conventional)	108 =	3%
Simple mastectomy + McWhirter radiation	73 =	23%

Table 2. Primary breast cancer treatments. Loco-regional
recurrences 1969–1976: 319 patients.

Loco-regional recurrences:

– Total	38	12%
– Local alone	8	3%
– Local + general	30	9%
– St. III	13	36% of the recurrent patients

Treatments:

Modified radical mastectomy + 0 : N–

Modified radical mastectomy + conventional radiation: N+
Preoperative radiation: operable st. III

Table 3. Primary breast cancer treatments. Loco-regional
recurrences 1973–1977: 390 patients.

Loco-regional recurrences:

– Total	44	11%
– Local alone	23	6%
– Local + general	21	5%
– St. III	10	23% of the recurrent patients

Treatments:

Modified radical mastectomy + 0 : N–

Modified radical mastectomy + parasternal radiation + chemotherapy: N+

Preoperative radiation and chemotherapy: st. III

Table 4. Primary breast cancer treatments. Loco-regional
recurrence rate: comparison of three treatment
regimens.

1. Radical mastectomy + radiotherapy:	3%
2. Modified radical mastectomy + radiation N+ only: ratio local/local + general I/3	12%
3. Modified radical mastectomy + chemotherapy N+ only: ratio local/local + general I/I	11%

85 p.c. of the local recurrences appeared in the first 18 post-operative months.

Table 3 shows the corresponding figures for the third regimen with a mean observation time of less than 3 years.

DISCUSSION

The time of observation of the two last regimens is too short to draw any conclusions regarding cure rate and survival.

As loco-regional recurrences are concerned, we observe that:

1. The lowest loco-regional recurrence rate is that of radical surgery associated with post-operative loco-regional radiation.
2. In both recent treatment regimens, modified radical mastectomy and elective loco-regional radiation or radiation to the parasternal area only resulted in an increased number of loco-regional recurrences.
3. Adjuvant systemic therapy-chemotherapy with or without hormonal manipulation and/or immunotherapy- decreases the number, or delays, generalised disease at the time of apparent loco-regional recurrence.
4. During the observation period apparent

isolated loco-regional recurrences appeared
to be amenable to good secondary cure by
excision and/or radiation.

5. Incidentally, we observed only one nodal
recurrence after modified radical mastectomy,
all others were scar or skin nodules

REFERENCES

1. M. Barkay, Le cancer du sein: mammectomie
simple suivie de radiothérapie selon
McWhirter et amputation du sein suivie de
radiothérapie tangentielle. Résultats et
évaluation. *Acta chir. belg*. 70, 681
(1971).

2. P. Mendes da Costa, W. Mattheiem and
G. Andry, Mastectomie radicale modifiée.
Acta chir. belg. 76, 423 (1977).

3. G. Andry, W. Mattheiem, J. C. Heuson and
G. Leclercq, Unpublished data.

New Drugs

New Cytotoxic Drugs for Breast Cancer and their Clinical Evaluation

S. K. Carter

Northern California Cancer Program, U.S.A.

Correspondence to S. K. Carter, Northern California Cancer Program,
P.O. Box 10144, Palo Alto, CA 94303, U.S.A.

Abstract—*The phase II testing of new drugs for breast cancer concerns itself with either analogues of existing known actives or new structures. The clinical strategy for analogues must differ in comparison with that for new structures. The analogue should be used in patients without prior exposure to the parent drug unless lack of cross resistance is being searched for. In a disease, such as breast cancer where combinations are so successful, this causes tactical problems. The response rate for an analogue must be evaluated against the background of what the parent structure can accomplish. Examples for anthracyclines, vince alkaloids and alkylating agents will be discussed. Among the new agents mentioned are neocarzinostatine, M-AMSA, Gallium NO_3 and Penta-methylemelamine.*

The success of combination chemotherapy has had an impact on drug development for breast cancer especially as related to the strategy for clinical evaluation. A new drug for breast cancer can no longer be evaluated in patients who have not been exposed to prior cytotoxic therapy. It is an established fact in cancer chemotherapy that patients who have failed on cytotoxic treatment will be less likely to respond to secondary drug treatment. This is due to aspects, such as a more extensive disease picture, with resultant poorer performance status along with compromise of bone marrow function. Therefore, a new drug in phase II evaluation will have to be more effective today than it would have had to be twenty years ago, in order to pass this critical hurdle.

The many active structures in breast cancer offer a great possibility for analogue development. The clinical evaluation of an analogue is different than that for a new structure (Table 1) (1).

Table 1. A new balance in breast cancer could improve the therapeutic index in the following way.

---

1) Increased efficacy

2) Diminished acute toxicity

3) Diminished chronic toxicity

For an analogue, activity per se is not the critical endpoint. The analogue must be shown to have a superior therapeutic index when compared to the parent structure. If the parent structure is part of a highly active combination then the testing of the analogue becomes complicated. It would be illogical to test the analogue after exposure to the parent structure in a combination unless a lack of cross resistance was being tested for. The substitution of the analogue for the parent structure into the combination causes several difficulties in interpretation. One major problem is that such a substitution requires a phase III study design to give a meaningful answer. In addition there is the concern about the pharmacologic interactions which could mask an effective single agent.

One of the most active areas for analogue development is with anthracyclines. Adriamycin is perhaps the most active single agent in breast cancer and is part of a wide range of combination studies (2). Since maintenance treatment with adriamycin is limited by the risk of cardiomyopathy many analogues are being tested in hopes that they will be less cardiotoxic. Before a new analogue can be evaluated for diminished cardiac damage in breast cancer, it must demonstrate efficacy at least comparable to that of adriamycin. In previously untreated patients adriamycin gives a response rate of about 40%. In previously treated patients this falls to about 25%. In the phase II evaluation of a new anthracycline, previously untreated patients can no longer ethically be utilized (Table 2).

An appropriate phase II population in breast cancer would be patients failing on a non-anthracycline containing combinations such as CMF, CMF + prednisone, or CMF + vincristine and prednisone. In this population a response rate of 25% would be required for further testing if lessened cardiomyopathy were the rationale for the study. If the rationale were increased efficacy, then a 40 to 50% response rate would be required unless

Table 2. Phase II strategy for adriamycin analogue in breast
cancer.

Prior therapy with

CMF
CMFP   Progressive
CMFVP   ─────────────────────────────────▶ Anthracycline
CFP   disease

Endpoint

Response rate

1) 20-30% if cardiac toxicity major thrust

2) 35-50% if efficacy major thrust

the new drug exhibited a more favorable acute toxicity pattern.

Among the analogues with the most clinical data available is rubidazone, a benzoylhydrazone derivation of daunorubicin. In experimental tumor systems rubidazone is more active than daunorubicin, but is not more effective than adriamycin. Rubidazone is less toxic than adriamycin and similar to daunorubicin in cardiac toxicity studies in the hamster. In other in vitro and in vivo animal tests, rubidazone is less toxic than either daunorubicin or adriamycin (3). Studies in the rabbit cardiac toxicity model (4) indicate that rubidazone does cause cardiac toxic effects, but at a higher total dose (mg/m^2) than adriamycin. This could be deceptive in predicting toxicity for man since much higher doses are used in a single course of rubidazone treatment when compared with adriamycin (5-7).

The first clinical studies with rubidazone were performed at the Hopital Saint-Louis in Paris. These studies were restricted to acute leukemia and reported results showed 11 of 24 patients with CR in ALL and 17 of 32 patients with CR in AML, including 12 responders among 18 patients without prior chemotherapy. The dose schedule had been 3.5 mg/kg (110-185 mg/m^2) daily for 4-7 days to obtain a total dose of 20-25 mg/kg (750 mg/m^2). As many as three doses of chemotherapy could be repeated at the point of bone marrow aplasia if blast cells persisted.

Rubidazone is clearly active in adults with acute leukemia. In a phase I and II trial at the M.D. Anderson Hospital 13 of 39 patients achieved complete remission with 11 occurring after only a single course. With the optimal dose of 450 mg/m^2 as a single one hour infusion repeated every 2 to 3 weeks complete remission was seen in 8/13 (62%) (8). The median time to CR was 29 days with a range of 19 to 69 days. Seven patients achieved CR in less than 30 days and 10 by day 36. The median duration of remission was 3 months with a range of 1 to 6 months. The median survival of complete responders was 8 months, from the onset of rubidazone therapy. These patients were heavily pretreated with a number of previous chemotherapeutic regimens ranging from 1 to 6 with a median of 2. In addition, 29 patients had received prior anthracycline chemotherapy

with adriamycin in doses ranging from 40 to 270 mg/m^2.

Cardiac toxicity was manifested by fatal congestive heart failure in 3 cases (8%). All had received prior adriamycin with the total dose range being 135 to 270 mg/m^2. The cumulative rubidazone doses in the 3 cases were 1,750 to 2,600 mg/m^2. An additional 4 patients had decrease in QRS voltage greater than 30% at cumulative rubidazone doses of 450 to 1,465 mg/m^2. All but 1 had received prior anthracycline.

In addition 12 patients (31%) developed an acute reaction consisting of fever and chills in 9, mild to generalized urticaria in 8, wheezing in 2, flushing in 2, and postural hypotension in 2. These symptoms occurred with the first dose of rubidazone even in patients who had not received prior adriamycin. Antihistamines were shown to ameliorate the reactions.

In solid tumors rubidazone must be given at a much lower dose than can be given to induce remissions in adult leukemia (9). At Wayne State (10), good risk patients received 150 mg/m^2 every 3 weeks and poor risk patients 120 mg/m^2. At these doses no responses were observed in 16 cases with squamous cell carcinoma of the lung. In 26 patients with colorectal cancer only one response was seen (4%) with a duration of 15 weeks. The major nonhematologic toxic effects consisted of anorexia (28%), nausea (40%), vomiting (17%), alopecia (15%), and fever and chills (5%). One possible cardiac toxicity was seen after 720 mg/m^2 total dose in a patient with previous radiation to the mediastinum and a history of arteriosclerotic heart disease. Myelosuppression was the dose limiting toxicity.

Two studies have evaluated rubidazone in breast cancer in the U.S. At M.D. Anderson (11) 14 patients were treated with 13 being evaluable but with no response being observed. At the Mayo Clinic (12) a randomized study was performed comparing rubidazone with adriamycin in 38 women with advanced disease who had failed prior chemotherapy. The rubidazone dose was 150 mg/m^2 Q 4 weeks compared to 60 mg/m^2 for adriamycin. No responses were observed with rubidazone, but 4 (21%) patients achieved a response with adriamycin.

Another area of current analogue study in breast cancer is the vinca alkaloids. Both

vincristine and vinblastine have response
rates of about 20% when used alone (2).
Vincristine is the vinca included in all
widely used combinations because of its lack
of marrow toxicity although its neurologic
side effects can be troubling. A new vinca
alkaloid chosen for diminished neurologic
toxicity should demonstrate at least a 20%
response rate in phase II study. It should
be remembered that vinblastine would meet
these qualifications, and is not cross-
resistant to vincristine. A vinca alkaloid
which is not limited by neurologic toxicity
would most likely be limited by marrow toxicity. Therefore, a new vinca alkaloid
analogue should be compared to both vincristine and vinblastine before widespread phase
III studies are undertaken.

Vindesine is desaceytyl vinblastine amide
sulfate. It is a chemically derived structural analogue of vinblastine sulfate. In
experimental tumors it has an activity spectrum similar to that of vincristine sulfate.
At the Memorial Sloan-Kettering Cancer Center
(13), a phase I trial was performed in 69
adult patients, using either a single dose
every 7-14 days, or daily injections × 5-10
days. The drug was shown to exhibit both
neurologic toxicity and myelosuppression.
The neurologic toxicity manifests itself as
paresthesias, asthenia, myalgia and hypore-
flexia. Despite the fact that it was a
phase I study, evidence of activity was
exhibited in leukemia, lymphoma and testicular neoplasms.

A phase II study in solid tumors has been
reported by Smith et al. (14) from the Royal
Marsden Hospital. Fifty patients were treated
including 23 with advanced breast cancer.
The dose schedule was 3 mg/m^2/wk by i.v.
bolus. In the 23 breast cases (of which 21

were evaluable) two achieved complete
response and four partial responses. Thus
the overall response rate was 29%. Five
other patients achieved a measurable response
so that in all 52% of evaluable patients
improved. Six of these 11 patients had
received no previous chemotherapy. Leukopenia (below 3000) was seen in nearly half
the patients with thrombocytopenia being
rare. Peripheral paresthesias were common
occurring in 19 patients (40%) and resembling
clinically the neurotoxicity associated with
vincristine. Nausea and vomiting was uncommon and transient. It appears that the
spectrum of toxicity lies between that of
vincristine and vinblastine and that the drug
has activity in breast cancer. Whether its
therapeutic index in combination will prove
superior to the earlier vincas remains to
be established.

An example of the complexity of the vinca
alkaloid analogue evaluation problem can be
illuminated by a recent report about 5-day
infusions of vinblastine in treatment of
refractory advanced breast cancer (15). This
study, by M. D. Anderson, was suggested by
the short plasma half life of the drug. When
vinblastine was given at a dose of 1.5-2
mg/m^2/day as a continuous 5-day intravenous
infusion to 25 patients, partial responses
were seen in 8 (42%), and stable disease 9
patients (47%). These patients were all
heavily pretreated. Four of 8 patients, who
had received prior conventional dose schedules of vinca alkaloids, responded including
two who had progressed on single intermittent
i.v. doses of vinblastine. Such data should
be kept in mind in attempting to determine
the ultimate clinical role for a drug such
as vindesine.

Similar strategies can be elucidated for

Table 3. Phase II strategy for a new alkylating agent in breast
cancer.

Prior therapy with

| AV or AF or AFM | Progressive disease → | New alkylating agent |

Endpoint

1) Response rate 20-30% if acute toxicity less

2) Response rate 30-50% if efficacy endpoint

Table 4. Phase II strategy for new fluorinated pyrimidine in
breast cancer.

Prior therapy with

| Adriamycin + cytoxan or adriamycin + vincristine | Progressive disease → | New fluorinated pyrimidine |

Endpoint Response rate

1) 20-30% if acute toxicity less

2) 30-50% if efficacy endpoint

analogues in the area of alkylating agents
(Table 3) and fluorinated pyrimidines
(Table 4).

One alkylating agent analogue being studied
in the U.S. is ifosfamide. Its chemical
structure differs from cyclophosphamide in
that the two functional chlorethyl groups are
not attached to the same nitrogen. In
experimental tumors it is more active than
cyclophosphamide (16). Early clinical trials
revealed that larger doses of ifosfamide
could be given and that the dose limiting
toxicity was hemorrhagic cystitis rather
than myelosuppression (17,18). At M. D.
Anderson (19) they took a phase II approach
of substituting ifosfamide for cyclophosphamide in their FAC regimen which included
5-fluorouracil and adriamycin. With the
ifosfamide combination (FAI) they observed
that 8 of 49 (16%) evaluable patients
achieved complete remission and 24 (50%)
achieved partial remission. With their
standard FAC regimen in 117 evaluable patients
the complete response rate was 16% and the
partial response rate 56%. Therefore, the
response rates were nearly identical as were
the duration of remission and overall survival. In the FAI group 25% of the patients
had hematuria, while none of the patients in
the FAC group had urinary complications.
Nausea and vomiting were more severe with
the ifosfamide combination. They concluded
that ifosfamide in combination with 5-FU and
adriamycin was more toxic than, and not
superior to, cyclophosphamide.

A variety of new structures are currently
under clinical evaluation in the United
States. Among these are neocarzinostatin,
M-AMSA, Gallium No$_3$, and pentamethylmelamine.

Neocarzinostatin (NCS) is a polypeptide
antibiotic isolated from the culture filtrate
broth of streptomices carzinostaticus. The
drug has had extensive clinical study in
Japan with indications of activity in acute
leukemia and gastrointestinal cancer, but
has just recently entered clinical evaluation
in the United States (20). The precise
mechanism of action has not been established
although its main locus of activity appeared
to be DNA, in which it causes both single
and double stranded breaks (21). At the
Sydney Farber Cancer Institute (22) a phase
I study was undertaken using an i.v. bolus
daily × 5 schedule. In this study 96
patients were treated at doses ranging from
500 to 2250 units/m^2/day repeated at four
week intervals. Myelosuppression, particularly thrombocytopenia, was clearly the
dose-limiting toxicity with the "MID" being
2250 units/m^2/d × 5. The thrombocytopenia
induced by NCS occurred in an erratic manner.
When it did occur it tended to be delayed,
sometimes protracted, and cumulative with
repeat doses. The occurrence of severe
protracted thrombocytopenia after NCS administration was seen in approximately 10% of
the patients treated.

NCS can cause an acute reaction manifested
by a severe rigor soon after drug administration which is anaphylactoid in nature.
Gastro-intestinal toxicity was mild. Antitumor activity was observed in hepatoma and

hematologic malignancies. On the other
hand, the activity in lung and colorectal
seemed limited.

M-AMSA is methanesulfon-m-anisidine,
4^1-(a-Acridinylamino)-. It was rationally
synthesized by Bruce Cain from New Zealand
during an investigation of the structure-
antitumor relationships of a series of bis-
quarternary salts and a series of 4^1-(9-
Acridimyl)-amino methanesulphonalides (23,26).
M-AMSA is active against a wide spectrum of
mouse tumors including L1210 leukemia (T/C
180-290%), P-388 leukemia (T/C 354-541%),
B-16 melanoma (T/C 217-243%) spontaneous
C3H mammary adenocarcinoma and CD8F$_1$ mammary
tumor. The drug binds to DNA through inter-
calating which may be its mechanism of
action. The drug has documented antiviral
activity and is also immunosuppressive in
mice.

In phase I study giving the drug as a
single dose every 28 days, the dose-limiting
toxicity was leukopenia (25). Thrombocytopenia was uncommon. Phelebitis was the major
nonmyelosuppressive toxic effect. This could
be circumvented by diluting the drug in 500
of 5% dextrose in water and infusing the
drug over one hour. The recommended dose
for phase II on this schedule was 120 mg/m^2.
Responses in this phase I study were seen in
patients with ovarian cancer and lymphoma.

At Mt. Sinai Hospital (26) in New York
City, M-AMSA was given at doses ranging
from 10 to 120 mg/m^2 every 3 weeks. Toxicity
was limited primarily to leukopenia with
relative platelet sporing. Myelosuppression
was not cumulative for up to 7 courses.
Responses were seen in Hodgkin's disease,
chronic lymphocytic leukemia, non-Hodgkin's
lymphoma and esophageal cancer even though
it was a phase I study. The recommended
dose for phase II is 120 mg/m^2 for good risk
patients dropping to 90 mg/m^2 for those with
prior drug exposure.

Gallium nitrate is an anhydrous salt
produced by the reaction of nitric acid and
gallium, a naturally occurring heavy metal.
It was chosen for clinical study based on
the activity in the Walker 256 carcinosarcoma.
In a phase I study at M.D. Anderson Hospital
(27) the drug was given on a daily × 3
schedule at doses ranging from 15 to 1350
mg/m^2. Forty of the patients were given 117
courses of drug. Renal toxicity was the most
frequent side effect and was dose-limiting.
Acute renal failure, as manifested by a
sudden development of anuria associated with
azotemia, hyperkalemia, vomiting, and change
in sensorium, occurred in ten patients during
11 of 38 courses given at doses ≥ 300 mg/m^2/
day. It was fatal in four cases. The
hematologic toxicity was mild and was manifested mainly by a hemoglobin drop. Gastro-
intestinal toxicity was mild and mainly
nausea and vomiting was manifested. The
antitumor activity in the phase I study was
minimal. While the renal toxicity appears
prohibitive, it needs to be remembered that
the same was true of cisplatinum diammine
dichloride in early studies.

Pentamethylmelamine (PXM) is a monodemethy-
lated derivative of hexamethylmelamine (HXM).

It has been developed for clinical trials because of its greater solubility and consequent suitability for parental administration. The experimental activity of pentamethylmelamine is similar to that seen with HXM. PXM has shown activity against the MX-1 breast xenograft which is one of the xenograft systems now utilized by the NCI. PXM is also active against $CD8F_1$ mammary tumors when tumor size on the final evaluation day was small, but not when large.

REFERENCES

1. S. K. Carter, The clinical evaluation of analogues I, The overall problem. *Cancer Chemotherapy and Pharmacology* 1, 69 (1978).

2. S. K. Carter, Integration of chemotherapy into combined modality treatment of solid tumors VII adenocarcinoma of the breast. *Cancer Treatment Reviews* 3, 141 (1970).

3. R. Maral, G. Posinet and G. Jolles, Etude de l'activite antitumorale experiementale d'un nouvel antibiotique semi-synthetique: la rubidazone (22050 R.P.). *CR Acad Sci (D)* 275, 301 (1972).

4. R. S. Jaenke, An anthracycline antibiotic-induced cardiomyopathy in rabbits. *Lab. Invest.* 30, 292 (1974).

5. J. Bernard, C. Jacquillat, M. Boiron, et al, Cinquante-sept observations de leucemies aigues. Essai de tratment par un derive semi-synthetique de la daunorubicine: le 22050 R.P. *Nouv Presse Med* 1, 2149 (1972).

6. C. Jacquillat, M. Weil, M. F. Gemon, et al, Treatment of acute myeloblastic leukemia with R.P. 22050. *B Med J* 4, 468 (1972).

7. C. Jacquillat, M. Weil, M. F. Gemon, et al, A new agent active in the treatment of acute myeloblastic leukemia: 22050 R.P. *Recent Results in Cancer Research* (Mathe, G. Pouillart, P., and Schwarzenberg, L. Eds). New York, Springer-Verlag, Vol. 43, p. 155 (1973).

8. R. S. Benjamin, M. J. Keating, K. B. McCredia, G. P. Bodey and E. J. Freireich, A phase I and II trial of rubidazone in patients with acute leukemia. *Cancer Research* 37, 4623 (1977).

9. R. J. Fraile, M. K. Samson, T. R. Buroker, A. O'Bryan, L. H. Baker and V. K. Vaitkevicius, Clinical trial of rubidazone in advanced squamous cell carcinoma of the lung and adenocarcinoma of the large intestine. *Cancer Treatment Reports* 62, 1599 (1978).

10. J. S. Kovach, M. M. Ames, M. L. Sternad and M. J. O'Connell, Phase I trial and assay of rubidazone (NSC 164011) in patients with advanced solid tumors. *Cancer Research* 39, 823 (1979).

11. S. S. Legha, R. S. Benjamin, A. V. Buzdar, G. N. Hortobagyl and G. R. Blumenschein, Rubidazone in metastatic breast cancer. *Cancer Treatment Reports* 63, 135 (1979).

12. J. N. Ingle, D. L. Ahmann, H. F. Bisel, J. Rubin and L. K. Kvols, Randomized phase II trial of rubidazone and adriamycin in women with advanced breast cancer. *PAACR-ASCO* 20, 427 (1979).

13. V. E. Currie, P. P. Wong, I. H. Krakoff and C. W. Young, Phase I trial of vindesine in patients with advanced cancer. *Cancer Treatment Reports* 62, 1333 (1978).

14. I. E. Smith, D. W. Hedley, T. J. Powles and T. J. McElwain, Vindesine: a phase II study in the treatment of breast carcinoma, malignant melanoma, and other tumors. *Cancer Treatment Reports* 62, 1427 (1978).

15. H. Y. Yap, G. R. Blumenschein, G. N. Hortobagyl, C. K. Tashima and T. L. Loo, Continuous 5-day infusion vinblastine in the treatment of refractory advanced breast cancer. *PAACR-ASCO* 20, 334 (1979).

16. N. Brock, Pharmacological studies with ifosfamide - a new $OXa2$ phosphorine compound. In *Proceedings of the 7th International Congress of Chemotherapy*, Prague, 1971 (Edited by M. Hajzlar, M. Semonsky and M. Meek), Munich, Urban and Schwarzenberg, pp. 748 (1972).

17. W. Scheef, Problems, experience and results of clinical investigators with ifosfamide. In *Proceedings of the 7th International Congress of Chemotherapy*. Prague, 1971 (Edited by M. Hejzlar, M. Semonsky and M. Meek), Munich, Urban and Schwarzenberg, pp. 797 (1972).

18. D. N. Bremner, J. St. C. McCormick and J. W. W. Thomson, Clinical trial of isophosphamide (NSC-109724) - results and side effects. *Cancer Chemotherapy Reports* 58, 889 (1974).

19. A. U. Buzdar, S. S. Legha, C. K. Tashima, H. Y. Yap, G. N. Hortobagyl, E. M. Hersh, G. P. Blumenschein and G. P. Bodey, Ifosfamide versus cyclophosphamide in combination drug therapy for metastatic breast cancer. *Cancer Treatment Reports* 63, 115 (1979).

20. S. S. Legha, D. D. VonHoff, M. Rozencweig et al, Neocarzinostatin, (NSC) 157365) a new carcinostatic compound. *Oncology* 33, 265 (1976).

21. T. A. Beerman, I. H. Goldberg, DNA Strand scission by the antitumor protein neocarzinostatin. *Biochem. Biophys. Res. Commun.* 59, 1254 (1974).

22. T. W. Griffin, R. L. Comis, J. L. Lokich, R. H. Blum and G. P. Canellos, Phase I and preliminary phase II study of neo-carzinostatin. *Cancer Treatment Reports* 62, 2019 (1978).

23. B. F. Cain, G. J. Atwell and R. N. Seelye, Potential antitumor agents 12. 9-anilo-acridines. *J. Med. Chem.* 15, 611 (1972).

24. B. F. Cain and G. J. Atwell, The experimental antitumor properties of three cogeners of the adridylemethanesulpharanilide cansal series. *Eur. J. Cancer* 10, 539 (1974).

25. D. D. VonHoff, D. Howser, P. Gormley et al, Phase I study of M-AMSA using a single-dose schedule. *Cancer Treatment Reports* 62, 1421 (1978).

26. M. A. Goldsmith, S. Bhardwad, T. Ohnuma,
    E. M. Greenspan and J. F. Holland, Phase
    I study of M-AMSA in patients with solid
    tumors and leukemias. *PAACR-ASCO* 20, 344
    (1979).

27. A. Y. Bedekian, M. Valdiviesco, G. P.
    Bodey, M. A. Burgess, R. S. Benjamin,
    S. Hall and E. J. Freireich, Phase I
    clinical study with gallium nitrate.
    Cancer Treatment Reports 62, 1449 (1978).

Vindesine as a Single Agent and in Combination with Adriamycin in the Treatment of Metastatic Breast Carcinoma

**I. E. Smith[1], R. C. Coombes[2], B. D. Evans[3], H. T. Ford[4],
J-C. Gazet[4], C. Gordon[5], J. A. McKinna[1] and T. J. Powles[4]**

[1]The Royal Marsden Hospital and Institute of Cancer Research, London and Surrey
[2]The Ludwig Cancer Research Institute, Sutton, Surrey
[3]The Royal Marsden Hospital, London
[4]The Royal Marsden Hospital, London and Surrey, The Combined Breast Clinic,
St. Georges' Hospital, London
[5]The Royal Marsden Hospital, Surrey

Correspondence to I. E. Smith, The Royal Marsden Hospital, London, U.K.

Abstract—*An overall response rate of 28.5% was achieved for vindesine in a
dose of 3 mg/m² i.v. weekly in the treatment of 21 patients with advanced
breast carcinoma. The major dose limiting toxicity was leukopenia, but this
was never severe. Neurotoxicity was also seen in 40% of patients but again
this was rarely severe. As a result of this study, a controlled randomised
combination chemotherapy trial was started in patients with advanced breast
cancer, comparing vindesine and adriamycin with vincristine and adriamycin.
Response rates are so far similar, but severe neurotoxicity has so far
been seen more commonly with the vincristine than with the vindesine combination. The trial is proceeding.*

INTRODUCTION

Vindesine, a semi-synthetic vinca alkyloid
derived from vinblastine, was introduced into
clinical practice on the basis of a wide
range of activity against experimental
animal tumours, and little neurotoxicity
(1). Twenty-one patients with advanced
breast cancer were therefore treated with
this drug as a single agent, as part of a
larger phase 2 study also involving other
tumours. The aim of this study was to
assess whether vindesine might be as active
as vincristine in the treatment of breast
cancer, with less neurotoxicity. Based on
the results of this study (described below)
a subsequent control randomised trial of
vindesine compared with vincristine in
combination with adriamycin in the management
of patients with advanced breast cancer has
recently been set up. The results of the
completed phase 2 study, and preliminary
results from the randomised trial are reported
below.

MATERIALS AND METHODS

Twenty-three patients with histologically
proven metastatic breast cancer were entered
into a phase 2 study between June 1977 and
February 1978. On the basis of phase 1 data
(1) vindesine was given at an initial weekly
dose of 3 mg/m² by i.v. bolus injection.
The dose was increased by 1 mg. weekly as
toxicity allowed.

Subsequently a control randomised clinical
trial of vindesine compared with vincristine
in combination with adriamycin in the treatment of advanced breast cancer was started
in October 1978 using the following dose
schedules: vindesine 5 mg. i.v. days 1 and
8 with adriamycin 40 mg/m² i.v. day 1 and
8; or vincristine 2 mg. i.v. days 1 and 8
with adriamycin 40 mg/m² days 1 and 8; each
regimen was repeated at 28 day intervals as
toxicity allowed.

In all patients objective response was
defined according to UICC criteria (2).

RESULTS

Of the 23 patients with advanced breast
cancer entered into the phase 2 study, 21
are assessable for response. Six achieved
an objective response (28.5%), including 2
complete responses (9.5%). Five other
patients achieved a measurable improvement
in tumour, but less than that required to
fulfil the criteria for partial response.
Five of the six patients achieving a response
had received no previous chemotherapy.
Response by site is shown in Table 1.

Details of toxicity from vindesine in all
47 patients entered into the full phase 2
study have already been reported (3). The
major dose limiting toxicity was leukopenia
but this was never severe. Peripheral paras-
thesiae were common, occurring in 19 patients
(40%) but symptoms were usually milder than
those associated with vincristine and only

I. E. Smith *et al.*

Table 1. Vindesine as a single agent in advanced breast cancer: response by site.

Site	Total	Responders
Soft tissue	14	5
Nodes	7	4
Lung	11	4
Bone	5	1
Marrow	3	0
Liver	2	0

Table 2. Comparative response rates of vindesine-adriamycin and vincristine-adriamycin in advanced breast cancer.

	Total	Responders
Vincristine/ADR	14	9
Vindesine/ADR	11	8

Table 3. Comparative neurotoxicity of vindesine-adriamycin and vincristine-adriamycin.

	Total	Neurotoxicity	
		Mild	Severe
Vincristine/ADR	14	2	4
Vindesine/ADR	11	0	2

slowly progressive in most patients. Neurotoxicity severe enough to stop treatment occurred in only 4 patients.

Twenty-five assessable patients have so far been entered into the control randomised combination chemotherapy trial. Fourteen have been randomised to receive vincristine and adriamycin, and of these 9 have achieved an objective response (64%). Eleven have been randomised to receive vindesine and adriamycin and of these 8 have achieved an objective response (73%) (Table 2).

Neurotoxicity associated with each of these regimens is shown in Table 3.

Six of the 14 patients receiving vincristine and adriamycin have reported neurotoxicity, including 4 severe enough to discontinue therapy. Two of the 11 patients receiving vindesine and adriamycin have reported neurotoxicity, both of these severe enough to require discontinuing treatment. These differences are not statistically significant. The trial is continuing.

DISCUSSION

The 29% response rate for vindesine as a single agent in the treatment of advanced breast cancer is slightly better than that previously described for vincristine or vinblastine (4), although the numbers were small and it is important to note that most of the responders had received no previous chemotherapy.

The second point to emerge from the study was that, although vindesine was an agent which caused neurotoxicity, it was our clinical impression that this was less severe and less rapidly progressive than one might have anticipated with vincristine also given in a weekly dosage. Furthermore, we hoped that a further reduction in vindesine-associated neurotoxicity might be seen if the drug were given less frequently than at weekly intervals.

For these reasons, a control randomised trial comparing the 2 vinca alkyloids given in combination with adriamycin in the treatment of advanced breast cancer seemed justified. Although this trial remains in its early stages, preliminary results are encouraging. The vindesine-adriamycin combination seems at least as effective as that of vincristine-adriamycin in the treatment of advanced breast cancer. Furthermore the lower incidence of neurotoxicity with vindesine, compared with vincristine so far noted is encouraging. We emphasise that these data are preliminary and no definite conclusions can be drawn at this stage; nevertheless we are encouraged and the trial is continuing.

ACKNOWLEDGEMENTS

We wish to thank the nursing staff of the Royal Marsden Hospital for their help and care in the management of the patients

described in this study. We also thank
Miss T. K. Berry for her skill and efficiency
in the preparation of the manuscript.

REFERENCES

1. R. W. Dyke, and R. L. Nelson, Phase I
   anti-cancer agents. Vindesine (desacetyl
   vinblastine amide sulfate). *Cancer Treatm.
   Rev.* 4, 135 (1977).
2. J. L. Hayward, and R. D. Rubens, Assessment of response to therapy in advanced
   breast cancer. *Br. J. Cancer* 35, 292
   (1977).
3. I. E. Smith, D. W. Hedley, T. J. Powles,
   and T. J. McElwain, Vindesine: A phase
   II study in the treatment of breast
   carcinoma, malignant melanoma and other
   tumours. *Cancer Treatm. Rep.* 62, 1427
   (1978).
4. S. K. Carter, Integration of chemotherapy
   into combined modality treatment of solid
   tumours. VII. Adenocarcinoma of the
   breast. *Cancer Treatm. Rev.* 3, 141 (1976).

A Phase II Study of Mitomycin C in Refractory Advanced Breast Cancer. A Multi-centre Pilot Study

A. T. van Oosterom*, T. J. Powles**, E. Hamersma***, I. E. Smith**** and E. Engelsman***

*Department of Radiotherapy and Medical Oncology, University Hospital, Leiden, The Netherlands
**Division of Medicine, Royal Marsden Hospital, Sutton, Surrey, U.K.
***Division of Medicine, Netherlands Cancer Institute, Amsterdam, The Netherlands
****Division of Medicine, Royal Marsden Hospital, Fulham Road, London, U.K.

Correspondence to A. T. van Oosterom, Department of Radiotherapy and Medical Oncology, University Hospital, Rijnsburgerweg 10, Leiden, The Netherlands

Abstract—*A phase II study of Mitomycin C was carried out in 40 patients from four centres in the Netherlands and the U.K. with histologically proven metastatic breast cancer, refractory to hormonal therapy and conventional chemotherapy.*

Treatment was given by intravenous bolus injection of 12 mg/m² of the drug and repeated every 21 days as toxicity allowed. The response rate in 32 evaluable patients was 28% (2 C.R. and 7 P.R.).

Thrombocytopenia occurred in 14 patients (43%), but leucopenia in only 1 patient. Nausea and vomiting were mild and occurred in only 38% and 31% of patients respectively, for only one day after injection. There was no other toxicity.

It is concluded that Mitomycin C is a clinically active cytotoxic agent for the treatment of metastatic breast cancer with low toxicity and may be useful for inclusion in combination chemotherapy schedules.

INTRODUCTION

The Mitomycin antibiotics derived from streptomyces caespitosus were discovered by Hata et al. in 1956 (1) and mitomycin C with antitumour properties was isolated by Wakaki in 1958 (2). The cytotoxic activity of this agent has been attributed, at least in part, to its ability to alkylate D.N.A. (3,4).

Since then, there have been several reports of responses of metastatic breast cancer to Mitomycin C with response rates ranging up to 40% (5,6). Although these response rates are encouraging the drug is not widely used in the treatment of breast cancer, perhaps because of reported high toxicity associated with daily injections of the drug (7).

We have therefore reexamined this drug, in a phase II study, give as a single injection every 3 weeks.

MATERIALS AND METHODS

Forty patients from four centres in the Netherlands and the U.K. with histologically proven metastatic breast cancer were included in this study. All patients had previous chemotherapy with cyclophosphamide (or chlorambucil), methotrexate and 5 fluorouracil; 26 of the patients had also had vincristine and adriamycin, 8 had been treated with vindesine, 6 with mithramycine.

None of the patients had had previous endocrine therapy in the two months prior to starting treatment with mitomycin C. The expected survival was at least 3 months.

Mitomycin C (Kyowa, Tokyo, Bristol Myers, Europe) was given intravenously 12 mg/m² as a bolus injection into a running infusion every three weeks as toxicity allowed.

Patients were considered evaluable for response if they had received at least two courses of treatment and were assessed at day 42. Evaluation was carried out according to the UICC criteria of response (8) and the records of all patients were subsequently reviewed by an extramural observer.

Thirty-two patients were evaluable for response, with a total of 55 different sites of disease.

RESULTS

Forty patients were entered into the study between February 1978 and March 1979. Eight were not assessable for response: 3 were excluded because of insufficient duration of treatment, 3 because of death not directly related to disease progression or drug toxicity, and 2 were lost to follow-up.

Two patients achieved a complete remission (C.R.), 7 a partial remission (P.R.), 7 showed no change in disease and 16 had progressive disease.

The response according to site of disease is shown in Table 1.

The median duration of response for patients with C.R. was greater than seven months (from

Table 1. Responses by anatomical site of involvement.

	CR.	PR.	NC.	PD.
Soft tissue	3	7	5	9
Visceral	-	4	5	6
Bone	-	2	9	5

5 months to 9+ months); and for patients with a P.R., greater than $4\frac{1}{2}$ months (> two-twelve months) and no change for > 13 weeks (2-5 months).

Eight of twelve patients with painful bone metastases reported a subjective decrease in their bone pain 2-3 days after the first injection, but recalcification of lytic lesions could be demonstrated in only two of these patients.

All patients tolerated the first two cycles at the full dosages. Nausea and vomiting were not major problems occurring in only 12 patients (38%) and 10 patients 31%) respectively. When these problems occurred they were transient and stopped within 24 hours after treatment.

The major toxicity observed was thrombocytopenia, which occurred in 14 patients (44%). This occurred after the second to the sixth course (median: fourth course) and necessitated postponing the treatment for one week. Treatment was then discontinued in six patients because of progression of the disease. Five of the remaining eight patients who four weeks later were given a further injection developed prolonged thrombocytopenia requiring at least a two week more delay before further treatment. Somewhat surprisingly, only one patient developed neutropenia requiring postponement of the scheduled dosage.

No renal, hepatic nor neurological toxicity attributable to mitomycin C occurred. In particular no evidence was seen for synergistic cardiotoxicity between mitomycin C and adriamycin in the 26 patients who had previously had up to over 600 mg/m^2 adriamycin, as described by Buzdar et al. (9).

DISCUSSION

The observed response rate of 28% for mitomycin C in metastatic breast cancer is slightly less than reported elsewhere in the literature. Most of the patients in this study, however, had far advanced disease and had already been previously treated with a variety of cytotoxic agents and were therefore often in a poor general state with diminished bone marrow reserve.

One of the striking features of mitomycin C was its low incidence of side effects, and most patients considered the drug to be considerably more tolerable than previous chemotherapeutic agents. The subjective bone pain relief experienced by several patients with advanced bony metastases was also gratifying.

The dose limiting feature with mitomycin C used in the schedule described here was

thrombocytopenia. This occurred in a significant number of patients, was cumulative and required increasing intervals of four later six weeks between courses after the first two to six courses.

It is our impression that the overall response rate and relative lack of general toxicity suggest that mitomycin C may be a useful agent in combination chemotherapy for breast carcinoma, however, in such combinations either a lower dosage or a more prolonged interval, perhaps six weeks, would seem appropriate.

REFERENCES

1. T. Hata, S. Nomura and I. Umezawa, Antitumor activity of antibiotic G 253. *Antimicr. Agents and Chemother*. 5, 542 (1956).
2. S. Wakaki, H. Marumo and K. Tomioka, Isolation of new fractions of antitumor mitomycins. *Antibiot. Chemother*. 8, 228 (1958).
3. V. N. Iyer and W. Szybalski, A molecular mechanism of Mitomycin C action: linking of complementary DNA strands. *Proc. Nat. Acad. Sci*. (Wash) 50, 355 (1963).
4. V. N. Iyer and W. Szybalski, Mitomycin C and Porfiromycin: Chemical mechanism of Activation and Cross-linking of DNA. *Science* 145, 55 (1964).
5. S. K. Carter, Mitomycin C. Clinical Brochure. *Cancer Chemother. Rep*. 1, 99 (1968).
6. S. K. Carter, Integration of Chemotherapy into combined modality treatment of solid tumors VII: Adenocarcinoma of the breast. *Cancer Treat. Rev*. 3, 141 (1976).
7. W. Frank and A. E. Osterberg, Mitomycin C an evaluation of the Japanese reports. *Cancer Chemother. Rep*. 9, 114 (1960).
8. J. L. Hayward, P. P. Carbone, J. C. Heuson, S. Kumaoka, A. Segaloff and R. D. Rubens, Assessment of response to therapy in advanced breast cancer. *Cancer Philad*. 39, 1289 (1977).
9. A. U. Buzdar, S. S. Legha, C. K. Tashima, G. N. Hortobagyi, H. Yong Yap, A. N. Krutchik, M. A. Luna and G. R. Blumenschein, Adriamycin and Mitomycin C. Possible synergistic cardiotoxicity. *Cancer Treatment Rep*. 62, 1005 (1978).

Hydroxy-9-Methyl-2-Ellipticinium (NSC 264-137) in 52 Cases of Osseous Metastases from Breast Cancer

P. Juret, Y. Le Talaer, J. E. Couette and T. Delozier

Centre Francois Baclesse, Cedex 14021, Caen, France

Correspondence to P. Juret

Abstract—An analysis of 52 patients with osseous metastases from breast cancer treated with Hydroxy-9-Methyl-2-Ellipticinium is reported. All patients had previously received endocrine therapy including castration followed by tamoxifen to premenopausal and tamoxifen alone to postmenopausal. 22 patients had also received cytotoxics prior to H9M2E treatment. In 6 patients radiological recalcification were obtained with a maximum duration of 18 months plus in one patient.

A main characteristic of this drug is the lack of haematogical toxicity a property which makes it useful in case of insufficient bone marrow function due to metastatic involvement or to therapeutic marrow suppression.

INTRODUCTION

Ellipticine is an alkaloid present in various plants growing in the islands of the Indian and Pacific oceans. Several derivatives of this compound were synthetized and some of them were found to be active against experimental tumors (1,2) and acute myeloblastic leukemia (3,4) but not against solid tumors.

As previous reported a new derivative, Hydroxy-9-Methyl-2-Ellipticinium (H9M2E thereafter) has proved to be effective against some solid tumors, mainly thyroid and breast cancer, and especially in bone metastases (5,6).

The principal advantage of this compound is the lack of hematological toxicity when the patients are given 80-100 mg/m^2 weekly. Patients with severe marrow aplasia might then be treated with this compound.

MATERIAL AND METHODS

52 patients included in this phase II trial had osteolytic metastases from breast cancer resistant to prior systemic treatment modalities. All patients had received endocrine therapy as first treatment of advanced disease including castration in premenopausal followed by tamoxifen and tamoxifen alone in post-menopausal patients. In 2 patients treatment was combined with hypophysectomy.

Twenty-two consecutive patients had previously received cytotoxic therapy including CMF and various alkylating or antimetabolic agents. These patients received H9M2E at time of relapse or progression or in case of discontinuation due to impairment of white cell or platelet counts.

The remaining 23 patients received H9M2E as first treatment after relapse to endocrine therapy.

The drug was administrated through slow intravenous perfusion diluted with isotonic glucose perfusion. The usual dose was 100 mg/m^2 in one weekly perfusion. Treatment was continued until progression.

RESULTS

It is known that in case of osseous metastases the assessment of an objective remission (as well as progression) is difficult. Recalcification of osteolytic lesions are generally not evaluable before 3 months after start of treatment. Other criteria of evaluation of the therapeutic effect consist of Tc^{99} phosphate uptake and biological markers (CEA, alkaline phosphatase calciuria).

In the present study radiological changes are the only criteria taken into account: an objective regression is hereby defined as a recalcification of osteolytic area during H9M2E therapy. The length of remission is calculated from the time of radiological recalcification without appearance of new metastatic lesions. Likewise the end of the remission is defined as the length of time from recalcification to decalcification or the appearence of new metastatic sites.

Defined under these conditions 6 objective regressions were observed in the 52 patients which respectively lasted 4, 6, 8, 12, 14+ and 18+ months. Two of these patients are presented in Figs. 1 and 2. In 2 of these 6 patients remissions were also observed in other organs (liver metastases and a tumor in the contralateral breast). In 3 of these

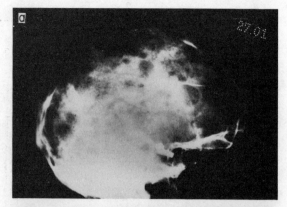

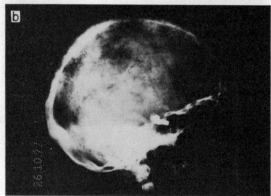

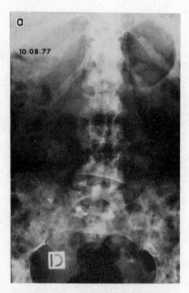

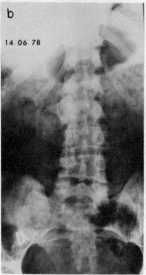

Fig. 1. (a) (January, 27, 1977), 48 years –
Previously treated with hormones and
chemotherapy – Hypophysectomy in
January 1976 – X-ray of the skull
prior to H9M2E.
(b) (October, 26, 1977) The same
patient after 9 months of treatment
with H9M2E.

patients H9M2E was given as first treatment
after endocrine therapy and in the last 3
patients after relapse on CMF treatment. In
all 6 patients relief of pain were reported.

Toxicity of H9M2E as reported (6) mainly
consist of minor gastrointestinal side
effects (nausea, vomiting), tongue myco-
sitis, dryness of mouth, cramps, phlebitis
at the side of injections and fatigue. In
3 of the 52 patients treatment had to be
discontinued due to side effects. One
patient who was still in remission after
12 months of therapy died from renal insuffi-
ciens. Autopsy could not be obtained. With
respect to its toxic characteristics the
lack of hematological toxicity of H9M2E must
be emphasized when given at a weekly dose of
80-100 mg/m^2.

DISCUSSION

In this phase II trial treatment with H9M2E
induced remission in 6 out of 52 patients
with osseous metastases from breast cancer.
Three of these patients were resistant to
both hormonal and cytotoxic therapy and the
other 3 patients were given H9M2E as first

Fig. 2. (a) (October, 8, 1977) 49 years –
Previously treated with hormones –
X-ray of the lumbar column.
column.
(b) (June, 14, 1978) The same
patient after 8 months of treatment
with H9M2E.

treatment after relapse or progression
on endocrine therapy. An important characteristic of this compound is the lack of
hematological toxicity when given as in this
trial at a weekly dose of 100 mg/m^2. It
therefore appears to be a useful therapeutic
alternative in case of bone metastases from
breast cancer resistant to cytotoxic or
endocrine therapy or in case of severe bone
marrow suppression.

REFERENCES

1. J. B. Le Pecq, C. Gosse, N. Dat-Xuong,
and C. Paoletti, Deux nouveaux dérivés
antitumoraux: 1'hydroxy-9-méthyl-2-ellip-

ticinium (acétate) et l'hydroxy-9-diméthyl-2, 6 ellipticinium (chlorure). Action sur la leucémie L 1210 de la souris. *C.R. Acad. Sc. Paris D.* 281, 1365 (1975).

2. J. B. Le Pecq, C. Gosse, N. Dat-Xuong, S. Cros, and C. Paoletti, Antitumor activity of 9-hydroxy-ellipticine (NSC 210 717) on L 1210 mouse leukemia and the effect of route of injection. *Cancer Res.* 36, 3067 (1976).

3. G. Mathé, M. Hayat, F. De Vassal, L. Schwarzenberg, M. Schneider, J. R. Shlumberger, C. Jasmin, and C. Rosenfeld, Methoxy-9-ellipticine lactate III. Clinical screening: its action in acute myeloblastic leukemia. *Rev. Eur. Et. Clin. Biol.* 15, 541 (1970).

4. B. M. Ansari, and E. N. Thompson. Methoxy-9-ellipticine lactate in refractory acute myeloide leukemia. *Post-grade Med. J.* 51, 103 (1975).

5. P. Juret, A. Tanguy, A. Girard, J. Y. Le Talaer, J. S. Abbatucci, N. Dat-Xuong, J. B. Le pecq, and C. Paoletti, Preliminary trial of 9-hydroxy-2-methyl ellipticinium (NSC 264-137) in advanced human cancers. *Eur. J. Cancer* 14, 205 (1978).

6. P. Juret, A. Tanguy, A. Girard, J. Y. Le Talaer, J. S. Abbatucci, N. Dat-Xuong, J. B. Le Pecq, and C. Paoletti, L'acétate d'hydroxy-9-méthyl-2-ellipticinium (NSC 264-137). Etude toxicologique et thérapeutique chez 100 cancéreux. *La Nouv. Presse Méd.* 8, 1495 (1979).

Trioxifene Mesylate (LY 133314) : A New Antiestrogen which Inhibits Growth Hormone Secretion in the Rat*

B. Arafah, A. Manni and O. H. Pearson

*Department of Medicine, Case Western Reserve University, School of Medicine,
Cleveland, Ohio*

Correspondence to O. H. Pearson

Abstract—*A new antiestrogen drug, Trioxifene mesylate (TM) (LY 133314), was
found to markedly suppress serum growth hormone (GH) levels in the rat.
Studies with this drug in 4 women with stage IV breast cancer have shown that
it suppresses arginine-stimulated GH secretion, but there was no significant
change in serum GH levels measured during the day and night. TM also blunted
the arginine-induced rise in serum glucagon levels. It had no effect on
serum prolactin and thyrotropin levels, but induced a moderate suppression
of serum gonadotropin levels. TM induced tumor regression and arrest of
disease in 2 previously untreated women with stage IV breast cancer, but
had no effect in 2 women whose disease was in relapse after tamoxifen-
induced remissions. This preliminary study suggests that Trioxifene has less
effect in suppressing GH secretion in women than in the rat.*

INTRODUCTION

The introduction of nonsteroidal antiestrogens has provided a major advance in
the treatment of hormone responsive breast
cancer. Up to 50% of postmenopausal patients
with stage IV breast cancer have been found
to respond to tamoxifen (1). Significant
palliation with tamoxifen could be obtained
in women who have previously undergone complete surgical hypophysectomy and in whom
serum prolactin (PRL) and growth hormone (GH)
were undetectable under provocative stimuli,
but with measurable estrogen levels (1).
These observations strongly suggest that
estrogens play a major role in the growth of
hormone responsive breast cancer in humans.
However, surgical hypophysectomy can induce
further remissions in two thirds of patients
who initially respond to tamoxifen then
relapsed and in one fourth of patients who
failed antiestrogen treatment (2). These
results suggest that pituitary hormones,
possibly the lactogenic hormones, PRL and
GH, may be implicated in stimulating tumor
growth in some patients with breast cancer.
It is possible that suppression of GH and
PRL secretion might provide a medical hypophysectomy when combined with an antiestrogen.
Effective suppression of PRL with ergot
drugs has yielded unsatisfactory results (3),
possibly because GH secretion was not
affected.

Trioxifene mesylate, the mesylate salt of
{3,4-dihydro-2-(4-methoxyphenyl)-1-naptha-
lenyl}-{4-(2-(1-pyrrolidinyl)ethoxy)-phenyl}
methanone has been found to possess potent
antiestrogenic activity in the rat.

In addition, it significantly reduces circulating GH levels in the unrestrained,
unanesthesized rat at a dose of 1-4 mg/kgm/
day (unpublished observations, Lilly Research
Laboratory). We were interested in testing
this drug in women with breast cancer, since
in addition to being a potent antiestrogen,
it has the potential of suppressing GH
secretion.

MATERIALS AND METHODS

Trioxifene mesylate (LY 133314), whose
structural formula is shown in Fig. 1, was
studied at the Lilly Research Laboratory and
found to possess potent antiestrogenic
activity. It caused a dose related inhibition of the estrone stimulated uterotropic
response of the immature mouse. It has a
high affinity for the estrogen receptor
approximately equal to that of estradiol. In
addition to being a potent antiestrogen,
Trioxifene mesylate was found to significantly
reduce circulating GH levels in the unrestrained, unanesthesized rats at doses of
1-4 mg/kgm/day (Fig. 2).

Five postmenopausal women (54 to 79 years
old) with metastatic breast cancer were
selected for a trial of Trioxifene mesylate
because they appeared to be suitable candidates for endocrine ablative treatment, but
whose disease did not seem so aggressive as
to jeopardize a possible response to standard
endocrine or chemotherapy if the experimental
drug failed. Informed consent was obtained
from all patients. Two patients who had

*Supported by grants from the U.S.P.H.S., RR-80 and CA-05197-19, and from the American Cancer
Society, Inc., PDT-48U.

TRIOXIFENE MESYLATE

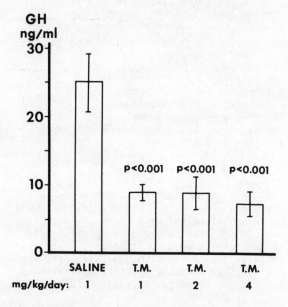

Fig. 1. The structural formula of Trioxi-
         fene mesylate.

Fig. 2. GH levels in the rat during treat-
         ment with Trioxifene mesylate (TM)
         at a dose of 1,2 and 4 mg/kgm/day
         for 14 days.

relapsed after a long remission with tamoxifen, were included in the study to determine
whether further benefit might be obtained.
One patient was previously treated with
estrogens with an unevaluable response while
2 patients had received no previous systemic
therapy. Trioxifene mesylate was given in
2 or 3 divided doses of 1 to 4 mg/kgm/day
and was continued for a minimum period of
2 months, except in one patient where it
was discontinued after 10 days because of
the development of hypercalcemia.

Before treatment was initiated and
repeatedly thereafter, all patients were
admitted to the Clinical Research Center and
had detailed physical, radiological and
laboratory evaluation including complete
blood and platelet counts, liver function
tests, blood chemistries as well as urinaly-
sis. In addition the following endocrine
studies were performed: serum thyroxin and
cortisol measured by standard radioimmunoassays and serum triiodothyronine resin
uptake was performed by standard technique.
Serum glucagon (4), PRL (5), GH (6),

gonadotropins, FSH (7) and LH (8) and
thyrotropin (TSH) (9) were measured by
specific radioimmunoassays. A standard
arginine stimulation test was performed
using 30 gms of arginine infused intravenously over 30 minutes. Insulin tolerance
test was done using 0.1 units/kgm intravenously.

Remission is defined as complete or
partial (> 50%) regression of dominant,
measurable lesions, or recalcification of
osteolytic lesions with no progression elsewhere and no new lesions appearing for at
least 3 months. No progression is defined
as < 50% reduction or < 25% progression of
measurable lesions with no new lesions
appearing for at least 3 months. Failure is
defined as > 25% progression of measurable
lesions or appearance of new lesions after
an adequate trial (at least 2 months).

RESULTS

Table 1 summarizes the clinical response
to Trioxifene mesylate in 4 patients. One
patient obtained complete regression of skin
and soft tissue metastatsis lasting 7+ months.
One patient has shown no progression of bone
metastasis after 6+ months of treatment.
Two patients in relapse after tamoxifen
therapy had progressive diseasse after 2
months of treatment with Trioxifene mesylate.
One patient with bone metastasis treated at
a dose of 2 mg/kgm/day developed symptomatic
hypercalcemia within 10 days of treatment.
Symptoms improved with return of serum
calcium to normal levels within 3 days following withdrawal of the drug and fluid therapy.
Subsequently, this patient was treated with
tamoxifen which she is tolerating well with
no significant side effects.

There was no significant effect of Trioxifene mesylate therapy on the basal or the
sleep related rise in serum GH levels in
all 4 patients when studied on 6 to 9 different occasions in each patient at a varying
dose of 1 to 4 mg/kgm/day (Table 2).

However, there was a moderate decrease in
the arginine-stimulated GH release in 3
patients that was noted first within one
week of treatment with a dose of 1.5 mg/kg/
day or more with no further appreciable
decrease when the studies were repeated on
6 to 9 occasions with different dosages up
to 4 mg/kg/day. Figure 3 shows a typical
response in one patient at two different
dosages, 1.5 and 4 mg/kg/day. The fourth
patient who had a minimal decrease in
arginine stimulated GH release did not have
any significant change in GH secretion following insulin induced hypoglycemia.

A moderate reduction in the arginine
stimulated glucagon release was also noted
in 3 patients. This was first detected one
week after initiation of treatment with a
dose of 1 mg/kgm/day. Minimal further reductions were noted when the dose was raised
up to 2 mg/kgm/day, but increasing the dose
thereafter did not alter the response.
Figure 4 shows such a response in one
patient when treated with Trioxifene mesylate

Table 1. Clinical results of trioxifene mesylate (TM) therapy.

Patient	Site of metastasis	Response to TM	Duration of treatment (months)	Estrogen receptor (fm/mg)
1.	Skin and soft tissue	Complete regression	7+	91.
2.	Bone	No progression	6+	ND
3.	Bone	Progression	2	ND
4.	Lymph node	Progression	.2	3.

ND = not done

Table 2. The effect of trioxifene on diurnal GH levels.

Patient no.	Rx mg/kgm/day	Duration on Rx (weeks)	18:00	20:00	22:00	Time 24:00	02:00	04:00	06:00
I	0	0	<1	<1	1.1	<1	3.4	<1	<1
	1.5	1	1.2	<1	1.4	1.9	<1	4.0	1.1
	2	2	<1	<1	4.7	8.4	<1	1.9	<1
	4	3	<1	1	1.1	<1	1.4	3.3	1.6
II	0	0	1.1	-	15	1.3	1.3	-	-
	1.5	1	9.5	1.1	10	1.8	2.0	3.4	20
	2.5	1	4.5	2.4	1.0	5.9	<1.	-	3.0
	3.5	2	6.2	3.0	2.4	<1	2.4	<1	18.7
III	0	0	1.9	2.3	2.3	1.9	1.5	-	-
	1	4	<1	1.7	1.1	2.3	3.4	3.5	1.0
	1.2	2	1.2	3.9	2.2	5.1	1.8	-	-
	1.5	2	1.0	6.7	6.2	<1	1.9	3.1	6.8
IV	0	0	1.4	2.5	3.3	2.0	6.1	5.0	1.4
	1	4	1.0	1.0	8.1	1.2	2.9	7.2	3.2
	2	4	1.3	1.1	5.6	1.4	4.3	3.9	3.9
	0	8	<1	1.3	7.2	<1	3.9	4.6	3.2

at a dose of 1 and 2 mg/kgm/day.

All 4 patients had a significant reduction in gonadotropin levels first noted after one week of treatment with a dose of 1 mg/kgm/day. Further reductions in gonadotropin levels were noted with time even when the dosage was reduced (Fig. 5).

Serial vaginal smears for cornification effect were performed on one patient showing atrophic inflammatory vaginal epithelium prior to Trioxifene mesylate therapy and subsequently showed moderately high cornification counts after 3 and 6 months of treatment (Karyopyknotic Index of 25 and 54).

In all 4 patients there was no significant effect on PRL or TSH measured through the night on 6 to 9 different occasions with variable dose of 1 to 4 mg/kgm/day. There was a tendency for a slight increase in serum thyroxin level associated with a decrease in serum T_3 resin sponge uptake and no significant change in the free thyroxin index.

Serum cortisol levels were not affected.

No significant effects were noted on liver function tests, blood chemistries, platelet or blood counts. Trioxifene mesylate was well tolerated by all 4 patients at all doses given (1–4 mg/kgm/day) with no undesirable side effects.

DISCUSSION

Trioxifene is a new, nonsteroidal anti-estrogen drug which was found to reduce serum GH levels in the unrestrained, unanesthesized rat. Preliminary studies of this drug in women with stage IV breast cancer have shown that, although it was able to blunt the arginine-induced rise in serum GH, it had no discernable effect on serum GH levels measured at various times of the day and night. The drug also partially suppressed the arginine-induced rise in serum glucagon

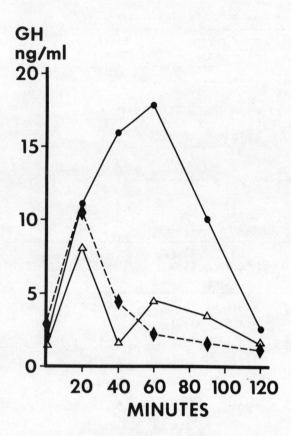

Fig. 3. Serum GH level during an arginine
         stimulation test in one patient
         before (o——o), and while on
         Trioxifene mesylate, 1.5 mg/kgm/day
         (△——△) and 4 mg/kgm/day (◊---◊).

levels. Trioxifene had no influence on prolactin and TSH levels measured during the day
and night. Thus, the striking suppression
of GH secretion induced by Trioxifene in the
rat was not obtained in women under the conditions tested.

Trioxifene induced objective tumor regression and arrest of disease in 2 previously
untreated women with stage IV breast cancer.
The drug induced no antitumor effects in
2 women who had relapsed after tamoxifen-
induced remissions. Further clinical trials
are needed to evaluate the effectiveness of
Trioxifene as an antitumor agent in women
with hormone-responsive breast cancer.

REFERENCES

1. A. Manni, J. E. Trujillo, J. S. Marshall,
   J. Brodkey and O. H. Pearson, Antihormone
   treatment of stage IV breast cancer.
   Cancer 43, 444 (1979).
2. A. Manni, O. H. Pearson, J. Brodkey and
   J. S. Marshall, Transsphenoidal hypophysectomy in breast cancer: evidence for an
   individual role of pituitary and gonadal
   hormones in supporting tumor growth.
   Cancer (1979) (in press).
3. O. H. Pearson and A. Manni, Hormonal control of breast cancer growth in women and

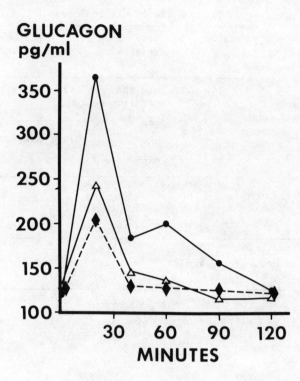

Fig. 4. Serum glucagon level during an
         arginine stimulation test in one
         patient before (o——o) and during
         Trioxifene mesylate therapy at
         1 mg/kgm/day (△——△) and 2 mg/kgm/
         day (◊---◊).

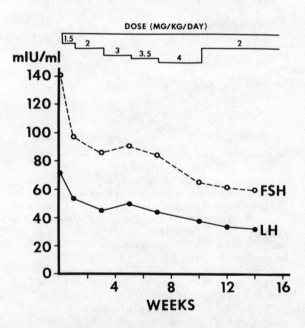

Fig. 5. Serum gonadotropin levels in one
         patient during treatment with
         Trioxifene mesylate at different
         doses from 1.5-4 mg/kgm/day. Each
         point represents the mean of 6-8
         determinations.

rats. In *Current Topics in Experimental Endocrinology* (Edited by L. Martini and V. H. T. James), Vol. III, p. 75. Academic Press, New York (1978).

4. G. R. Faloona and R. H. Unger, Glucagon. In *Methods of Hormone Radioimmunoassay.* (Edited by B. M. Jaffe and H. R. Behrman), p. 317. Academic Press, New York (1974).

5. Y. N. Sinha, F. W. Selby, U. J. Lewis, and W. P. VanderLaan, A homologous radio-immunoassay for human prolactin. *J. Clin. Endocrinol. Metab.* 36, 509 (1973).

6. D. W. Schalch and M. L. Parker, A sensitive double antibdy immunoassay for human growth hormone in plasma. *Nature (Lond.)* 203, 1141 (1964).

7. A. R. Midgley, Radioimmunoassay for human follicle stimulating hormone. *J. Clin. Endocrinol. Metab.* 27, 295 (1967).

8. S. Raiti and W. T. Davis, The principles and application of radioimmunoassay with special reference to the gonadotropins. *Obstet. Gynec. Survey* 24, 289 (1969).

9. A. E. Perkary, J. M. Hershman and A. F. Parlow, A sensitive and precise radio-immunoassay for human thyroid-stimulating hormone. *J. Clin. Endocrinol. Metab.* 41, 676 (1975).

ACKNOWLEDGEMENT

The authors wish to thank Dr. Richard W. Dyke of the Eli Lilly Company for supplying this new drug for our studies. We also wish to thank the Staff of the Clinical Research Center, Edward Burkett and Roberto Salazar for their technical help and the Administrative Coordinator, Mrs. Mary D. Wu.

Estrogen-linked Cytotoxic Agents of Potential Value for the Treatment of Breast Cancer

G. Leclercq, N. Devleeschouwer, N. Legros and J. C. Heuson

Clinique et Laboratoire de Cancérologie Mammaire, Service de Médecine,
Institut Jules Bordet, 1000 Brussels, Belgium

Correspondence to G. Leclercq

Abstract—*The potential therapeutic value of 13 estrogen-linked cytotoxic agents has been analysed in vitro (11 nitrogen mustard, 1 adriamycin and 1 aziridine derivatives). They may be subdivided into 3 classes according to the extent of substitution by cytotoxic groups of the two oxygen function of their estrogen moieties (E_2, DES, HEX or E_1) by the cytotoxic agent. In Class A both are substituted, in class B only one and in class C none (no. drugs per class: A = 5; B = 3; C = 5). The nitrogen mustard derivatives were represented in each class; the adriamycin and the aziridine ones were in class B and C respectively. Drugs of class A and B were devoid of significant affinity for cytoplasmic estrogen receptors (ER). In contrast, interaction with ER occurred with the drugs of class C. Assessment of the action of these compounds on the growth of two breast cancer cell lines MCF-7 (ER +) and Evsa-T (ER -) revealed a marked inhibitory effect on the former line. This observation suggests a participation of ER in the cytotoxic action of these drugs.*

INTRODUCTION

The interest of using estrogens linked with cytotoxic agents relies on the principle that such drugs might bind to estrogen receptors (ER) in target tissues including breast cancer and thereby concentrate in these tissues. This might improve the specification and reduce the systemic toxicity.

We have initiated a screening program for assessing the potential value of such drugs (1). Thirteen drugs have already been analysed. They may be subdivided into 3 classes according to the extent of substitution by the cytotoxic groups of the two oxygen functions of the estrogen moieties (hydroxyl functions for estradiol, hexestrol and diethylstilbestrol; hydroxyl and cetonic functions for estrone). In class A both are substituted, in class B only one and in class C none. Drugs with only one oxygen function substituted by a cytotoxic agent were also included in class A when the second function is substituted by another group. This classification relies upon the fact that these two oxygen functions are required in the free state for maximum binding to ER.

The present paper analyses the binding affinity of these drugs for the cytoplasmic ER. Potential antitumor efficacy of those having significant affinity are also investigated by testing their effect on the growth of human breast cancer cell lines either containing (MCF-7) or lacking (Evsa-T) the receptors (2).

MATERIALS AND METHOD

1. Chemicals

(2, 4, 6, 7) ^{3}H-estradiol-17β(^{3}H-E_2) $\sim$ 100 Ci/m M, was purchased from the Radiochemical Center Amersham, England; estradiol (E_2) and estrone (E_1) from Sigma chemical Co., St. Louis, Mo.; nafoxidine was supplied by Upjohn Co., Kalamazoo, Mich.; ORG 4333 by Organon, Oss, The Netherlands.

Cytotoxic linked estrogens were from the following origins: Ha compounds: Dr. H. Hamacher, B.G.A. Berlin, Germany; Leo compounds: Leo A.B. Helsinborg, Sweden; E_1-aziridine: Organon, Oss, The Netherlands; E_2-adriamycine: Farmitalia, Milan, Italy, E_2-mustard: U.S. National Cancer Institute; ICI 85, 966: Imperial Chemical Industries, Macclesfield, U.K.

2. Growth Medium

Earle's minimal essential medium, fetal calf serum and L-glutamine were purchased from Gibco, Glasgow, Scotland; penicillin and streptomycin from Difco, Detroit, Mich.; gentamicin from Schering Co., Kenilworth, N.J.

3. Cells

MCF-7 cells were supplied by Dr. M. Rich

(Michigan Cancer Foundation), Evsa-T cells
by Dr. M. E. Lippman (U.S. National Cancer
Institute). Cytoplasmic ER determinations
(3) confirmed the presence of receptors in
MCF-7 cells only; ER concentration estimated
in several experiments revealed values ranging from 110 to 200 fmoles/mg cytosol protein
which are close to those previously reported.
Growth of the MCF-7 cells was also confirmed
to be very sensitive to the inhibitory
effect of the antiestrogen nafoxidine (4).
This effect was shown to be reversed by 11-
Chloromethylestradiol (ORG 4333), estradiol
and estrone, the former estrogen being the
strongest antagonist of nafoxidine (5). In
contrast, Evsa-T cells appear insensitive
to nafoxidine and estrogens.

4. Apparent Binding Affinity of Cytotoxic-linked Estrogens to Cytoplasmic ER

The apparent binding affinity of cytotoxic-
linked estrogens was measured by evaluating
their ability to inhibit the binding of
^{3}H-E$_2$ to cytoplasmic ER from immature rat
uterus or DMBA-induced rat mammary tumors
(1,6,7). It was expressed by the relative
concentration of compound and unlabeled
estradiol or estrone (controls) required to
achieve 50% of the ^{3}H-E$_2$ binding.

5. Cell Culture

MCF-7 and Evsa-T cells were grown in
Falcon plastic flasks (75 sq cm) containing
Earle's minimal essential medium (MEM) supplemented with 0.6 mg L-glutamine/ml, 40 μg
gentamycin/ml, 100 U penicillin/ml, 100 μg
sireptomycin/ml and 10% fetal calf serum. At
confluency, cells were removed by trypsini-
sation (trypsin 0.05%, EDTA 0.025%) and
adjusted to 200,000/ml in the growth medium
supplemented with charcoal stripped fetal
calf serum (0.5% charcoal, 0.005% dextran in
1.5 ml medium/ml serum; overnight incubation
at 4°C). Cells were then plated in 35 mm
Petri dishes containing this medium and
cultured at 37°C in a humidified 95% air
5% CO$_2$ atmosphere. After 24 hours cytotoxic-
linked estrogens (solvent: ethanol at the
final concentration of 0.1%) were added to
the culture dishes. Forty-eight hours later
the medium was replaced by fresh medium
containing these drugs. The culture was
then pursued for an additional 72- hour
period before harvest. At this time, the
cells were washed twice with 2 ml of Earle's
base before being suspended in 1.5 ml
trypsin-EDTA. Total DNA of collected cells
was precipated in 0.5N perchloric acid and
evaluated by the diphenyl-amine method of
Burton (8).

RESULTS

1. Apparent Binding Affinity of Cytotoxic-linked Estrogens

Analysis of Tables 1 and 2 reveals that

cytotoxic-linked estrogens of class A and
B are either devoid of apparent binding
affinity for ER or characterized by an
affinity roughly 1,000 to 10,000 times lower
than E$_2$. In fact, whether or not these compounds really bind to the receptors is not
clear. In such competition assays as used
here, very small contaminations of the drugs
by free estrogens (less than 1%) might produce a reduction of ^{3}H-E$_2$ binding of the
same order as a very weak binder. Moreover,
in the case of 3 of the drugs (EM, Leo 299
and 275) additional studies revealed their
progressive degradation into high affinity
compounds including most probably free E$_2$
(6,7). Such a degration process may also be
responsible for the observed reduction of
^{3}H-E$_2$ binding.

Table 3 shows that the two bialkylating
compounds Ha IV and Ha V of class C also
display an apparent binding affinity for ER
about 10,000 times lower than E$_2$. Their
affinity although very low was shown to be
due to the compounds themselves and not to
contaminating parent estrogens. Thus, in
contrast to E$_2$, diethylstilbestrol and hexestrol, Ha IV and Ha V were found to form very
stable complexes which were not displaced by
^{3}H-E$_2$ in exchange experiments (1).

In contrast, the three monoalkylating drugs
Ha VI, Ha VII and E$_1$-Azi of class C are
characterized by a relatively high apparent
binding affinity for ER (roughly 3 per cent
of their parent estrogen (E$_1$) for Ha V and
Ha VII; 7 per cent for E$_1$-Azi). Additional
exchange experiments (1) revealed that the
two nitrogen mustard derivatives Ha VI and
Ha VII formed more stable complexes than
their parent estrogen. Exchange by ^{3}H-E$_2$
occurred at a much slower rate than E$_1$ and
was even totally absent under certain conditions. In contrast E$_1$-Azi was found to
interact reversibly with ER in a similar
manner as E$_1$.

2. Effect of Cytotoxic-linked Estrogens on MCF-7 and Evsa-T Cell Lines

The effect of the compounds of class C,
all of which interacted with ER was tested
on the growth of MCF-7 and Evsa-T cells
(Table 4). Growth was estimated by measuring
the amount of DNA after 120 hours of culture
in the presence of the drugs at concentra-
tions of 10^{-8}, 10^{-7} and 10^{-6}M. These concentrations were chosen because they cover the
range reported to produce effects on MCF-7
cells with estrogens and antiestrogens (2).
In this regard, in our laboratory, 10^{-8}M
estradiol was found to slightly stimulate
growth (0-20%); nafoxidine at 10^{-6}M and
5×10^{-7}M was always inhibitory (60-80% and
40-60% respectively).

At the concentration of 10^{-6}M, all nitrogen
mustard derivatives inhibited growth of the
MCF-7 cells. The two bialkylating drugs
Ha IV and Ha V produced an inhibition effect
of about 35 to 40%; the monoalkylating ones
Ha VI and Ha VII produced a stronger inhibition (about 80 to 90%). At lower concentrations, all drugs were devoid of significant

Table 1. Apparent binding affinity of compounds of class A for cytoplasmic estrogen receptors.

Name	Apparent binding affinity (E_2 = 100)
Estradiol mustard	<0.01
ICI 85,966	<0.01
Leo 299 (Estracyt)	0.01
Ha I	<0.01
Ha II	<0.01

Inhibition curves of ^{3}H-E_2 binding to cytoplasmic ER: Ref. 1.

Table 2. Apparent binding affinity of compounds of class B for cytoplasmic estrogen receptors.

Name	Apparent binding affinity (E_2 = 100)	Structure
Leo 275	0.1 - 0.01	
Leo 298	<0.01	
Estradiol-Adriamycin	<0.01	

Inhibition curves of ^{3}H-E_2 binding to cytoplasmic ER: Ref. 1.

Table 3. Apparent binding affinity of compounds of class C
for cytoplasmic estrogen receptors.

	Name	Apparent binding affinity	
		(E_2 = 100)	(E_1 = 100)
	HA IV	0.01	
	Ha V	0.01	
	Ha VI	0.5	3
	Ha VII	0.5	3
	E_1-Azi	1	7

Inhibition curves of ^{3}H-E_2 binding to cytoplasmic ER: Ref. 1.

effect except Ha VII which markedly inhibited
growth at 10^{-7}M (45%). With regard to the
Evsa-T cells, only Ha VII was found to inhibit growth ($\sim$ 80%) at 10^{-6}M indicating that
these drugs had a weaker effect on this line
than on the MCF-7 one. Additional studies
showed that 10^{-8}M estradiol or 11-chloro-
methylestradiol failed to reverse the inhibition of the drugs on the MCF-7 cells (data
not shown).

The aziridine derivative (E_1-Azi) also
influenced the growth of the MCF-7 cells.
Concentrations of 10^{-8} and 10^{-7}M appeared
stimulating ($\sim$ 40%) whereas 10^{-6}M was slightly
inhibitory (23%). Nafoxidine at 5 × 10^{-7}M
was found to reverse the activating effect
of the drug; 10^{-8}M estradiol reversed its
inhibiting effect at 10^{-6}M (data not shown).

With regard to the Evsa-T cells, no effect
was observed at any concentration.

DISCUSSION

Among the estrogen-linked cytotoxic agents
investigated, interaction with ER appeared
only to occur in those of class C. Assessment of the action of these drugs on the
growth of the two breast cancer cell lines
MCF-7 (ER+) and Evsa-T (ER-) revealed a
marked inhibitory effect on the former line.
Furthermore, the nitrogen mustard derivatives,
having the highest apparent binding affinity
(Ha VI and Ha VII) produced the strongest
growth inhibition of the MCF-7 cells. This
observation supports the hypothesis of a

Table 4. Action of cytotoxic-linked estrogens on growth of cultured cell lines.

Compound	DNA (µg) ± S.D.							
	MCF$_7$ (ER+)				Evsa-T (ER−)			
	Control	10^{-8}M	10^{-7}M	10^{-6}M	Control	10^{-8}M	10^{-7}M	10^{-6}M
Ha IV	10,4 ± 1,4	10,0 ± 0,8 (96)[+]	9,4 ± 0,9 (90)	6,6 ± 1,3 (64)	22,6 ± 2,5	20,0 ± 2,1 (88)	19,6 ± 2,6 (87)	19,2 ± 2,3 (85)
Ha V	14,8 ± 0,5	13,6 ± 0,1 (92)	13,6 ± 1,8 (92)	9,1 ± 1,6 (62)	8,8 ± 1,0	10,0 ± 1,0 (114)	9,1 ± 0,8 (103)	9,5 ± 1,2 (108)
Ha VI	10,4 ± 1,5	10,5 ± 0,4 (101)	9,2 ± 0,7 (88)	2,4 ± 0,5 (23)	11,4 ± 0,8	13,2 ± 0,6 (116)	9,8 ± 0,8 (86)	12,6 ± 0,6 (110)
Ha VII	12,1 ± 1,8	12,7 ± 1,4 (105)	6,7 ± 1,2 (55)	1,2 ± 0,2 (10)	25,7 ± 2,5	26,1 ± 0,5 (102)	23,7 ± 2,9 (92)	4,5 ± 1,1 (18)
E$_1$-Azi	6,9 ± 1,0	9,5 ± 0,5 (138)	8,8 ± 1,3 (128)	5,3 ± 1,0 (77)	12,8 ± 0,8	12,8 ± 1,4 (100)	13,6 ± 0,8 (106)	12,0 ± 1,8 (94)

All experiments were performed in quadruplicate.

[+]Percent of control value.

participation of ER in the cytotoxic action of the drugs. However, estradiol and 11-chloromethylestradiol were unable to overcome their inhibiting effect which do not support the hypothesis. Nevertheless, the lack of sensibility could also be explained by the very stable interaction of these drugs with ER.

The aziridine derivative (E_1-Azi) either stimulated or slightly inhibited the growth of the MCF-7 cells depending upon the concentration used. It seems likely that ER mediated these effects since they were suppressed by nafoxidine and estradiol respectively.

In conclusion, estrogen-cytotoxic agents tested in the present study seemed to display a stronger inhibitory effect on estrogen sensitive than on autonomous cell lines. This difference suggests that these compounds may affect the former through a specific mechanism involving ER. A higher non specific sensitivity of this cell line towards cytotoxic drugs may however not be ruled out. Additional investigations are therefore needed to confirm the specific action of these drugs. Analysis of their effects on the growth of a variety of other cell lines either containing (9) or lacking ER (2) should be the first step to solve the problem.

ACKNOWLEDGEMENT

We wish to thank Drs. F. Arcamone (Farmitalia), H. Hamacher (B.G.A., Berlin, Germany), I. Konives (Leo), D. N. Richardson (Imperial Chemical Industries), O. Yoder and R. B. Ing (U.S. National Cancer Institute) and F. J. Zeelen (Organon) for the gift of the cytotoxic linked estrogens.

This work was supported by a grant from the "Fonds Cancérologique de la Caisse Générale d'Epargne et de Retraite", Belgium and by the contract No. 1-CM-53840 from the National Cancer Institute, Bethesda, Maryland.

REFERENCES

1. G. Leclercq and J. C. Heuson, Estrogen-linked cytotoxic agents of potential value for the treatment of breast cancer. Binding affinity for estrogen receptors. Proceedings of the symposium "Pharmacological Modulation of Steroid Action" (Turin, July 23-25, 1978). F. DiCarlo and W.I.P. Mainwaring Eds., Raven Press, New York (in press).
2. M. E. Lippman, G. Bolan and K. Huff, The effect of estrogens and antiestrogens on hormone-responsive human breast cancer in long-term tissue culture. *Cancer Res.* 36, 4595 (1976).
3. E.O.R.T.C. Breast Cancer Cooperative Group, Standard for the assessment of estrogen receptors in human breast cancer. *Europ. J. Cancer* 9, 379 (1973).
4. C. T. Zava, G. C. Chamness, K. B. Horwitz and W. L. McGuire, Human breast cancer: Biologically active estrogen receptor in the absence of estrogen? *Science* 196, 663 (1977).
5. N. Devleeschouwer, G. Leclercq, N. Legros and J. C. Heuson, Reversion of Nafoxidine inhibition on MCF-7 cells growth by three estrogens with different binding affinity for estrogen receptors. (Unpublished data).
6. G. Leclercq, J. C. Heuson and M. C. Deboel, Estrogen receptors interaction with Estracyt and degradation products, a biochemical study on a potential agent in the treatment of breast cancer. *Europ. J. Drug. Metab. Pharmacokinet.* 1, 77 (1976).
7. G. Leclercq, M. C. Deboel and J. C. Heuson, Affinity of estradiol mustard for estrogen receptors and its enzymatic degradation in uterine and breast cancer cytosols. *Int. J. Cancer* 18, 750 (1976).
8. K. Burton, A study of the conditions and mechanism of the diphenylamine reaction for the colorimetric estimation of dexocyribonucleis acid. *Biochem. J.* 62, 315 (1956).
9. L. W. Engel, N. A. Young, T. S. Tralka, M. E. Lippman, S. J. O'Brien and M. J. Joyce, Establishment and characterization of three new continuous cell lines derived from human breast carcinomas. *Cancer Res.* 38, 3352 (1978).

Anti-Tumour Potential of a New Luteinizing Hormone Releasing Hormone Analogue, ICI 118630

R. I. Nicholson*, K. J. Walker* and P. V. Maynard**

*Tenovus Institute for Cancer Research, Welsh National School of Medicine,
Heath Park, Cardiff CF4 4XX, U.K.
**Department of Obstetrics and Gynaecology, City Hospital, Nottingham, U.K.

Correspondence to R. I. Nicholson

Abstract—A new potent LHRH agonist, $|D\text{-}Ser(Bu^t)^6Azgly^{10}|$ LHRH (ICI 118630) was given at high concentration to intact female rats. Twice-daily administration of 5 µg ICI 118630 for 14 days significantly elevated plasma LH and FSH levels and decreased oestradiol concentrations. In addition the LHRH analogue decreased ovarian, pituitary and uterine weights and caused the regression of the majority of oestrogen receptor positive DMBA-induced mammary tumours. Vaginal smears taken before and during ICI 118630 treatment indicated a shift from a regular pattern of 4 day oestrous cycles to a dioestrus condition. The events are consistent with ICI 118630, on this treatment regime, producing the effects of a chemical castration.

INTRODUCTION

The initial treatment of premenopausal women suffering from advanced breast cancer is generally the surgical removal of the ovaries. However, only 30% of patients undergo objective remissions following this treatment. Thus it is important to select those patients who have a good chance of benefitting from the treatment.

The oestrogen receptor content of breast tumours is currently used in this context, although their detection is not necessarily a pre-requisite for a worthwhile response, some 40-50% of oestrogen receptor positive tumours failing to undergo objective breast tumour remissions (1).

The present communication, investigates the capacity of a new and potent luteinizing hormone releasing hormone (LHRH) analogue, ICI 118630 (D-Ser|Bu^t|^{6}Azgly^{10}-LHRH) to reduce ovarian function in the rat and hence growth of ovary-dependent dimethylbenz (a)anthracene(DMBA)-induced mammary tumours.

MATERIALS AND METHODS

1. Peptide

ICI 118630 was synthesised by solution methods (2) by Dr. A. S. Dutta, ICI Pharmaceuticals Division, Macclesfield, England. The purity of the sample was > 95% as assessed by paper electrophoresis, thin-layer chromatography and amino-acid analysis.

2. Animals

Mature virgin female Sprague-Dawley rats bred in the Institute were used throughout the study. The animals were housed in a 12 h light and 12 h dark environment and had access to feed and water ad lib. The peptide was dissolved in physiological saline and injected (100 µl) intramuscularly into the rear legs of rats. Blood samples were obtained as indicated in the appropriate figure and table legends.

The method of induction of DMBA-induced mammary tumours has been described previously (3) as have the plasma hormone assays for oestradiol (4), LH and FSH (5) and the procedure for the estimation of the oestrogen receptor content of tumour biopsy specimens (6).

RESULTS

Figure 1 shows the temporal effects of single and multiple injections of 5.0 µg ICI 118630 on plasma LH levels. Following each injection there was a rapid increase in immunologically reactive LH in the plasma which reached peak concentration at 1-2 h after administration of the LHRH analogue. The pattern of plasma LH release determined after 14 days of ICI 118630 treatment was qualitatively similar to that observed on the first day of treatment, although the quantity released was considerably lower. Nevertheless, plasma LH values determined at this time were significantly higher than those obtained in 3-week ovariectomized animals (Table 1). In addition, the synthetic analogue raised plasma FSH levels, but not to the values seen in the ovariectomized group.

It is also clear from Table 1 that long-term administration of 5.0 µg ICI 118630 twice-daily reduced the circulating concentration of oestradiol to that seen in

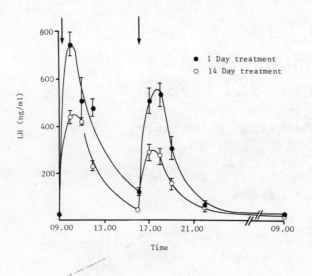

Fig. 1. Effect of ICI 118630 on plasma LH levels. Animals were administered ICI 118630 twice-daily for 1 day (●) or 14 days (o) and killed by exsanguination at the times indicated. The arrows indicate the times of injection of the LHRH analogue. Plasma LH values are the mean ± SEM of 5 animals. Data reproduced from the Br. J. Cancer (4).

oestrogen receptor status was known (Fig. 3b). Of the tumours examined four continued to grow during the treatment period and contained receptor concentrations of less than 12 fmol/mg cytosolic protein. The majority of tumours, however, regressed on ICI 118630 treatment and with the exception of one tumour, had receptor values in excess of 24 fmol/mg cytosolic protein. Despite these findings no significant correlation was found between the oestrogen receptor concentration of tumours at time zero and their response to 3 weeks of ICI 118630 treatment (Fig. 3b).

On cessation of ICI 118630 treatment a period of tumour regrowth was observed (Fig. 4b).

These tumours, however, retained a degree of hormone dependency and regressed after either ovariectomy or a further treatment period with the LHRH analogue (Fig. 4c).

DISCUSSION

It has been previously demonstrated that $|D-Ser(Bu^t)^6-Azgly^{10}|$ LHRH (ICI 118630) is a potent LHRH agonist, inducing ovulation in androgen-sterilized constant-oestrus rats after iv. injections of doses as low as 5 ng/rat (8). The results described in this paper, and elsewhere (4), indicate that, when administered at higher doses (0.5-5.0 μg bd.),

Table 1. Organ weights and plasma hormone levels in animals treated with ICI 118630. Groups of mature female rats were given twice-daily injections of 5.0 μg ICI 118630 for 14 days before exsanguination. Blood samples were removed 1 h after the final morning injection of ICI 118630. Levels are expressed as mean ± the range of values obtained and are compared to values determined in saline-treated controls and 3 week ovariectomized animals. The results are the mean of 6 animals per group. *Significantly different from control group (p < 0.05) in a Mann-Whitney U Test. Data reproduced from Br. J. Cancer (4).

	Organ weights (mg/g initial body weight)			Plasma hormone levels		
	Ovaries	Pituitary gland	Uterus	LH (ng/ml)	FSH (ng/ml)	Oestradiol (pg/ml)
Control	0.42 (0.29-0.61)	0.041 (0.032-0.050)	2.03 (1.58-2.55)	48 (20-145)	905 (583-1211)	32.8 (11.1-64.5)
ICI 118630 (5.0 μg bd.)	0.19* (0.13-0.29)	0.031* (0.025-0.048)	0.67* (0.56-0.73)	522* (443-805)	2631* (2229-2913)	8.2* (3.2-14.3)
Ovariectomy	–	0.035 (0.029-0.049)	0.68* (0.52-0.89)	315* (119-444)	3202* (1931-3727)	8.7* (3.5-26.0)

ovariectomized rats and decreased ovarian, pituitary and uterine weights. Vaginal smears taken before and during the treatment period indicated a shift from a regular four-day pattern of oestrous cycles to a continuous dioestrus condition, with little evidence of vaginal cornification (Fig. 2).

Figure 3 shows the effect of twice-daily administration of ICI 118630 on the growth of DMBA-induced mammary tumours (Fig. 3a) whose

ICI 118630 reduces ovarian weights and prevents normal oestrous cycles in mature rats. In addition, twice-daily administration of the drug promoted substantial tumour regressions in the majority of oestrogen receptor positive DMBA-induced mammary tumours, although no overall correlation was observed between the quantity of receptor and the degree of tumour regression produced (Fig. 3, refs. 9,10). These observations taken in

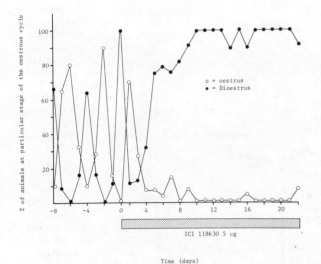

ICI 118630 5 µg

Time (days)

Fig. 2. Effect of ICI 118630 vaginal smears.
Vaginal smears were taken as scheduled in the figure. The stage of
the oestrous cycle was assessed by
the presence of various cell types
in the smears (7) and were classified as follows: oestrus; the
smear consisting of cornified cells
only; metoestrus, presence of leucocytes dispersed with the cornified
cells; dioestrus, the smears consisting mainly of leucocytes; pro-
oestrus, presence of epithelial
cells with marked nuclei. Only the
oestrus (o) and dioestrus (•) conditions are illustrated. The results
are plotted as the percentage of
animals in a particular stage of
the cycle and represent the sequential data from 12 animals.

conjunction with the findings that ICI 118630
when administered to intact animals decreases
uterine weights and plasma oestradiol levels
to values seen in ovariectomized rats,
suggests that the compound may act by elicit-
ing a chemical castration and thus depriving
the tumour tissue of oestradiol (10).

On cessation of ICI 118630 treatment some
tumour regrowth was observed. These tumours,
however, retained their hormone-dependency
and regressed following the removal of the
ovaries or in response to a second treatment
period of ICI 118630. Duplication of these
events in premenopausal women would potentially be of two-fold value in the treatment
of advanced breast cancer. Firstly, to
initiate regression of ovary-dependent tumours
and secondly, in doing so, to predict the
response of such tumours to oophorectomy and
subsequent endocrine therapy. Obviously,
these possibilities await clinical evaluation.

ACKNOWLEDGEMENTS

The authors are grateful to ICI Ltd.,
Pharmaceuticals Division for the opportunity
to study the LHRH analogue; to Dr. G. V.
Groom, Mr. B. G. Brownsey and G. Evans for
hormone assays; to Professor K. Griffiths
for his constructive criticism and advice;
and to the Tenovus Organization and ICI Ltd.
for financial support. K. J. Walker is the
recipient of a joint Tenovus and ICI Scholarship.

REFERENCES

1. W. L. McGuire, P. P. Carbone and E. P.
   Vollmer (Eds.). In Estrogen Receptors
   in Human Breast Cancer. Raven Press,
   N.Y. (1975).
2. A. S. Dutta, B. J. A. Furr, M. B. Giles
   and B. Valcaccia, Synthesis and biological activity of highly active α-aza-
   analogues of luliberin. *J. Med. Chem.*
   21, 1018 (1978).
3. R. I. Nicholson and M. P. Golder, The
   effect of synthetic anti-oestrogens on
   the growth and biochemistry of rat
   mammary tumours. *Europ. J. Cancer* 11,
   571 (1975).
4. P. V. Maynard and R. I. Nicholson, Effects
   of high doses of a series of new lutein-
   izing hormone-releasing hormone analogues
   in intact female rats. *Br. J. Cancer* 39,
   274 (1979).
5. G. V. Groom, The measurement of human
   gonadotrophins by radioimmunoassay.
   J. Reprod. Fertil. 57, 273 (1977).
6. R. I. Nicholson, P. Davies and
   K. Griffiths, Tamoxifen binding in
   mammary tumours in relation to response.
   Rev. Endocrine Related Cancer, Supplement April, ICI Publications (UK) p. 307
   (1978).
7. R. R. Fox and C. W. Laird, In *Sexual
   cycles in reproduction and breeding
   techniques in laboratory animals* (E. S.
   Hafez, ed.) p. 107, Lea and Febiger,
   Philadelphia (1970).
8. A. S. Dutta, B. J. A. Furr, M. B. Giles,
   B. Valcaccia and A. L. Walpole, Potent
   agonist and antagonist analogues of
   luliberin containing an azaglycine resi-
   due at position 10. *Biochem. Biophys.
   Res. Comm.* 81, 382 (1978).
9. R. I. Nicholson, E. Finney and P. V.
   Maynard, Activity of a new LH-RH analogue,
   ICI 118630, on the growth of rat
   mammary tumours. *J. Endocrinol.* 79,
   51P (1978).
10. R. I. Nicholson and P. V. Maynard,
    Anti-tumour activity of ICI 118630, a
    new potent luteinizing hormone-releasing
    hormone agonist. *Br. J. Cancer* 39, 268
    (1979).

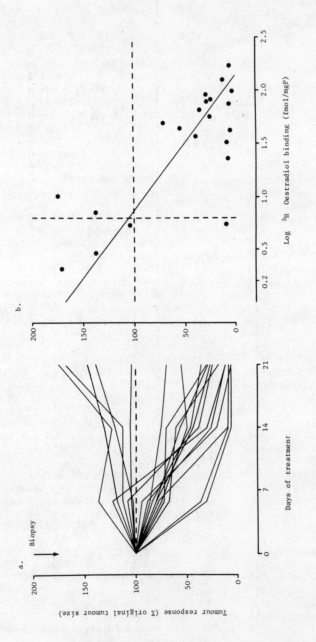

Fig. 3. Effect of ICI 118630 on the growth of rat mammary tumours: correlation with their oestrogen receptor status. When tumours reached an approximate size of 1.5 cm mean diameter a small portion (100 mg) of each tumour was removed under ether anaesthesia and assayed for oestrogen receptors (6). The remainder of the tumour was left *in situ* and the animals treated for 3 weeks with 5.0 μg ICI 118630 twice daily. (a) Tumour growth patterns of ICI 118630 treated animals. (b) Relationship of tumour size following 3 weeks of ICI 118630 treatment and the logarithm of the oestrogen receptor content of the tumours at time zero.

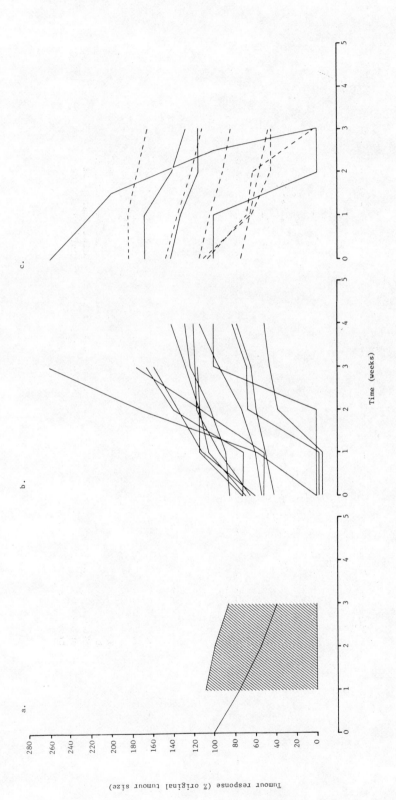

Fig. 4. Growth patterns of tumours in animals after cessation of ICI 118630 treatment. (a) Animals bearing DMBA-induced mammary tumours were administered 5 µg ICI 118630 twice-daily for 3 weeks. The results are the mean ± the range of values of 13 tumours. (b) Tumour regrowth after the cessation of ICI 118630 treatment. (c) Secondary effects of either ovariectomy (———) or 5.0 µg ICI 118630 twice-daily (----) treatment on tumours growing after initial drug withdrawal.